Sickle Cell and the Social Sciences

Sickle cell disease (SCD) is a severe chronic illness and one of the world's most common genetic conditions, with 400,000 children born annually with the disorder, mainly in Sub-Saharan Africa, India, Brazil, the Middle East and in diasporic African populations in North America and Europe. Biomedical treatments for SCD are increasingly available to the world's affluent populations, while such medical care is available only in attenuated forms in Africa, India and to socio-economically disadvantaged groups in North America and Europe.

Often a condition rendered invisible in policy terms because of its problematic association with politically marginalized groups, the *social* study of sickle cell has been neglected. This illuminating volume explores the challenges and possibilities for developing a social view of sickle cell, and for improving the quality of lives of those living with SCD. Tackling the controversial role of screening and genetics in SCD, the book offers a brief thematic history of approaches to the condition, queries the role of ethnicity and includes a discussion of how the social model of disability can be applied, as well as featuring chapters focusing on athletics, prisons and schools.

Bringing together a wide range of original research conducted in the USA, the UK, Ghana and Nigeria, *Sickle Cell and the Social Sciences* is anchored in the discipline of sociology, but draws upon a diverse range of fields, including public health, anthropology, social policy and disability studies.

Simon Dyson is Professor of Applied Sociology and Director of the Unit for the Social Study of Thalassaemia and Sickle Cell at De Montfort University, Leicester, UK.

Routledge Studies in the Sociology of Health and Illness

For more information about this series, please visit: www.routledge.com/
Routledge-Studies-in-the-Sociology-of-Health-and-Illness/book-series/RSSHI

Sickle Cell and the Social Sciences

Health, Racism and Disablement

Simon Dyson

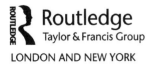

Routledge
Taylor & Francis Group

LONDON AND NEW YORK

First published 2019 by Routledge

2 Park Square, Milton Park, Abingdon, Oxon, OX14 4RN

605 Third Avenue, New York, NY 10017

Routledge is an imprint of the Taylor & Francis Group, an informa business

First issued in paperback 2020

British Library Cataloguing-in-Publication Data
A catalogue record for this book is available from the British Library

Library of Congress Cataloging-in-Publication Data
Names: Dyson, Simon, author.
Title: Sickle cell disease and the social sciences / Simon Dyson.
Description: Abingdon, Oxon ; New York, NY : Routledge, 2019. |
Includes bibliographical references and index.
Identifiers: LCCN 2018056906| ISBN 9781138298392 (hardback) |
ISBN 9781315098685 (e-book)
Subjects: | MESH: Anemia, Sickle Cell–ethnology
Classification: LCC RC641.7.S5 | NLM WH 170 | DDC 616.1/527–dc23
LC record available at https://lccn.loc.gov/2018056906

ISBN: 978-1-138-29839-2 (hbk)
ISBN: 978-0-367-70267-0 (pbk)

Typeset in Times New Roman
by Wearset Ltd, Boldon, Tyne and Wear

Contents

Figures

Tables

Acknowledgements

I would like to thank the following for permissions to use/adapt previously published materials: Elsevier, for Table 1.2; Whiting and Birch for Tables 1.3 and 1.4; *The Lancet*, Elsevier for Table 1.6; the World Health Organization for Figure 7.1. Some of the ideas developed in Chapter 3 were originally published as Dyson, SM (2018) "Assessing Latour: The case of the sickle cell body in history". *European Journal of Social Theory*. Copyright [2018] by permission of SAGE Publications.

I would like to thank Karl Atkin, Bob Carter, and Todd Savitt for supporting the publication of the book. Thank you to Tom Williams, Todd Savitt, and Scott Grosse for their generosity in reading and commenting on individual chapters, and making many helpful suggestions. I would especially like to thank Bob Carter and Oliver Harris for their ongoing academic support through our reading group, for their friendship, and for reading and commenting on the entire draft book. They both embody an intellectual openness and generosity of spirit that give one hope in such dark, mean-spirited times. I alone take responsibility for errors and weaknesses in the line of argument.

Thank you to my two African PhD students, Jemima Dennis-Antwi of Ghana, and Bolanle Ola of Nigeria, for allowing me to accompany you in your learning. I would like to thank Funso Balogun and Ayoola Olajide for facilitating photographs from Lagos State, Nigeria.

Thank you to university colleagues with whom I have shared sickle cell discussions over the years, including Elizabeth Anionwu, Karl Atkin, Maria Berghs, Sangeeta Chattoo, Peter Chimkupete, Lorraine Culley, Sue Dyson, Mark Fowler, Richard Hall, Dave Hiles, Carlton Howson, Mavis Kirkham, Viv Rolfe, Momodou Sallah, Iain Williamson, Scott Yates and the late Dave Rowley.

Thank you to all the members of the Sickle Cell Society; the Organization for Sickle Cell Anaemia Research (OSCAR); the Sickle Cell and Thalassaemia Association of Nurses, Midwives and Allied Health Professionals (STANMAP); the UK Forum on Haemoglobin Disorders; the Global Sickle Cell Disease Network, and past members of Worldwide Initiative on Social Studies of Hemoglobinopathies (WISSH) for your support.

Thank you to the many members of the sickle cell community who have helped me, including Myrle Blaine, Keith Chambers, Ajay Dattani, Kye Gbangbola,

Baba Inusa, John James, Vanita Jivanji, Tony Mason, Annie McDonald, Rachel McFee, Vanetta Morrison, Asa'ah Nkohkwo, Philip Nortey, Comfort Okolo, Patrick Ojeer, Esther Onolememen, Kalpna Patel, Suzi Raybould, Cecilia Shoetan, Leon Smith, Jacqueline Simpson, Iyamide Thomas, Miriam Williams and the late Neville Clare, Kevin Dunkley, Sonia Lindsay, Comfort Ndive and Ade Olujohungbe. Thank you to Leicester OSCAR, especially Carol King, and to the late Erskine Cave, Richard Fenton and Winston Nurse, all of whom started me on my sickle cell journey at a community seminar in 1986.

Finally, I would like to thank all my family. My wife Sue, for her enduring love, her patience with me, and for allowing me to share the joy of welcoming three grandchildren into the world: Nina, Toby and Henry. In thanking my adult daughters, Rehana and Ingrid, a scene from the popular TV series *The Simpsons* (Season 8, Episode 5, *Bart after Dark*) is instructive. Homer is confronted on his doorstep by the Reverend Lovejoy, and other concerned citizens of Springfield, about yet another one of Bart's moral misdemeanours. Homer groans and rolls his eyes "This is not about Jesus, is it?" he complains. "Homer, *everything* is about Jesus," replies the Reverend. I am familiar with that groan and that roll of the eyes. It is the one Rehana and Ingrid developed as children when I broached a conversation. "Dad, it's not about sickle cell, is it?" And I write here what I said to them. In the end, *everything* is about sickle cell.

Introduction

The late Jamaican-born sociologist Stuart Hall once described sickle cell as an emblematically black disease (Hall, 2003). By this, I understand him to have meant that, within our language system, sickle cell has become associated with specific other concepts. Concepts derive their meanings from their place in relation to other concepts in the same system (a bit like when we say *table*, we have learned to associate *table* with *chair*, as if intuitively). Within such systems, certainly in North America and Europe, we have been led to an association of sickle cell and black as if this were common sense. Furthermore, because cultural systems in the USA and Europe are partly comprised of the ideational resources of racism, it is a short step for sickle cell to be associated with the range of negative, racist connotations of being black in those nations (see Bediako and Moffitt, 2011). However, this is *not* the story that is told by our genes.

Genes associated with sickle haemoglobin are found most extensively, but not exclusively, in peoples of African, Caribbean, Middle Eastern, Indian, and Mediterranean descent (Serjeant and Serjeant, 2001). We can see straight away that this list of continents, sub-continents and regions indicates diverse geographic associations of sickle cell well beyond Africa. This means that sickle cell need not necessarily indicate recent African ancestry. Indeed, the US anthropologist Frank B. Livingstone produced a compendium including the frequencies of sickle cell genes, as reported in hundreds of twentieth-century studies. Some of the highest rates were not in Africa at all, but in the Eastern province of Saudi Arabia, and in parts of India (Livingstone, 1985).

There are two competing sets of theories about the origins of sickle cell. The recently revitalized uni-centric model suggests the gene mutation leading to sickle cell occurred once, about 7,300 years ago, either in the Sahara (when the so-called *Green Sahara* was lush and fertile), or in West/Central Africa at the edge of the forest canopy, and subsequently spread from this single origin (Shriner and Rotimi, 2018). The multi-centric model suggests the gene arose on five separate occasions in different geographical locations yielding five main haplotypes (haplotype: the gene encoding sickle haemoglobin is found on chromosome 11, but there are other groupings of genes close by on that chromosome, which are often inherited together with sickle cell. Haplotype refers to which of these different groupings is inherited alongside the gene associated with sickle cell, that is, the chromosomal context of the gene encoding sickle cell.) Four sickle cell haplotypes are said to have originated in Africa, and are referred to as Senegal, Benin, Central African and Cameroon haplotypes. However, a fifth haplotype arose in India (Serjeant and Serjeant, 2001) (see Figure I.1).

However, irrespective of the resolution to this debate, the tale of sickle cell in the Indian contexts remains to be written (Chattoo, 2018). Indeed, the tale of (possible) Indian origins, ecological habitats and social meanings needs to be written if we are to escape the mind-set that only looks for connections to Africa (Singer, 1954) as the starting point for understanding sickle cell in India. Furthermore, as we shall see further in Chapter 3, the Benin haplotype is found extensively in contemporary Mediterranean populations, and therefore reference to recent migration to Europe from Africa (whether in the twentieth century, or even the seventeenth century with the trade in enslaved Africans) is not necessary in order to make sense of the presence of the sickle cell and related genes in white-skinned peoples (Lehmann and Huntsman, 1974; Dyson, 2005, 2007). In genomic terms, it would therefore be a misconception in the extreme to describe sickle cell anaemia as a black disease. However, there are examples where, drawing on such racialized notions, enrolling sickle cell has proved efficacious in helping people feel secure within racialized identities (Bediako *et al.*, 2007) and in advancing claims to citizenship rights, for example, in the USA in the Civil Rights era (Tapper, 1999) or in early twenty-first-century Brazil (Creary, 2018).

The key to understanding the link between people, geography and sickle cell lies in the mosquito-borne disease malaria. Briefly, the sickle cell gene is thought

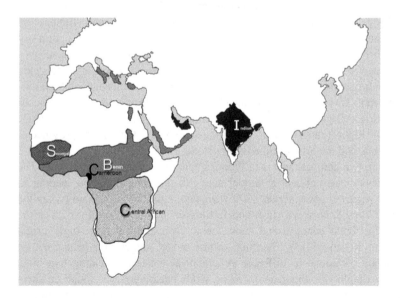

Figure I.1 Multicentric five-haplotype theory of origins of sickle cell.
Source: Adapted from Tony Allison.

to be a human genetic adaptation to help protect against malaria. More specifically, being a genetic carrier of the sickle cell gene (note a genetic carrier, not having the disease itself) confers profound protection in infancy against severe and fatal cerebral malaria (a malaria caused by the protozoan parasite *Plasmodium falciparum*) (Allison, 1954). Those who live in malarial environments build up some environmental resistance to malaria, but infants under two years are very vulnerable to malaria, lacking this environmental protection. It was the South African medical scientist Anthony Allison who first published on the close similarities between the distribution of the sickle cell gene and the distribution of falciparum malaria in Africa (see Figure I.2).

Note, however, the relative absence of malaria and the sickle cell gene in parts of the map. These have to do with latitude, altitude, and solitude. *Latitude:* on the map, the malarial belt finishes somewhere south of the Zambezi River. The mosquitoes that carry the protozoan parasite causing malaria have greater difficulty surviving in colder climes further away from the equator. *Altitude:* one unshaded part of the malaria map corresponds to the area of the Kenyan highlands. Mosquitoes are less likely to survive at colder higher altitudes, and so one would anticipate lower levels of sickle cell in groups living in the highlands than on lower altitudes by the coast or inland lakes. *Solitude:* as mosquitoes need warm shallow pools of water for their larvae to hatch, one might anticipate that in desert areas, such as the contemporary Sahara Desert, sufficient rainfall to create pools may only occur when there is a shift in usual weather patterns. (Indeed, a greater vulnerability to malaria as parts of the world become hotter and wetter than previously and expose populations not used to malaria to that deadly disease is just one consequence of climate change we may reasonably anticipate in the future.) Thus desert regions show less prevalence of the sickle cell trait, with the notable exception of oases (where, of course, there is both

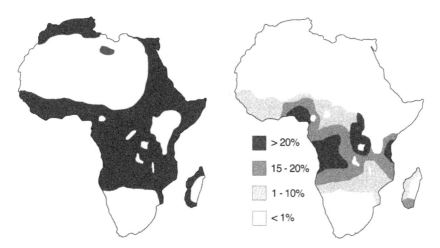

Figure I.2 Distribution of *Plasmodium falciparum* malaria and sickle cell in Africa.
Source: Tony Allison.

water and more concentrated human population). For example, the association of oases with sickle cell has been noted in Egypt (El-Beshlawy and Youssry, 2009; Moez and Younan, 2016) and in Al-Qatif and Al-Hasa in Eastern Saudi Arabia (El-Hamzi *et al.*, 2011). There is another sense of the term solitude which throws light on the issue, and that is the solitude of the nomad compared to the increased density of human populations when they become agriculturalists and live in settlements, and this is discussed further in Chapter 3. It is the concepts of *altitude*, *latitude*, and *solitude* (in the sense both of deserts and of isolated humans) that materially influence malaria, and hence sickle cell, and *not* the concept of negritude (blackness). It is insights such as these that are examined further in this book.

The structure of the book

Chapter 1 outlines key features of sickle cell, at first, in a basic form. However, beneath each of these simplifications lie several layers of scientific complexities. This raises some questions for relationships between doctors and scientists, on the one hand, and people living with sickle cell disease (SCD), on the other. Which simplifications are appropriate and who decides this? This also raises questions about whether science should be democratic, and, if so, what form this might take.

Chapter 2 attempts to link biology, ecology and sociology in a coherent explanation of sickle cell. Two works published in the same year influenced this chapter. One is the developmental biology of Steven Rose, which takes the view that there is one material world but several different ways to know that world: one ontology, many epistemologies (Rose, 1997: 91). The other is the sociological work of Ray Pawson (Pawson and Tilley, 1997), which takes a critical realist approach to practical sociological research. Both texts turn on the phrase "it depends": much depends on context, and knowledge is therefore tentative, provisional and conditional. The phrase "it depends" is very appropriate in trying to understand the manner in which genomic, biological, ecological and collective contexts are all important for how we understand sickle cell. Sickle cell emerges out of what DeLanda (2016) calls assemblages of humans and non-humans, folded into one another at different scales, each with their histories, their emergent powers and their virtual possibilities for the future.

Chapters 3 and 4 are concerned with histories of sickle cell. Medical histories of sickle cell tend to focus on a series of key published medical papers: the first description of sickled cells under the microscope (Herrick, 1910); the first use of the term sickle cell anaemia (Mason, 1922); the paper proposing that sickle cell is a molecular disease (Pauling *et al.*, 1949); the medical trial that proved the efficacy of giving newborn infants with sickle cell anaemia daily penicillin (Gaston *et al.*, 1986); the study that showed hydroxyurea reduced the frequency of sickle cell painful episodes in some people living with SCD (Charache *et al.*, 1995), or the one that established that strokes in children with sickle cell could be prevented through blood transfusions (Adams *et al.*, 1998). By contrast these two chapters look at the different ways in which sickle cell becomes (in)visible, and why this matters for the sickle cell experience. The protagonists of this history are not restricted to human beings, nor, among humans, only to the medical and scientific communities. Rather, the protagonists considered are more diverse in terms of species, social stratification and global geographical spread. Chapter 3 is a less anthropocentric history of sickle cell, acknowledging non-humans such as mosquitoes, malaria parasites, water, plants and forests. Chapter 4 is a narrower history, being at once more anthropocentric, concentrated primarily on the USA, and focused on the historically and culturally specific racialized assumptions in the US cultural system. The contrast is deliberate, since issues discussed in the latter chapter go some way to buttressing a world-view I term *primordialism*. By primordialism, I mean the tendency to think of human bodies as fixed, passing down genetic sameness through generations (thus conflating the concepts of genetic, inherited and innate) with a separately conceived environment from which humans have sprung, but which is at their disposal.

The damaging consequence of such primordialism is the subject of many of the subsequent chapters, beginning with Chapter 5. Chapter 5 concerns those who are genetic carriers of the sickle cell, who are often referred to as having sickle cell trait. The chapter concerns how and why sickle cell screening of student athletes in the USA came about. In doing so, the chapter illustrates how struggles over human social and financial interests become linked to struggles over primordialist views. It is the first of several chapters to assess how sickle cell trait comes to have social and political consequences.

Chapter 6 examines the life-and-death consequences of the misuse of sickle cell trait. In particular, it looks at the manner in which sudden deaths of black people, in contact with state officials, are accounted for by the prison and police authorities. This accounting is contradictory: deaths where the person has sickle cell trait are attributed to this carrier state rather than to use of conductive electrical devices, pepper spray, restraint equipment, restraint techniques, violence, or positional asphyxia. Deaths where the person has the far more serious sickle cell disease occur with the authorities ostensibly taking little or no interest in preventing the death. The chapter critically evaluates the concept of institutional racism, finds this concept wanting as an analytical tool for explaining and changing the situation, and suggests alternative ways of framing both an understanding of, and challenges to, these unnecessary deaths.

Chapter 7 reviews the history and consequences of the way that sickle cell has been framed within discourses to do with race, ethnicity and immigration, noting how primordialist views share key beliefs with some foundational components of fascist ideology, a key contemporary concern given the growing reality of migration in the face of climate change. Starting with a rejection of the idea of distinct races as having a material basis, the chapter considers the manner in which ethnicity was used as a tool to help target sickle cell screening, especially in the UK and the USA. The chapter suggests that although North American and European societies continue to frame sickle cell in terms of ethnicity, the implementation of universal sickle cell screening tends to produce realities undermining this framework.

Antenatal or prenatal screening for sickle cell is the focus of Chapter 8. This finds us at the intersection of several issues to do with gender, disability rights, new reproductive technologies and state surveillance of population health. Globally, such screening is undertaken with varying degrees of directedness. In liberal democracies, such screening may be presented to the pregnant mother as offering informed reproductive choice. However, this chapter questions whether people are able to actualize those choices, and thus questions liberal notions of freedom as well as the assumptions of primordialism. Meanwhile there is a lack of correspondence between technical professional knowledge of being a sickle cell carrier and lay understandings of sickle cell trait, missing the possibility that ambiguity may in some instances represent accuracy (Morton, 2017).

Chapters 9 through 11 consider virtual possibilities of the sickle cell experience, recognising, contrary to primordialism (which takes humans, formed in history, as fixed) that what human sickle cell bodies could be, their species-being, is withdrawn because it is in the future (Morton, 2017). Chapter 9 discusses newborn screening for sickle cell disease. Such newborn screening, coupled with basic treatment, is an effective life-saving intervention for sickle cell disease, and such technology is affordable even in resource-poor settings such as parts of Sub-Saharan Africa. The example of the newborn screening programme in Kumasi, Ghana, is used in order to make the point that culture is not a static entity and that beliefs in supernatural causes of sickle cell may be eroded if a cohort of young people living with SCD can be shown to be flourishing, once a newborn screening programme has been in place for several years. This Ghanaian example indicates a possible future with the enhanced survival of infants with SCD globally, and this future might entail millions surviving with SCD who currently die.

Chapter 10 draws on important insights from the social model of disability and the sociological theory of stigma. The chapter draws on work undertaken in Nigeria, the country with the largest sickle cell population measured in absolute numbers. Mental and physical health is not simply a product of having sickle cell disease, but may be a consequence of discriminatory attitudes, structural barriers to good education and employment opportunities, and lack of enabling social policies. This Nigerian example indicates a possible future with enhanced flourishing of young people and adults with SCD globally, a flourishing which could enable those living with SCD to take control of sickle cell organizations and begin themselves to determine the direction of research and policy.

Chapter 11 considers the author's own work in trying to link academic research to social policy, written with respect to the example of sickle cell in schools. In the UK, research showed that young people with SCD were not well supported at school. Teacher knowledge and awareness of sickle cell proved insufficient to improve reported experiences of young people with SCD. This chapter describes the creation of a *Guide to School Policy on Sickle Cell*, produced as an open education resource in 2011, and then adapted for use, with varying degrees of success and failure, in the USA, Nigeria, Brazil, and Sierra Leone. When, despite the positive framing proposed in Chapters 9–11, people with SCD continue to endure pain, fall ill, and be disabled by their bodies, they are merely exhibiting the future of all human bodies (Morton, 2017).

This book is the culmination of a lifetime spent advocating the merits of social scientific approaches to sickle cell (see also Dyson and Atkin, 2012). This has often been to the puzzlement of medical, clinical and basic science colleagues who do not necessarily see the vast repertoire of social science approaches and diverse philosophies that could usefully be brought to bear on sickle cell. It has also sometimes bewildered social science colleagues who fret about the narrowness of my research interests. Hopefully this may go some way to explain myself. If not, no matter. The most important thing is to try to prepare the ground for a day when those living with SCD, people from the Global South, and those with indigenous knowledge (Todd, 2016), who understand sickle cell through its entanglements with ancestors, non-humans, climate and place, are extensively involved in leading such studies. This book aspires to do just that job of ground-clearing. Let us see.

1 Sickle cell and the complications of science

This first chapter introduces the basics of sickle cell for the non-specialist reader. It starts from the types of information devised for public health consumption, but then notes ways in which this information has been simplified. For example, the chapter covers the following differences:

- between sickling and "normal sickling";
- between sickling considered as a blockage of sickled cells versus sickling as a set of complex physiological interactions;
- between concepts of genotype and phenotype;
- between the focus on sickle cell painful crises as the emblematic symptom of sickle cell and other major sickle cell complications;
- between theoretical probability in patterns of inheritance and empirical occurrence.

The gap between popular community health education and science has been explained in various ways: as a response necessary to account for the technical ignorance of "the public", or as impartial professionals protecting the public from the overwhelming complexity of reality. The chapter concludes by identifying the need for change in the way scientific practice is understood by scientists themselves, in order to move beyond the militaristic-paternalistic sounding model of "public engagement" that currently dominates the relationship between professionals, scientific knowledge and the people.

Sickle cell disease/sickle cell disorder (SCD)

Sickle cell disease/sickle cell disorder (SCD) is an umbrella term denoting a family of severe, inherited, chronic illnesses. The form that is found most frequently is called sickle cell anaemia, accounting for perhaps 70 per cent of SCD. But there are a number of other forms of SCD. One set is where the gene encoding sickle haemoglobin (haemoglobin S) is inherited together with a gene encoding another haemoglobin variant (haemoglobins C, D or E, for example). For instance, haemoglobin SC disease accounts for around 20 per cent of sickle cell disease. Still further types are where a gene associated with sickle cell is co-inherited with a form of thalassaemia. Thalassaemias are associated with a reduction in the *quantity* of the key oxygen-carrying component of red blood cells, haemoglobin, while hae-moglobin variants, which include sickle cell, represent a *qualitative* change in the type of haemoglobin produced. The main conditions in sickle cell disease are listed in Table 1.1.

Sickle cell disease is the term of choice for clinicians. By contrast, some community-based organizations use the phrase sickle cell disorder (Clare, 2007). Three reasons appear to underlie this choice of words. First, "disease" has implications of contagion, of being transmissible from person to person. My own early work on community awareness of sickle cell tried to underscore the idea that sickle cell is not caught like coughs or colds, but is a genetic condition inherited from both biological parents (Dyson, 1997). In this sense, using the word disorder tries to prevent inaccurate connotations of the word disease. Creary (2018) cites a Brazilian activist discursively reclaiming SCD as a "true black health issue", precisely to distance it from HIV as an infectious disease, HIV/AIDS being ascribed, in racist discourses, to the black body (Sabatier, 1988). Second, part of the ideology of racism is that black people are reduced to *only* their bodies (Shilling, 1993) with allegedly limited interior psyches (Skeggs, 2014). Furthermore, such bodies are viewed through a racist lens as inherently diseased (Savitt, 2002). Since sickle cell might be partially described as a blood disease, this makes it vulnerable to being negatively linked to the infamous Tuskegee Syphilis study on African-American men. In this study, men with syphilis or "bad blood" were permitted to die or go blind without treatment when that became available, in order for junior public health doctors to trace the (alleged) natural history of the disease (Reverby, 2000). The third reason is that sociologists, drawing upon insights of the social model of disability (about which more in Chapters 10 and 11), may choose the term disorder (Atkin and Ahmad, 2001). This is because one tenet of disability rights is to assert that dis-ability is not an illness. A disease implies possibility of cure by a doctor, and the social model of disability criticizes medical models that seek cure or rehabilita-tion for disabled peoples (Oliver, 1998). Terming sickle cell a disorder has at least the potential to frame the issue as one of disablement: re-focusing on the rights of the disabled person concerned and changes to the collective environ-ment. Re-framing the issue still further to emphasize the agency of the person

Table 1.1 Basic classification of sickle cell disease/sickle cell disorders

	Genotype notation
Sickle cell anaemia	HbS/S
Haemoglobin SC disease	HbS/C
Sickle beta-zero thalassaemia	HbS/β^0
Sickle beta-plus thalassaemia	HbS/β^+
Haemoglobin sickle cell/D-Punjab	HbS/D-Punjab
Haemoglobin sickle cell/E	HbS/E
Haemoglobin sickle cell/O-Arab	HbS/O-Arab

with sickle cell produces terms like "sickle cell warrior", in use at the time of writing in US community-based organizations. How something is referred to initiates our process of understanding and provides our first clue to which framings of sickle cell require resisting.

Sickle cell symptoms

Sickle cell is referenced as the first molecular disease. A single change at the molecular level produces an altered form of haemoglobin (Pauling *et al.*, 1949). Haemoglobin is the protein in our red blood cells that gives blood its red appearance. One of its tasks is to carry oxygen from the lungs to the rest of the body. The delivery of oxygen takes place in blood vessels (capillaries) which, at their narrowest, may be less than the width of a red blood cell. In people with usual adult haemoglobin (called haemoglobin A, abbreviated to HbA), the red blood cells remain sufficiently flexible to enable them to squeeze through the capillaries and transfer their oxygen. However, in people with sickle cell anaemia, a majority of the haemoglobin is sickle haemoglobin (called haemoglobin S or HbS). When the cell is not oxygenated, the haemoglobin no longer remains in solution but crystallizes into long twisted chains (a process called *polymerization*). Like a rigid stick within a balloon, these chains of haemoglobin distort the cell membrane into peculiar elongated shapes. When such chains are formed rapidly, the red blood cell becomes crescent-shaped like a sickle (the ancient agricultural tool for harvesting grasses). However, the particular shape depends partly on the speed with which the chains of haemoglobin stack up, and holly-leaf and granular forms are also possible (Serjeant and Serjeant, 2001: 64).

A *simplified* account would continue as follows. In contrast to usual red blood cells which are flexible and can squeeze through narrow blood vessels, sickle-shaped cells are rigid, and may create a log-jam in the capillaries, depriving that part of the body of oxygen. However, the dynamics of polymerization are generally too slow to result in sickling while the red blood cells are in the capillaries and *vaso-occlusion* (vaso-, to do with the blood vessels, and occlusive, concerned with closure or blocking) is not just related to this. The blockage of capillaries is not exclusively due to sickling but to a multicellular collaboration with the lining of the blood vessels (called the *endothelium*), and sickling occurs in conjunction with other physiological mechanisms (Eaton and Bunn, 2017). This is addressed more fully a little later in this chapter.

The consequence of these complex physiological processes is a symptom emblematic of the sickle cell experience: a sickle cell painful episode (vaso-occlusive episode). Such episodes are often referred to as a "sickle cell crisis". The resultant pain may be mild, moderate or excruciating and may last minutes, hours or days. Painful episodes may be emblematic of sickle cell illness, but this draws attention away from other issues. The red blood cells are continually destroyed prematurely (*haemolysis*), the person is anaemic, and chronic fatigue is a neglected symptom of SCD. The cumulative effect of sickled red blood cells and periodic denial of oxygen is long-term damage to tissues and the possibility of organ failure. The consequences of SCD are thus far more extensive than acute painful sickle cell crises.

All parts of the body require oxygen delivered by red blood cells, so clearly anything that disrupts that process may produce pain at multiple sites in the body and, over time, may produce damage to tissues and organs. SCD is thus not just a blood disorder but a systemic disorder: it is the underlying mechanism that generates effects in nearly every part of the body. This diversity in empirical symptoms generated through underlying mechanisms partially explains why SCD remained hidden from the medical profession for so long (Wailoo and Pemberton, 2006).

Since SCD is a systemic disorder, people with SCD may experience acute or chronic pain in any part of the body. They may experience a truly daunting range of symptoms: strokes caused by bleeds or blockages; silent strokes; loss of the spleen (or splenic function) leading to vulnerability to infections; severe anaemia; acute chest syndrome; hand-foot syndrome; leg ulcers, necrosis (*necrosis*: death of body tissue) of the shoulders or hip joints, visual or hearing problems, damage to the kidney or the liver, among many other symptoms and complications (Serjeant and Serjeant, 2001). There are also other types of sickle cell crises other than acute painful episodes. A splenic sequestration crisis involves red blood cells becoming trapped in the spleen, leading to a painful enlargement of the spleen, and constituting a medical emergency. Education of parents to recognize this is part of the newborn screening for sickle cell discussed further in Chapter 9. An aplastic crisis involves parvovirus B19 and the collapse in the production of red blood cells. Understandably, much focus is on the immediacy of the acute painful sickle cell crisis, but SCD is also a progressive disorder: repeated infarctions damage key organs over time, and people living with SCD can be faced with the challenges of long-term organ damage.

Nor is the acute sickle cell painful crisis the only source of sickle cell-related pain. In addition to acute pain, people with SCD experience chronic pain and neuropathic pain, that is, pain caused by damage to the central nervous system, which then renders the person hypersensitive to future pain (Ballas *et al.*, 2012). One study in the USA suggests that in people with SCD nearly one-third describe sickle cell pain every day; over 50 per cent report pain on more than half of the days; and only one in seven rarely experience chronic pain (Smith *et al.*, 2008). However, we also need to be cautious that people with SCD in a US social environment of relative poverty and racism do not necessarily stand for the global experience of people with SCD in other settings. With respect to both range of symptoms and types of pain, and to physical and collective environments, the sickle cell illness experience is about more than acute painful episodes.

Treatment for sickle cell disorders

The treatment for sickle cell disorders reflects in turn the wide range of clinical symptoms that can affect people living with SCD. It has been suggested that only specialist sickle cell centres can adequately provide comprehensive care for people with SCD, so extensive is the spectrum of medical, psychological and social care required (Serjeant, 2006). Such comprehensive care can lead to significantly less use of emergency departments and to reduced health care costs (Ballas, 2009).

The pain associated with a sickle cell crisis can be excruciating, and has been described as "like hammering inside your bone", "being set on fire continuously" and that "labour is a piece of cake [compared] to this" (cited in Coleman *et al.*, 2016: 196). Pain scales, in which patients are invited to rate their pain on a scale of 1–10, with ten representing the worst pain imaginable, are said by people living with SCD not to reflect the severity of their pain experience. The title of the painting by the Haitian artist living with SCD, Hertz Nazaire, "Ten Redefined", suggests that even ten on the scale is insufficient to adequately describe sickle cell pain. For me, the most evocative expression of such pain is when a person with SCD reportedly spoke of their SCD pain in terms of how many years of life they would trade to be rid of their current pain.

In well-resourced settings, treatments for a sickle-cell painful crisis may include use of opioid painkillers. Treatment protocols and consensus approaches are developed by the National Institutes of Health (NIH) in the USA (NIH, 2014: 34), and the National Institute for Health and Care Excellence (NICE) in the UK (NICE, 2012). The latter recommends treating a sickle cell painful crisis as a medical emergency and that analgesia be given within 30 minutes of presentation. The issue of relief for the extreme pain of sickle cell has been the subject of antagonism between people with SCD and health service providers. In societies where racist stereotypes still abound, access to the most powerful analgesics, such as morphine, are sometimes denied to people with SCD (Maxwell *et al.*, 1999). For example, in the USA, opiates are given to African-American hospital patients for pain at significantly lower rates than they are given to white patients (Pletcher *et al.*, 2008). In the USA, specialist sickle cell acute care units have been associated with higher dosing of opioids for acute painful episodes in adults with SCD compared to practice in emergency room admissions, with improved pain outcomes and decreased hospitalizations (Molokie *et al.*, 2018). Historically, many sickle cell patients, both in the USA and the UK, have complained that they were treated as recreational drug users by health staff when they asked for pain relief (Hill, 1994; Maxwell *et al.*, 1999; Anionwu and Atkin, 2001; Rouse, 2009). Interestingly at varying times across the twentieth century some clinicians either eschewed completely (Konotey-Ahulu, 1996), or sought to minimize the use of opioids (Serjeant and Serjeant, 2001) in favour of the approach of the holistic physician who knew their patient well and could work with them to identify and avoid factors liable to trigger a sickle cell crisis. Indeed, the earliest physician involved in treating a cohort of patients with SCD, Lemuel Diggs of Memphis, Tennessee, is reported not to have used opiates, as, in his view, they had little effect on the most severe sickle cell pain (Nollan, 2016).

There are established guidelines on treatment for those with sickle cell disease (Sickle Cell Society, 2018). This is not to say that this necessarily translates into optimal care. Indeed, a further source of tension between those with SCD and health professionals is the lack of knowledge of non-sickle-cell-specialists, such as family doctors, or accident and emergency staff, who may be reluctant to administer pain relief quickly enough or at all (Anionwu and Atkin, 2001). In the UK, this lack of competency is illustrated through a number of high profile cases. These include Sarah Mulenga, a university student with SCD who died when ambulance staff refused to take her to hospital (BBC, 2013b); three-year-old Obed-Edom Bans, who, despite having a medical card stating he had SCD, was sent away from a walk-in health centre, and subsequently died of meningitis (*Evening Standard*, 2010); five-year-old Emmanuel Akinmuyiwa, who died of cardiac arrest when a junior doctor ignored a consultant's instructions, which included requesting a blood test for level of anaemia (*Birmingham Mail*, 2014); and three-year-old Johan Pambou, who died from pneumococcal septicaemia after failing to receive the relevant vaccine, despite four letters from the consultant to the family doctor requesting the vaccination be carried out (*Birmingham Mail*, 2017). Distressingly, even in a health system free at the point of use and funded through general taxation, these incidents still occurred. In other health systems the situation may be further complicated.

In the USA, the highest quality care is available to those who can afford high levels of insurance. A large number of people are uninsured, or under-insured, and many rely on the Medicaid system. This causes problems. For example, Medicaid might only cover three days of hospitalization but a sickle cell crisis might require a longer stay in hospital. Doctors may not wish to risk their insurance liability in order to treat sickle cell patients for any non-sickle cell illness, as sickle cell can complicate treatments for other conditions. Historically in the USA, children with SCD might be able to obtain treatment, but not uninsured adults. Hence, what is already a challenge in terms of psychological adjustment during the transition between paediatric and adult services, becomes a matter of even greater concern. Medicine, it has been long established, has a moral as well as a technical dimension (Parsons, 1951). This may be illustrated through moral attributions to paediatric patients. "Good" patients can be rewarded with the delay of transition beyond 18 years old by their sympathetic provider so they can continue their care in a paediatric setting. Troublesome or unpopular "bad" patients can then effectively be punished merely through the application of usual routines (transfer out of paediatric care at standard age).

In many other countries affected by SCD, health insurance schemes may be embryonic and payment for health services at the point of usage may be the norm. The more tenuous credibility of medicine for those with a chronic illness in resource-poor parts of Africa was brought home to me through watching a short drama led by a person living with SCD, Olivier Mmounda à Nyam, originally from the Cameroon, at St Bartholomew's Church in Leeds in 2009. The humour of the drama derived from the fact that, whether the person with SCD consulted a herbalist, a spiritual healer, or a medical doctor, the key feature of the encounter was the request for payment. As will be noted further in Chapter 10, recurring financial costs of SCD treatment may change the nature of the social relationships between someone living with SCD and their family.

Inheritance of sickle cell disorders

If both partners have sickle-cell trait, then *in each and every pregnancy* there is a one in four chance that they will have a child with sickle-cell anaemia; a one in four chance they will have a child with usual haemoglobin; and a one in two chance that they will have a genetic carrier, that is a child with sickle-cell trait. In Table 1.2 someone with only usual haemoglobin is denoted HbAA; someone who is a genetic carrier is denoted HbAS, and someone with sickle cell anaemia (the most common form of SCD) is denoted HbSS.

There are important differences between the terms sickle cell disease, sickle cell anaemia, and sickle cell trait that have lent themselves to misunderstandings and misinformation (see Chapters 4–6). Sickle cell disease or sickle cell disorder (SCD) refers to the whole group of clinically significant conditions in which the sickle cell gene is present (see Table 1.1). As we have seen, sickle cell anaemia is the main form of SCD, in which the person inherits the gene encoding sickle haemoglobin (HbS) from both biological parents.

There are other types of SCD, in which, in addition to haemoglobin S from one parent, the person inherits another haemoglobin variant (C, D-Punjab, E or O-Arab) from the other parent. Note that, unlike haemophilia, for example, the pattern of inheritance is not sex-linked so both women and men are equally likely to be sickle cell carriers or to have SCD. When inherited alongside haemoglobin S, haemoglobins C, D-Punjab, E or O-Arab produce sickle cell disease, for example, haemoglobin SC disease. A person might also inherit co-inherit beta-thalassaemia.

Sickle beta-thalassaemias are types of sickle cell disease in which the person inherits sickle haemoglobin from one parent, and a gene associated with beta-thalassaemia from the other. Beta-thalassaemia is associated with reduction in the *quantity* of the beta-chain part of the haemoglobin molecule produced.

Table 1.2 Pattern of inheritance of sickle cell anaemia

Gene inherited from mother who is sickle cell genetic carrier (HbAS)	Gene inherited from father who is sickle cell genetic carrier (HbAS)	
	β^A	β^S
β^A	AA Person has usual adult haemoglobin *(homozygous)*	AS Person is sickle cell genetic carrier [Person has sickle cell trait] *(heterozygous)*
β^S	AS Person is sickle cell genetic carrier [Person has sickle cell trait] *(heterozygous)*	SS Person has sickle cell anaemia (the most common form of sickle cell disease) *(homozygous)*

Source: adapted from Dyson (2005: 6).

A haemoglobin molecule comprises two alpha and two beta chains, and a reduction in or lack of production of either of these chains affects the capacity to produce haemoglobin. A discussion of the effects of co-inheritance of alpha-thalassaemia is deferred until Chapter 2. For the time being, we can note that these sickle beta-thalassaemias may be of variable severity (sickle beta-plus types) or just as severe as sickle cell anaemia itself (sickle beta-zero types). In any case, these compound types of SCD create considerable scope for misunderstanding the differences between sickle cell disease, sickle cell anaemia, sickle cell trait, and sickle cell carrier.

First, people who carry one copy of the gene encoding adult haemoglobin (haemoglobin A) and one copy of the gene associated with sickle cell (haemoglobin AS) are sickle cell genetic carriers (HbAS). They may be referred to as "having" sickle-cell trait or, alternatively, as "being" sickle cell carriers. The term "trait" may refer to a genetically determined characteristic. However, the word "trait" is also derived from the word "trace", which means having a small quantity of something, plausibly a small quantity of sickle haemoglobin. Between 20 per cent and 45 per cent of the haemoglobin of sickle cell carriers is sickle haemoglobin (Serjeant and Serjeant, 2001: 482). The phrase "sickle cell trait" is thereby open to interpretations, and community members have erroneously understood that a sickle cell carrier might go on to develop the disease, or else have a milder form of the disease. There is room for legitimate confusion when faced with medical descriptions of sickle cell trait as simultaneously a medical diagnosis and a healthy carrier state (Dyson *et al.*, 2016a).

In the past, these ambiguities were amplified owing to a particular laboratory procedure. The sickle solubility test entails adding a small amount of blood to a test tube containing a reagent and a buffer. In blood where cells have sickle haemoglobin, the mixture is opaque. Bold black lines marked on a white card cannot then be seen through the cloudy mixture. On the other hand, in samples without any sickle haemoglobin, the lines can be seen as the mixture remains clear. Unfortunately, this procedure can only identify someone as "sickle positive" and thus fails to distinguish between those with sickle cell anaemia and those with sickle cell trait. It can only note that the blood contains some haemoglobin S. Historically, reports that someone was "sickle positive" meant it was uncertain if the person had SCD (whether sickle cell anaemia or a compound type) or had sickle cell trait. Moreover, in terms of testing of blood in anticipation of genetic counselling, the sickle solubility test identified neither carrier states of other variant haemoglobins (C, D, E, etc.) nor beta-thalassaemia carriers.

Third, a person may be referred to as "having sickle cell". This ambiguous term might equally refer to a person who has sickle cell anaemia (haemoglobin SS); is a genetic sickle cell carrier (haemoglobin AS); or has a heterozygous compound condition (for example, haemoglobin SC disease, see Table 1.3). The technical language of genetics may lead to further confusion. A person who has haemoglobin AA and a person who has sickle cell anaemia (haemoglobin SS) are equally referred to as homozygous (that is they carry only *one* type of the possible variation on the gene – either haemoglobin A from both parents, or

Table 1.3 Pattern of inheritance of haemoglobin SC disorder

Gene inherited from parent who is sickle cell genetic carrier (HbAS)	Gene inherited from parent who is haemoglobin C genetic carrier (HbAC)	
	β^A	β^C
β^A	AA Person has usual adult haemoglobin *(homozygous)*	AC Person is haemoglobin C genetic carrier [Has haemoglobin C trait] *(heterozygous)*
β^S	AS Person is sickle cell genetic carrier [Person has sickle cell trait] *(heterozygous)*	SC Person has haemoglobin SC disease (the second most common form of sickle cell disease) *(heterozygous)*

Source: adapted from Dyson and Boswell (2009: 18).

haemoglobin S from both parents). By contrast, a person who inherits different alleles (allele: a possible variation on a gene) from each parent is heterozygous. However, this could be someone who is a sickle cell carrier (haemoglobin AS) or someone who has a form of sickle cell disease based on co-inheriting haemoglobin S and one of the other clinically significant haemoglobin variants (C, or D-Punjab, to cite but two examples). In such cases, both the carrier and the person with sickle cell disease are heterozygous.

Fourth, any ambiguity in terminology is crucial in encounters between clients and professionals. A lack of clarity may stem from the indeterminate nature of the diagnostic test itself, or may derive from lack of understanding on the part of either professional and/or the person, of phrases, such as "having sickle cell" or "being sickle positive".

A further possibility is that, even where someone is living with a form of SCD, this does not mean they have had a definitive medical diagnosis. Where there is newborn screening for SCD, for example in the USA, many European countries and Brazil, nearly all children with SCD will be identified at birth. In countries without such newborn screening, a person may not know they have SCD, even when those symptoms are severe (see Tamedu, 2005). In Jamaica, instances have been reported of people, presumably with milder types of SCD, reaching adulthood without realizing that they have sickle cell disease (Serjeant and Serjeant, 2001).

Finally, the emergence of SCD into public policy focus is associated in the USA with the Civil Rights Movement and the 1972 Sickle Cell Anemia Control Act. The improved citizenship status of African-Americans was reflected in the introduction of comprehensive sickle cell centres (Tapper, 1999) but also saw controversies in which confusion between SCD and sickle cell trait was erroneously incorporated into policy decisions and legislation (Duster, 2003). Furthermore, early medical case studies failed to distinguish between sickle cell anaemia, other forms of SCD, and sickle cell trait (Konotey-Ahulu, 1996: 362–363). This is discussed further in Chapter 4, but we can note for now that the legacy of medical and policy misinformation was itself used as a resource by African-American women living in poverty to dissociate themselves from (technically accurate) public health education messages about sickle cell trait and reproductive risk (Hill, 1994). Thus, although the distinction between different forms of SCD and between SCD and sickle cell trait is material and real, the subtleties of such distinctions have provided the basis for discrimination, both intentional and unintentional, of both people living with sickle cell trait and those living with SCD.

Distinguishing sickle cell anaemia, sickle cell disease and sickle cell trait

The sickle solubility test is no longer the first line of testing for variant haemoglobins such as sickle cell, and more sophisticated laboratory techniques are now in operation, including haemoglobin electrophoresis, iso-electric focusing, high performance liquid chromatography and mass spectrometry, in addition to DNA analysis (APHL/CDC, 2015). These techniques rely on separating out variant haemoglobins from one another based on differences in electrical charge (iso-electric focusing); differences in atomic weight and charge (high performance liquid chromatography) or differences in atomic weight (mass spectrometry).

So, for example, basic haemoglobin electrophoresis operates by virtue of the fact that adult haemoglobin (HbA) differs in electrical charge from sickle haemoglobin (HbS), and from other variant haemoglobins, such as haemoglobin C. A small amount of blood is deposited on gel or paper. Different haemoglobin molecules have different electric charges and, when an electric current is introduced, the molecules move at varying speeds across the medium. Consequently, over time, the different haemoglobin types will show up in bands at different points of the medium. The control locations to recognize different bands will differ depending upon whether the medium is alkaline or acid. A schematic diagram of haemoglobin electrophoresis is provided in Figure 1.1. In Figure 1.1, haemoglobin A moves fastest, haemoglobin S at an intermediate rate and haemoglobin C moves the slowest. In the first row of Figure 1.1, a person with only adult haemoglobin exhibits a band only at the known control location for haemoglobin A. Likewise a person with sickle cell anaemia (the third row of Figure 1.1) has only sickle haemoglobin, and exhibits a band only at the location for haemoglobin S. From this we can interpret the second row of Figure 1.1 as someone with bands corresponding to both sickle and usual adult haemoglobin, in other words, someone who is a sickle cell carrier (has sickle cell trait, HbAS).

Meanwhile, haemoglobin C exhibits a different electrical charge from either sickle or adult haemoglobin, moves at yet another differing rate across the medium, and corresponds to another control location. From this we can see that (row 4 of Figure 1.1) a person can have bands denoting both haemoglobin A and

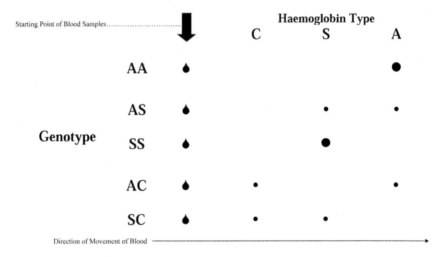

Figure 1.1 Schematic representation of haemoglobin electrophoresis.

Source: Adapted from Dyson and Boswell (2009: 20).

haemoglobin C, and is a haemoglobin C carrier. Finally (row 5 of Figure 1.1), someone may exhibit bands at points corresponding to haemoglobin S and to haemoglobin C. Such a person has haemoglobin SC disease, the second most common form of SCD, and one not definitively identifiable through a sickle solubility test.

The sickle cell solubility test remains useful, however, as bands corresponding to haemoglobin D and haemoglobin S may be difficult to differentiate, and the sickle solubility test may be required to distinguish between the two. Just as importantly, haemoglobin electrophoresis does not identify beta-thalassaemia trait. Thus, basic haemoglobin electrophoresis cannot rule out sickle cell disease, since it cannot identify the various forms of sickle cell disease called sickle beta-thalassaemia. Later in the chapter, we will return to the issue of the capacity of sickle haemoglobin to be differentially mobile in electrical fields, as this capacity also illustrates important subtleties in discussing the genetic inheritance of sickle cell.

Sickling and "normal sickling"

An internet search of images for sickle cell reveals a relative lack of pictures of people living with SCD, but rather an extensive focus on the sickle shape of the red blood cell and the role of that distorted shape in blocking blood vessels. These two factors tend to be the mainstay of community health education lessons on sickle cell: the sickle-shaped red blood cells block the capillaries at the point at which oxygen is delivered to the tissues. The diagrams show that this is possible because the capillaries may be less than the width of a red blood cell. The flexible membrane of the usual elliptical-shaped red blood cell easily squeezes through such a narrow space, but the rigid, sickled, cell cannot pass so readily and may become stuck. In this simplified account, the blockage that ensues from the clumping together of the sickled cells is what (purportedly) leads to that part of the body being denied oxygen for a period of time, with the result that the person suffers pain in the part of the body affected: the sickle cell painful episode. A consequence of such presentations is that it foregrounds the *shape* of the cell in being the initiating factor behind such blockages and the primary cause as the *physical* phenomenon of blocking. This ignores the process of what has been called normal sickling (Embury *et al.*, 1994).

The usual rate of the flow of arterial blood travelling to deliver oxygen to parts of the body is very rapid. Indeed, it is faster than the time taken for the molecules of haemoglobin to stack together into long twisted chains, and to distort the red blood cell membrane into its elongated crescent shapes. Usually, by the time that the red blood cell has sickled, it has already passed through the narrow capillaries and is back in the venous side of the circulation, in veins that are wider than the width of a blood cell, blood vessels that it therefore cannot physically block (Eaton and Hofrichter, 1994; Eaton and Bunn, 2017). This process of normal sickling, in which the red blood cell sickles, and (mostly) unsickles when re-oxygenated by the lungs, should give us pause for thought about standard health communications about sickling and what is lost in this process of simplification. Thus, most of the time, in someone with SCD, their red blood cells (comprising 90 per cent haemoglobin S in each cell) sickle after deoxygenation, and unsickle when re-oxygenated. By contrast, someone who has sickle cell trait might have around 40 per cent haemoglobin S in each red blood cell and in most situations this is insufficient for the molecules of sickle haemoglobin to form into twisted rods and to sickle the cell.

Such simplifications are in stark contrast to the plethora of publications that analyse the physiology of sickling, publications that implicate a much wider range of interacting factors. Such factors include:

- how the sickling and unsickling of red blood cells result in loss of water, with the red blood cells becoming ever denser (the haemoglobin more concentrated), resulting in irreversibly sickled cells (Rucknagel, 2001);
- how the blood becomes more viscous (thicker), slowing the rate of blood flow;
- how the membranes of the sickle cells become "sticky" with a tendency to clump together;
- how the endothelium (the lining of the blood vessels) becomes inflamed, further increasing the tendency of red blood cells to adhere to this lining as well as to each other;
- how this inflammation of the lining releases adhesive substances, substances themselves implicated in the process of clotting;
- how the usual functions that enable the walls of the endothelium to relax and widen are prevented from happening (Kato *et al.*, 2007);

- how these adhesive factors may increase the rate of rupturing of the red blood cells (Chen *et al.*, 2011);
- how other components of blood – platelets and white blood cells – are also implicated in the physiological processes generating sickle cell vaso-occlusive episodes.

Thus, rather than a physical shape (sickle) and a mechanical process (blocking), we have a complex series of dynamic biological processes: these processes are complex, dependent on context, interactive and cumulative. This complexity surpasses the truism that "sickle cells cause a blockage". It is even possible to suggest that the emblematic sickle cell shape taken on by the red blood cells is as much a *consequence* of such processes as an initiating cause. To summarize, the more prevalent simplifications of science, presented in community health education, emphasize the shape of the cell (sickle) and the mechanism of blockage. This tends towards a successionist version of causality. A (simple) successionist explanation is of the nature that one variable produces a consequence, A causes B, sickled cells cause a blockage. A generative notion of causality would stand in contrast to the successionist one described (see Pawson and Tilley, 1997).

Too often science confuses constant conjunction (A always appears alongside B) with causation. Nor is a mechanistic notion of causation sufficient (when A is introduced, B occurs). By contrast, a philosophical tradition termed critical realism takes a generative view of causation (when A is introduced, B tends to occur, but only if context C applies, and countervailing tendency D is not operating). UK philosopher Roy Bhaskar (2008 [1975]) uses the metaphor of a spark and gunpowder as an illustration of these ideas. Their conjunction does not always result in an explosion because the gunpowder may be damp; the gunpowder may be incorrectly compacted; the ratio of ingredients may be awry; the spark may be too brief; a vacuum may exist, and so on. What is missing is context. The notion of generative causality is perhaps best encapsulated in the formulation suggested by Pawson and Tilley (1997) of context-mechanism-outcome. A mechanism is a tendency (if A, then usually B). But this recognizes that while the tendency is usual, it depends upon the context. A context may enable or disable a mechanism and the outcome may or may not be produced. Or a countervailing tendency may cancel out the initial tendency.

A generative notion of causality would note that, in explaining an event such as a sickle cell crisis, there has to be a capacity, an enabling of that capacity, an absence of countervailing tendencies, several layers of context, and an understanding of which of several mechanisms in operation are the significant ones. Many, though not all, of these mechanisms are of the physiological level described, but in Chapter 2 we consider further the nested levels of causality – ecological and collective – implicated in understanding the sickle cell phenomenon. Even more importantly, if we stopped at a successionist model of causality for sickle cell, we might be content to note that people with sickle cell trait (HbAS) have some sickle haemoglobin, that their red blood cells can be made to sickle *in vitro* (see the sickle cell solubility test, discussed above) and conclude that there is a plausibility to claims that a person with sickle cell trait can exhibit sickling. As Chapters 5 and 6 show, there is a socio-political importance, as well as a biological one, to moving towards a generative notion of causality in understanding a sickle cell crisis, not least to challenge the simplifications that a sickle cell shape and mechanical blocking are the sole mechanisms in the *initiation* of physiological processes.

Genotype and phenotype

A key distinction in genetics is between a genotype and phenotype. *Genotype* refers to genetic information contained within each cell, passed on from biological parents to offspring. *Phenotype* refers to the observable physical structure and function of the organism concerned. Sociological engagements with genetics often seek to counter the perceived dangers of genetic reductionism. Genetic reductionism means reducing patterns in phenomena, for example, claimed variations in measured IQ between black and white peoples, to genetic explanations. In the case of race and IQ, such explanations have little scientific basis (see Lewontin *et al.*, 1984), and pervert the original intentions of IQ testing to help children catch up (Gould, 1996). Even the notion of general intelligence as a fixed, innate quantity arose only as an artefact of solving limitations of statistical tests, and expanded in response to anti-Semitic, anti-immigration, eugenic and racist social interests (ibid.). Thus, *political* claims are frequently smuggled in to accompany genetic claims: either that the phenomenon is unalterable because it is genetic, or that a genetic cause can be equated with a just outcome. Popular interpretations of genetics claim that genetic means we must accept the "the way things are" and that genetic equates with "natural" and "the way things are morally supposed to be". But being genetic does not make a phenomenon unalterable (see Lewontin *et al.*, 1982; Gould, 1996). Hence, as will be argued in Chapter 10, living with a genetic condition does not necessarily place limitations on the possible achievements of people living with SCD, even in the absence of a cure. Nor does a genetic cause logically dictate that a resulting distribution of life-chances is morally just (see Rose and Rose, 1986). But neoliberal social policy in the UK in which, for example, people with chronic illnesses of an unpredictable kind such as SCD are held to "fail" moral tests of employability, and are then denied both employment opportunities and adequate social security support in the absence of employment, effectively asserts this untruth. The usual reaction of sociologists is to regard genetic reductionism as a self-explanatory criticism: events and behaviours cannot be directly reduced to genes, but rather what happens in the world is an interaction between genes and the physical and collective environment. Indeed, this is the basis of criticisms outlined in Chapters 5 and 6, where it is argued that policies on sickle cell trait and athletes, and those in police contact are wrongly guided by such genetic reductionism.

From this, one might conclude that an accommodation between genetics and sociology could be reached by restricting genetic explanations to genotype and sociological explanations to how the phenotype emerges in social context.

However, this does a disservice to both disciplines. A gene is never actualized except in its environment, so a genotype, strictly speaking, exists only in the mind of the scientist who abstracts back to a genotype as a model based on regularities observed in phenotypes (Ingold, 2000).

Sociological studies of the public understanding of science have noted that many genetic scientists work with a homogeneous, passive notion of "the public" in which all people outside of scientists are characterized in the same undifferentiated manner: as ignorant of technical scientific matters, in this case, genetics (Kerr *et al.*, 1998). On the other hand, scientists are understandably keen to distance themselves from any negative consequences of genetic information, such as being discriminated against by the insurance industry or employers on the basis of such information (Kerr *et al.*, 1997). We shall see in Chapter 8 that a concept like "reproductive choice" enables clinicians to associate with the benefits of genetic information, but to withdraw from the difficult moral consequences such information brings.

Being held accountable for the unintended consequences of scientific information arguably lies behind scientists seeking to control which simplifications are communicated to which public and how. The issue, as the UK biologist Steven Rose (1997) notes, is that scientific discourse presents concepts such as proteins and molecules as coterminous with the real material world they model, as "facts" that are "out there" in nature, rather than as being theoretically strong models that adequately, but not completely, make sense of the world. Some scientists fail to recognize that we can neither directly nor wholly access the real world. Rather, constructing knowledge entails multiple small translations, that is, small adjustments at each link in a chain of relationships between scientists and things, adjustments that themselves alter the world (Latour, 2013). Failure to recognize how science is *actually* practised underpins a lack of self-understanding by some scientists of their own work and results in puzzlement when scientific "facts" fail to impress a discerning public (ibid.). In short, there are many gaps between scientific categories and the material world.

As we saw above, two crucial scientific categories with respect to genetic inheritance are the *genotype* (genetic information contained within every cell, passed from one generation to the next) and the *phenotype* (the physical structure and function of the organism that can be observed). Tables 1.2 and 1.3 on genetic inheritance follow the usual conventions by referencing patterns of inheritance in terms of genotype. In Table 1.2, the pattern is recessive (two copies of the variant gene are required to actualize the severe chronic illness). In other inherited illnesses, for example, Huntington's chorea, one copy of the variant gene is sufficient to actualize the condition and such patterns are said to be dominant (strictly, autosomal dominant, if the gene is on any other chromosome than the sex-linked chromosome).

However, the concepts recessive and dominant should properly refer to the *relationships* between the phenotype and the genotype (Griffiths *et al.*, 2002). Such a distinction has important implications for our understanding of sickle cell. Sickle cell is associated with a number of different phenotypic features at the level of the whole organism. These different features include: (1) the degree of resistance to malaria at the individual cell level; (2) the particular electrical charge of molecules as shown up in haemoglobin electrophoresis; (3) the expression of sickle haemoglobin, and the ultimate capacity of the cells to sickle; and (4) whether or not the person exhibits severe anaemia (Griffiths *et al.*, 2002).

Table 1.4 summarizes: (1) forms of inheritance; (2) a number of the possible relationships between genotype and phenotype; (3) a metaphorical explanation of such relationships; and (4) how these relationships underpin the different phenotypic features of sickle cell listed by Griffiths *et al.*

As well as the form of inheritance, we need to consider at what *scale* of the organism we are considering different effects. In terms of resistance to falciparum malaria, both people with sickle cell trait (HbAS) and those with sickle cell anaemia (HbSS) have sickle haemoglobin in their red blood cells (around 40 per cent and 90 per cent sickle haemoglobin respectively, illustrating the notion of *incomplete dominance*). The presence of sickle haemoglobin can inhibit the growth of the malarial parasites. Crucially, though, at the level of the whole organism, it is principally those with sickle cell trait that are afforded a degree of protection against death from falciparum malaria in early infancy. While resistance to malaria at the cell level may mean someone with sickle cell anaemia may also be less likely to contract malaria, at the level of the whole organism, they are extremely vulnerable to death from malaria (Williams and Obaro, 2011).

If we return to Figure 1.1, we can see an illustration of *codominance*. In the case of a sickle cell carrier (HbAS), in electrophoresis, both sickle (HbS) and usual adult haemoglobin (HbA) show up as distinct bands on the electrophoresis pattern.

Finally, if we consider the phenotypic feature of severe anaemia, this characteristic is inherited in a *recessive* manner. Thus, the anaemia is characteristic of someone with two copies of the sickle gene (HbSS) and not of a person with only one copy of the gene (HbAS). Such severe anaemia provides a different physiological context for the complex processes involved in sickling, and suggests that a generative notion of causality is necessary for understanding sickle cell symptoms, and not a successionist one that foregrounds only the sickle shape of cells. This becomes crucial in defending propositions that sickle cell trait is benign compared to sickle cell disease.

Theoretical probability and empirical occurrence

There are other extant simplifications in communicating the science of sickle cell to broader audiences, and these discussions are deferred until later chapters of the book. The subtle consequences of referring either to being a sickle cell carrier or to having sickle cell trait come more into focus when we consider debates as to whether sickle cell trait should be considered harmless or symptomatic, in Chapters 5 and 6, and when we consider antenatal screening for sickle cell in Chapter 8. Others are beyond the scope of this book. For example, the

Table 1.4 Relationship between genotype and phenotype in sickle cell

Form of inheritance	Description of relation between genotype and phenotype	Metaphor Think as if ...	Sickle cell example
Dominant	One allele dominates the alternative allele	One red plus one white equals white	Resistance to malaria at cellular level
Co-dominant	A cross between organisms with two different phenotypes produces offspring with a third phenotype in which both of the parental traits appear together	One red plus one white equals red-and-white striped	Tendency of adult and sickle haemoglobin to move at different rates in haemoglobin electrophoresis
Incomplete dominance	A cross between organisms with two different phenotypes produces offspring with a third phenotype that is a blend of the parental traits	One red plus one white, expressed less strongly, equals pink	Some sickle cell haemoglobin, some (context-dependent) capacity for the cell to exhibit a sickle shape
Recessive	Two copies of same allele required to actualize the characteristic	One red plus one white equals white, one red plus one red equals red	Haemolysis (destruction of red blood cells) and severe anaemia

standard genetic risk explained in genetic counselling is, where both biological parents are genetic carriers of a gene clinically relevant to SCD, for a 1-in-4 risk, in each and every pregnancy, of having a child with SCD. However, for reasons yet to be fully explained, the actual numbers of those born with SCD exceeds the 25 per cent expected by theoretical probability based on classic recessive patterns of inheritance. Such patterns are usually referenced back to Gregor Mendel, the nineteenth-century friar who crossed generations of peas, and first proposed the principles underpinning patterns of heredity. Less well known is that it appears that Mendel's original statistics seem to have fitted his model too perfectly, but that the mechanism of heredity he proposed had sufficient strength to allow him to ignore or otherwise adjust the empirical results *for clarity of public presentation* (Novitski, 2004). This hints that science consists of practices that build up *knowledge* rather than delve down into reality to reveal *truth* (Harman, 2018).

There is data suggesting that the numbers born with SCD exceed the expected Mendelian ratio of 25 per cent. One Brazilian study (in a non-malarial environment) noted that, when the other partner was AA, mothers who were sickle cell genetic carriers (AS) were more likely to transfer the gene than would be predicted by the classic Mendelian risk ratios (Duchovni-Silva and Ramalho, 2003). The deviation from the expected theoretical ratio is also reflected in epidemiological evidence, where actual numbers of newborns with SCD diverge from the proportion expected, based on a theoretical model called the Hardy-Weinberg Equation (Adamkiewicz and Piel, 2014; Piel *et al.*, 2016). One proposed explanation has been the practice of polygamy in parts of Africa. Where a husband has sickle cell trait and has children with SCD who die in infancy, this may accentuate the tendency to seek further wives who do not produce children with SCD (Konotey-Ahulu, 1980). Such deviations from the canons of science are usually shielded from public discussion. However, there is a more basic issue and that is the limits of what science can explain, and here we must distinguish theoretical probability from empirical occurrence.

A genetic risk of 1-in-4

In the early 2000s, I received an email from a genetic counsellor in Pakistan about a mother who had given birth to six children with beta-thalassaemia major. Beta-thalassaemia major is another severe inherited chronic illness, with inheritance based on the same 1-in-4 risk in each and every pregnancy of having a child with the major condition where both parents are genetic carriers for that condition: the same principle as underlies inheritance for sickle cell anaemia. Was there any way, the genetic counsellor wondered, to persuade the mother not to have further children? Quite apart from moral assumptions about what the mother should do, and the implication that the issue at stake was one of technical ignorance, the example does show up the importance of distinguishing between empirical occurrence and theoretical probability. The concepts of empirical occurrence and theoretical probability belong to different ways of thinking about the world. The English anthropologist Edward Evans-Pritchard (1976 [1937]) studied the Azande peoples of Central Africa. Famously, the Azande understood that someone seeking shelter from the sun under the grain stores built on wooden stilts might be killed if the building collapsed. They attributed such deaths to witchcraft. But this did not mean they failed to understand the science (that termites were progressively eating away the wooden stilts, leading the building to collapse). But science did *not* explain the particular conjunction of the particular person caught in a collapse at a particular time. That conjunction was in the realm of, for the want of a more adequate expression, magic or fate. Even if the mother in Pakistan had understood that the 1-in-4 chance applied to each and every pregnancy, the statistical numbers applying as if without memory of previous pregnancy results, and that having six affected children in a row was a 1-in-4096 chance, this scientific knowledge fails to explain why that particular woman had that conjunction of risk empirically happen to her. Science can explain theoretical probability but *not* empirical occurrence, which remains the province of magic, fate or divine will.

A teaching exercise on recessive inheritance I use with students illustrates the practical consequences of understanding empirical occurrence as well as theoretical probability (Dyson *et al.*, 1994). In this exercise students play the role of sickle cell genetic carriers (HbAS), represented by a coin, with heads denoting usual haemoglobin A (HbA) and tails representing sickle cell trait (HbS). Twenty students are asked to work in ten pairs and to have imaginary families of four children. They do this by means of each student in the pair tossing a coin where heads and tails represent the passing on of genes associated with usual adult haemoglobin (HbA) and sickle haemoglobin, (HbS) (Table 1.5). With the possibilities of the coin toss paralleling the chances of recessive genetic conditions, each coin toss has a 1-in-4 chance of throwing up the tails-tails combination that stands for "inheriting" HbS from both parents and having a child with sickle cell anaemia (HbSS).

Of course with 10 pairs role-playing the production of four children each we have a "population" of 40 children (a number chosen to ease the on-the-spot calculations of the educational facilitator). The ideal distribution would be 10 HbAA, 20 HbAS and 10 HbSS, and the first learning point is that this theoretical ideal distribution may well not be the empirical distribution created, though it is unlikely to differ too greatly. However, when we look within certain

Table 1.5 A learning exercise on patterns of recessive inheritance

	Heads (usual haemoglobin A)	*Tails (sickle cell trait)*
Heads (usual haemoglobin A)	Heads-heads represents HbAA (usual haemoglobin)	Heads-tails represents HbAS (sickle cell trait)
Tails (sickle cell trait)	Tails-heads represents HbAS (sickle cell trait)	Tails-tails represents HbSS (sickle cell anaemia)

"families" of four children, other learning points become possible. Few individual families of four will have the ideal theoretical distribution of one child with usual haemoglobin, two sickle cell trait and one sickle cell anaemia. Some of the projected families may have more than one child with sickle cell anaemia: a powerful illustration of the difference between theoretical probability and empirical occurrence. In many instances, the families will comprise only children with usual haemoglobin or sickle cell trait. When noting that, without specific blood testing, the sickle cell trait is indistinguishable, this allows students to understand how sickle cell can be passed through families over generations without being noticed. This learning point can be accentuated if asked to think about the tendency in the Global North to smaller families, and to report on only the first two children produced in the exercise. One actual participant reported becoming dispirited after three imaginary children in a row with HbSS (Dyson *et al.*, 1994), and though discussion of emotional responses is possible, this needs to be tempered with challenging disabling language such as associating children with sickle cell anaemia as "being unlucky" or "having a bad outcome". Of course the language of risk, in conjunction with prenatal screening for sickle cell, already implicitly frames the birth of a child with SCD as an undesirable outcome, and this is discussed further in Chapter 8.

There are other examples too where science is complicated, health education messages are simplified, and the link between the two warrants further scrutiny. The oversimplification that sickle cell protects against malaria is compared to more nuanced arguments about malaria and sickle cell as part of arguments developed in Chapter 2. Perhaps the most important is the tension between sickle cell alleles (being a sickle cell carrier) and having sickle cell trait, and whether to regard sickle cell trait as harmless or symptomatic. This is explored further in Chapters 5 and 6. Another simplification – the problematic and complex relationship between socially constructed ethnicity categories and human genomic variation – is examined in Chapter 7. Chapter 8 on antenatal screening takes up the complexities of genetic risk and reproductive decision-making.

Sickle cell and science

One issue at stake in this chapter has been the fact that science is complicated. By this is meant more than being complex, since folk knowledge can be of equal complexity to science. In this sense, complicated refers to the idea that many factors, both material (scientific instruments, transport and funding) and ideational (scientific theories, scientific communications, societal cultural systems) stand between researchers and the tentative or "remote" knowledge they generate (Latour, 2013; Delanda and Harman, 2017). These have been described as lengthy chains of reference that sustain the process of knowledge production (Latour, 2013). It has been extensively documented that this is what scientists actually do, contrasts directly with how some scientists account publicly for their work (Gilbert and Mulkay, 1984; Lynch, 1985; Latour, 1999), and confirms that scientific knowledge, and the material world we construct knowledge about, are not the same thing.

For Latour (2013), science depends not on direct access to the truth, as if the scientist could double-click a computer mouse and directly apprehend reality. Rather, Latour describes the *institution* of science, which depends on demonstrating an audit trail of what he terms "chains of reference". These chains of reference comprise all the practices and artefacts, linked together, which make the construction of scientific knowledge possible. We can illustrate this in the work of US/Swiss biophysicist Stuart Edelstein (1986) on the sickle haemoglobin molecule. In order to explain how molecules of sickle haemoglobin stack together, Edelstein has to marshal: technological artefacts (electron microscopes); measurements (the angle of 26 degrees at which molecules of haemoglobin stack together); scientific grants; human communications; use of transport; and models (treating the haemoglobin molecule "as if" a globe with the effect of the allele dependent upon a position at points of latitude and longitude). More recent scientific research depends also on non-humans: bacteria in gene editing and disabled sickle cell mice as animal models. Scientific knowledge is constructed through such complicated relations. Both methodological transparency and scientific knowledge depend on acknowledging these lengthy chains of reference in accounting for evidence.

It has been suggested that professions have "guilty knowledge" of their clients (Hughes, 1962). For example, doctor-patient confidentiality places a duty on doctors not to impart many types of knowledge *about* their client to others. But they may also harbour "guilty knowledge" that they do not impart *to* their client:

- that they are more concerned about long-term organ damage in hastening premature death than the current sickle cell crisis;
- that they know how many decades away from accessible clinical practice the latest technological sickle cell "breakthrough" lies;
- that they have exhausted their known repertoire in attempting to, for example, minimize adverse reactions to blood transfusions;
- that neither they nor other clinical sickle cell specialists know the answer to a particular challenge of SCD.

A further variation on this theme is the notion that scientists hold in trust the responsibility of protecting all others from the complexities of life, complexities that may be overwhelming or frightening (Dingwall, 2001). So we convey the message that HbAS is a genetic carrier of sickle cell, while knowing that several very rare types of "super-sickling" variants of haemoglobin S exist that result in HbAS genotypes having a form of SCD (see Table 1.6, a level of complexity greater than Table 1.1). The role of scientists and professionals in such situations comes to be custodians of which complexities should be bracketed for public consumption. This creates a problem, for it could be argued that those without technical scientific expertise are not in a position to make judgements about the directions of scientific endeavours. The complementary question might also be posed: why should scientists exercise the right to exclude the public from decisions about the priorities of science (Kerr *et al.*, 1997)? Since non-scientists

Table 1.6 Different types of sickle cell disease

Type of sickle cell disease	Characteristics
Severe sickle cell disease	
HbS/S (β6Glu > Val/β6Glu > Val) sickle-cell anaemia	The most common form of sickle-cell disease
HbS/β⁰ thalassaemia	Most prevalent in the eastern Mediterranean region and India
Severe HbS/β⁺ thalassaemia	Most prevalent in the eastern Mediterranean region and India; 1–5% HbA present
HbS/OArab (β6Glu > Val/β121Glu > Lys)	Reported in North Africa, the Middle East, and the Balkans; relatively rare
HbS/D Punjab (β6Glu > Val/β121Glu > Gln)	Predominant in northern India but occurs worldwide
HbS/C Harlem (β6Glu > Val/β6Glu > Val/β, β73Asp > Asn)	Electrophoretically resembles HbSC, but clinically severe; double mutation in β-globin gene; very rare
HbC/S Antilles (β6Glu > Lys/β6Glu > Val, β23Val–Ile)	Double mutation in β-globin gene results in severe sickle-cell disease when co-inherited with HbC; very rare
HbS/Quebec-CHORI (β6Glu > Val/β87Thr > Ile)	Two cases described; resembles sickle-cell trait with standard analytical techniques
Moderate sickle-cell disease	
HbS/C (β6Glu > Val/β6Glu > Lys)	25–30% cases of sickle-cell disease in populations of African origin
Moderate HbS/β⁺ thalassaemia	Most cases in the eastern Mediterranean region; 6–15% HbA present
HbA/S Oman (βᴬ/β6Glu > Val, β121Glu > Lys)	Dominant form of sickle-cell disease caused by double mutation in β-globin gene; very rare
Mild sickle-cell disease	
Mild HbS/β⁺⁺ thalassaemia	Mostly in populations of African origin; 16–30% HbA present
HbS/E (β6Glu > Val/β26Glu > Lys)	HbE predominates in south-east Asia and so HbSE uncommon, although frequency is increasing with population migration
HbA/Jamaica Plain (βᴬ/β6Glu > Val, β68Leu/Phe)	Dominant form of sickle-cell disease; double mutation results in Hb with low oxygen affinity; one case described
Very mild sickle-cell disease	
HbS/HPFH	Group of disorders caused by large deletions of the β-globin gene complex; typically 30% foetal haemoglobin
HbS/other Hb variants	HbS is co-inherited with many other Hb variants, and symptoms develop only in extreme hypoxia

Source: reprinted from *The Lancet* 376(9757): 2018–2031, with permission from Elsevier.

Notes
Genotypes that have been reported to cause sickle-cell disease are listed. All include at least one copy of the βˢallele, in combination with one or more mutations in the β-globin gene. HbS = sickle haemoglobin. HbA = haemoglobin variant A. HbE = haemoglobin variant E. Hb = haemoglobin.
Notations such as (β6Glu > Val/β6Glu > Val) represent the change in molecular structure of the variant haemoglobin in question.
Numerical references in the original table (Rees *et al.*, 2010: 2020) have been omitted.

themselves recognize the social interests and social conditions at play in knowledge production (Kerr *et al.*, 1998), exclusionary tendencies will tend to diminish trust in science. Instructive here is the work of Spanish archaeologist Pablo Alonso-González (2016). Ethnographic research showed that the more archaeologists attempted to legitimise their authority by claiming certainty of scientific facts, where only scientists were judged capable to decide, the more pseudo-archaeology proliferated. In contrast, acknowledging the work of amateurs restrained the growth of pseudo-archaeology by creating networks of trust between amateurs and professionals. Restoring trust between people and institutions is crucial (Latour, 2013), and creating such trust between scientists and doctors, on the one hand, and people with SCD and their communities, on the other, requires us to carry out sickle cell studies that include interested "amateurs" (used here in a strictly non-pejorative sense) in debates on the simplifications of sickle cell science.

Conclusion

In this chapter we have seen that sickle cell is a condition with multiple layers of complexity. This raises the question of the relationship between scientists and doctors, on the one hand, and people living with SCD and wider communities of interest, on the other. A simplistic model of the public understanding of science, in which the "general public" is held to be unable to understand the technical complexities of scientific information, which should then be hermetically sealed from public inspection, in my view, represents an inadequate conception of the relationship between science and people. For me, the lessons to be learned about this relationship are:

1   Doing science is (literally) complicated. Many transformations are involved (theoretical models, language concepts, scientific instruments, institutional arrangements, funding) between the material reality and the scientific knowledge. Material reality does not reveal itself to scientists, and they have neither direct nor complete access to it.
2   There is a difference between knowledge, and the material world that knowledge models (this is discussed further in Chapter 2).
3   Other modes of knowledge exist (theoretical probability is not empirical occurrence), modes that are not commensurate with science.
4   Scientists and social scientists should consult people living with SCD about research agendas and priorities as well as communicate research findings in accessible ways.
5   There are advantages to involving people with SCD in research processes (beyond passive participation in clinical trials), so that the boundary between doing science and practical wisdom is a permeable one.
6   Provided scientific communities act in accordance with points 1–5, only then it is reasonable to ask SCD communities to extend a certain level of trust in return. The alternative is an endemic lack of trust that undermines scientific endeavours around sickle cell (see Benjamin, 2011).

In Chapter 2, we look at the way in which different disciplines have tended to caricature one another, often linked to struggles for prestige within academic institutions, arguing that an understanding of sickle cell can be reduced to neither biology nor sociology.

2 Why genes are not "for" sickle cell

Introduction

It was noted at the outset of the book that sickle cell has come to be regarded as an emblem of being black. We further noted that racism acts like a language system, such that the concept black signals up other (usually negative) concepts within the cultural system. Sickle cell is part of this system, but plays an especially crucial part. The role of racist ideology is to attempt to fix meaning. As such, sickle cell represents the use of race/ethnicity categories as coded messages about biological inevitability and inalterability (Outram and Ellison, 2005). In other words, because sickle cell is genetic, and because sickle cell is linked, accurately or not, to being black, part of the unspoken logic of racism is as follows: sickle cell is black; sickle cell is biological-genetic; biological-genetic means something is given; being given means that it cannot be changed; if something is given and cannot be changed, it must be fair or just (the "natural" order of things). Sickle cell has thus been misappropriated as a key bridge in racist logic, providing a link between blackness, genetics and inequality as the (alleged) natural order of things.

It is arguably social science objections to genetic determinism and genetic reductionism that constitute part of the problematic interface of biology and sociology. However, biologists themselves have identified how particular socio-political claims, claims which do not follow logically at all from the evidence, have been smuggled into genetic "explanations" of human behaviours. Lewontin *et al.* (1982) pointed out, for example, that even if (and this is still an if) biology does contribute to an unequal distribution of social rewards and life chances, logically we are not thereby required to view the order so established as just or fair. Nor does a congenital origin dictate that the order of things is unchangeable (Rose and Rose, 1986). The UK social anthropologist Tim Ingold (2000: 385) suggests that genetic change is possible without a change in the form or behaviour of an organism, and that changes in form or behaviour are possible without genetic change. The UK sociologist Caroline New (2005) has advanced a critical realist conception of the sexes, which posits human sex dichotomism as real (and gender as culturally formed, imposed and resisted). In this view, the complex and lengthy biological pathways between generative structures (human sex dichotomism) may form a foetus whose features *tend to* cluster together around poles of female and male, but which also generate those with features on a continuum between the poles. The choice is not between a fixed biology and a fluid postmodern sociology, for plasticity is already within biology.

In this respect New brings together two important traditions, in biology and in sociology. One is the tradition of UK biologist Steven Rose (1997), whose developmental biological "lifelines" suggest complex biochemical pathways through which the parts of the genome may or may not be instantiated, or may be instantiated in different ways, thus emphasizing the plasticity through which genes influence our development. It could be said that Rose anticipated the problems of the Human Genome Project in that he noted that proteins and molecules, far from being Nature "out there" revealed to scientists, are concepts for thinking with, albeit strong concepts that work well in many circumstances.

This illustrates an important principle, namely, *that knowledge and what we have knowledge of are not the same phenomenon*. This idea has been expressed by the metaphor "the map is not the territory" (Latour, 2013). Likewise the concept of genotype represents the map, not the terrain. Since there is no specification of an organism independent of its environment, the genotype only exists in the mind of the genetic scientist who develops rules based on abstractions from the observed characteristics of the whole organism (Ingold, 2000). The fact that we cannot definitively say how many genes there are (Pennisi, 2003) suggests that genes, too, are scientific concepts that, however strong as conceptual tools for modelling the world, are not the same thing as the evolving reality they describe. This does not mean there is no material reality independent of human beings, but it does mean that we do not have direct access to this material reality (Delanda and Harman, 2017) and that other non-human entities (as well as human thought) are some of the inevitable mediators between human knowledge and material reality (Latour, 2013).

This chapter takes the issue of sickle cell as a particularly useful vehicle for illustrating that human variation and diversity of illness experience are produced at several analytical scales, from genomic, through organisms to environments. This delineation is central to the thinking of Rose (1997), who argues that genes are not "for" anything. But sometimes, issues become, in the words of the French anthropologist Claude Lévi-Strauss, *bonnes à penser*: either good-for-thinking-with or goods-for-thinking-with, depending upon the translation (Leach, 1970). And so it is with sickle cell, which has an ideological role in fixing meanings, from buttressing the views of extreme right-wing groups (Anionwu, 1993; Clare, 2007) to becoming incorporated into rhetoric with which state officials account for sudden deaths of black people in custody (Dyson and Boswell, 2009). We need to unfix these meanings. In order to unfix these meanings, we need to see how and why genes are not "for" sickle cell.

Genes and genomes

Sickle cell anaemia is cited by the World Health Organization as a monogenic (single-gene) disease (WHO, 2012). The variation between usual adult haemoglobin (haemoglobin A) and sickle haemoglobin (haemoglobin S) involves just one alteration in the molecular structure, with one amino acid valine replacing the usual amino acid glutamine at point six of the β-globin (beta-globin) chain (Ingram, 1957). But phenotypes of SCD are modulated by polymorphisms within the overall human genome not immediately related to the single mutation of the β-globin gene (Driss *et al.*, 2009). The sickle cell phenomenon is therefore not exhausted by the notion of a monogenetic disease.

The first factor to consider is that SCD refers to several different types of sickle cell disease. In the medical literature, the different types are often ascribed varying levels of severity (see Table 1.6). Thus, the particular haemoglobin variant co-inherited with the gene associated with sickle haemoglobin appears to play a part in sickle cell. Indeed, if SCD had not first become visible to the medical profession in the context of the historically-specific racialized poverty of its socially marginalized patients (Wailoo, 2001), it might be that we heard less about SCD as a homogeneous whole and more about individual sickle cell disorders, each in their own right.

The second factor about the gene associated with sickle haemoglobin is that there are other irregularities in gene locations nearby on the same chromosome (chromosome 11 of the human genome). Systematic variations in this chromosomal context have been used to propose the theory of a multi-centric origin for sickle cell. This multi-centric origin model at first laid claim to having identified three African haplotypes (Pagnier *et al.*, 1984), then an Indian one (Kulozik *et al.*, 1986) and subsequently one further African (Cameroon) haplotype (Lapouniéroulie *et al.*, 1992), and thus five different chromosomal contexts or haplotypes in total. The multi-centric theory thus proposes that the gene associated with sickle haemoglobin arose on five separate occasions and locations: Senegal, Benin, Cameroon, Central Africa and India. The Central African haplotype was formerly described as the Bantu haplotype after the family of languages spoken by the hundreds of diverse ethnic groups across Central Africa. The term is now less used, owing to its association with the pejorative racist classification of the twentieth-century regime of apartheid in South Africa. An alternative theory – of a single origin for the gene encoding sickle haemoglobin – has recently been reinvigorated by Shriner and Rotimi (2018). This single origin theory proposes one common ancestor, around 7,300 years ago, with possible locations in either the Green Sahara or the north-west sector of the West/Central African rainforest. The Green Sahara possibility (where between 7500 and 3500 BCE greater rainfall rendered the Sahara more fertile than before or today), is a cautionary reminder that place does not remain the same over time and so mutations in the human genome induced by malarial pressures may reflect historical rather than contemporary geography. It has been suggested that some haplotypes may be associated with less severe clinical effects. Shriner and Rotimi further suggest that the 20 haplotypes they identify do not map neatly onto the canonical five, and propose this may be confounding attempts to link haplotype to phenotype symptoms. There are social scientific challenges as well. For example, the Senegal haplotype is said to run a milder course than other African haplotypes. However, the US anthropologist Duana Fulwilley (2011) argues that this ascription of a milder course of SCD is made too readily. She suggests this draws attention away from other factors in the sickle cell experience in Senegal, including the adverse effects of economic structural adjustments forced on to Senegal by the global monetary community; the serial failure of politicians to act on promises to develop sickle cell services; and the complex basis for the effectiveness of the plant *fagara* as a local treatment: seemingly effective as much for its embeddedness in complex social relationships with local healers as for any direct pharmacological effects.

In an era in which we are promised personalized medicine based on precision genomics, it is also worth reflecting critically on the drivers of the Human Genome Project. Although genes associated with sickle cell are of huge significance (to the Global South), the focus on the human genome only arose when genes became linkable to putative multifactorial causes of cancer and heart disease (the major killers of the Global North), and hence of interest to venture capital (Martin, 1999). The upsurge in genomic medicine continues, and has become associated with notions of personalized medicine, that drugs could become tailored to suit unique genomes (or at least the genomes of wealthy individuals). Yet somehow sickle cell has been by-passed again. Without the need to sequence the whole genome, little research has explored the possible effects of which haplotypes a particular person with SCD may have inherited. For example, Benin/Benin would represent inheriting the same sickle cell haplotype from both biological parents, whereas Central African/Benin would represent inheriting the Central African haplotype from one, and the Benin haplotype from another. With five claimed haplotypes, a cross-tabulation yields 25 possibilities. This intermediate position, between the misleading notion of sickle cell as a monogenetic (singe-gene) disease, and extreme individualized genomics, has attracted comparatively little by way of research endeavours (Okumura *et al.*, 2016).

Even compared to the Senegal haplotype, the Indian haplotype has been described as yielding the mildest condition of all (Piel *et al.*, 2017). This is thought to be because the haplotype is associated with higher levels of foetal haemoglobin. Foetal, or baby haemoglobin, has a high affinity for oxygen (attracts oxygen especially strongly) and is the primary haemoglobin in the foetus from 6–12 weeks' gestation until the baby reaches 3–6 months old, before being replaced with adult haemoglobin. An increased level of residual foetal haemoglobin in adults with SCD is thought to produce a less severe form of SCD. However plausible this may seem, Indian researchers continue to note the possibility of severe SCD symptoms for those living with SCD on the Indian sub-continent (Jain *et al.*, 2016). This does draw attention to the work of Rose (1997), which argues that genes may only be expressed in the phenotype through lengthy biochemical pathways or what he terms "lifelines". In the next section of this chapter, we look at two examples of factors which have established, if complex, conditional and sometimes opposing, effects on sickle cell when considered at the level of the whole organism.

The organism

Sickle cell enjoys an important but complex relationship to *Plasmodium falciparum* malaria. The notion that the gene associated with sickle cell protects against malaria is an over-simplification, and mechanisms that may be protective when considered at the cellular level do not necessarily translate into greater protection when considered at the level of the organism as a whole. Those who do not inherit a gene encoding sickle cell at all and who only have usual adult haemoglobin (HbAA) are profoundly vulnerable to falciparum malaria. Those who inherit one copy of the gene associated with sickle cell (sickle cell genetic carriers, HbAS) are protected, not from contracting such malaria, but are relatively protected from death from such malaria in a key window between the ages of 2 and 20 months old. This is the window of vulnerability between maternal-acquired immunity waning, and environmentally-provoked immunity building up. Those who inherit a gene associated with sickle cell from both parents, most notably sickle cell anaemia (HbSS), may be less liable to contract malaria, but should they do so, they will be extremely vulnerable to early death from malaria (Williams and Obaro, 2011). Indeed, death from malaria is an important cause of death for an infant with SCD in Africa (McAuley *et al.*, 2010) and, overall, SCD may be responsible for at least 3–4 per cent of under-5 mortality in Sub-Saharan Africa (Modell and Darlison, 2008), and as much as 5–16 per cent according to some estimates (Grosse *et al.*, 2011). In such a situation, the prevalence of genes associated with sickle cell in the overall population increases, since those with sickle cell trait differentially survive, and also decreases, as most of those with SCD die prematurely. Eventually the population concerned establishes a balance between the early deaths from SCD (reducing the numbers with genes associated with sickle cell in the overall population) and the increased reproductive fitness of those who are sickle cell genetic carriers. Scientists refer to this as *balanced polymorphism*, and sickle cell is the canonical example, though science students living with SCD may well be distressed by statements in older textbooks that state that people with SCD do not live into adulthood (Anionwu and Atkin, 2001).

As we have seen, even with those who have inherited genes associated with sickle cell and have a form of SCD, there is considerable variation in the characteristics of the actual person. A higher proportion of foetal haemoglobin is associated with a reduced tendency of cells to sickle. However, the US Professor of Medicine, Martin Steinberg, has summarized the complexities in assessing the clinical severity of sickle cell (Steinberg, 2005). First, higher levels of foetal haemoglobin (HbF) may have different effects with regard to different SCD symptoms. Hence, for example, higher levels of HbF are associated with protective effects (promoting positive features or reducing negative effects) for some SCD symptoms but not others. HbF is protective in increasing survival, reducing painful episodes, decreasing splenic sequestration and lessening leg ulcers, but may have little discernible protective effects for stroke or pulmonary hypertension.

A key development in medical treatment of SCD has been the re-purposing of a cancer drug, hydroxyurea (hydroxycarbamide), in treating SCD and reducing the complications of sickle cell painful crises in some patients (Charache *et al.*, 1995). It works through promoting increased levels of foetal haemoglobin, though not all patients show benefits, as the distribution of haemoglobin F may be uneven between the red blood cells, leaving some cells unprotected from the damage of the long, twisted rods that can form with sickle haemoglobin. The efficacy of increased HbF with specific regard to reducing acute chest syndrome seems to depend on the HbF increase arising from treatment with hydroxyurea rather than inborn levels of HbF, again drawing attention to the context-dependent nature of causality.

A further example of SCD being modified by co-inheritance of other genes is the case of α-thalassaemia (alpha-thalassaemia) (Steinberg, 2005), where a person with SCD may co-inherit a deletion of one or two of the four genes encoding the α-globin chain. Again, the possible beneficial effects of co-inheritance of α-thalassaemia deletions do not all point in the same direction, depending upon which particular phenotype of SCD one considers. Thus, co-inheritance of an α-thalassaemia deletion is associated with a reduction in the prevalence of strokes and leg ulcers. Conversely, it may make splenic sequestration more likely. However, it may have different or even opposing consequences if one compares co-inheritance of α-thalassaemia in people with sickle cell anaemia (HbSS) compared to people with haemoglobin SC disease (HbSC). It may make painful sickle cell crises less likely in someone with HbSC, but have little effect (or even make things worse) with respect to painful episodes in someone with HbSS. Likewise, co-inheritance of α-thalassaemia may be associated with a reduction in the incidence of osteonecrosis (death of bone tissue, especially the shoulder and hip joints) in a person with HbSC, but an increased incidence in someone with HbSS (Steinberg, 2005).

There is also the possibility of epistatic interactions (epistasis: other genes that modify the effects of the gene in question) at the level of populations rather than individuals. Penman *et al.* (2009) put forward a thesis to explain why the sickle cell gene, which may have "out-competed" thalassaemia genes in West/Central Africa as the human genetic protection against severe malaria, remains relatively uncommon in Mediterranean populations. They suggest that in Mediterranean populations, which have considerable levels of genes encoding both α-thalassaemia and β-thalassaemia, the protection against malaria which α-thalassaemia and β-thalassaemia carriers both exhibit is still retained in those who co-inherit both α- and β-thalassaemia traits. Where this is the case, they argue, populations with a threshold level of α-thalassaemia and β-thalassaemia genes resist being supplanted by the sickle cell gene. Such complex interactions of different genes have been used to explain the emergence of sickle cell hotspots (small areas of the Mediterranean where the level of sickle cell in the population is as high as in West Africa, such as parts of Greece, Sardinia and Sicily), which remain over time but without spreading throughout the region (Penman *et al.*, 2012). The nature of the interaction of genes is different if one considers sickle cell trait rather than SCD. For example, there is negative epistasis between co-inheritance of sickle cell trait (HbAS) and α^+-thalassaemia, a combination that apparently cancels out the protective effect of HbAS. Studies in Kenya have shown that while both α^+-thalassaemia trait and sickle cell trait are strongly protective against severe malaria when inherited independently, when inherited in combination, this degree of protectiveness is lost (Williams *et al.*, 2005).

The physical environment

As we will see in Chapter 3, ecology played a vital role in the development of the sickle cell mutation. For those now living with SCD, the environment is an important source of variation in lived experience (Tewari *et al.*, 2015; Piel *et al.*, 2017). In the next two sections we look at the physical and social environments, although, as will become apparent, this distinction is merely a device to organize material, since humans help make (and destroy) the ecological environment, and non-humans are integral to the collective environment.

Sickle cell arose in the context of malaria, and while sickle cell trait offers partial protection against *Plasmodium falciparum* malaria, the said malaria is a major killer of infants with sickle cell disease. The danger falls in early infancy, between the waning of acquired immunity from the mother, and the development of environmentally-acquired resistance to *Plasmodium falciparum*. A child born outside of a malarial context, for example, in the process of parental migration from Sub-Saharan Africa to Northern Europe, but then threatened with sudden forced removal to a malarial environment (the word "removal" is important: it is not a "return") will not have developed any acquired immunity. Such is the case of a number of asylum seekers in the UK, where lawyers have argued that the removal of a child with SCD, born in the UK and thus without acquired immunity to falciparum malaria, would make the child extremely vulnerable if deported to a malarial country in which they had never lived (Dyson, 2009). For example, a father who fled persecution in Cameroon for protesting the unlawful execution of nine boys, and sought asylum in the UK, had twins born in the UK with SCD, and his British-born infants would have been endangered if forced to move to an area of endemic malaria in which they had themselves never lived (Word Press, 2008).

The weather is also a key determinant of the experience of living with SCD. In a maritime temperate climate, such as the UK, particular weather patterns in an urban environment have been associated with increased sickle cell hospital admission for acute pain episodes (Jones *et al.*, 2005). The particular conditions are windy weather and low humidity. Windy weather may be associated with rapid cooling of exposed skin, akin perhaps to the experience when exiting an unheated swimming pool. Meanwhile, low humidity may dry out mucous membranes which help protect from infection, infections to which, as previously outlined, those with SCD are especially vulnerable as repeated infarctions damage their infection-fighting organ, the spleen.

The weather plays a causal role in different ways when we consider different SCD symptoms. In the USA, higher monthly temperatures were significantly associated with both lower pain intensity and pain frequency for people living with SCD (Smith *et al.*, 2009). A study in Northern Nigeria found three peaks for occurrences of vaso-occlusive sickle cell crises in relation to both the rainy season and the Harmattan, a dry dust wind that blows over West Africa from the Sahara. Winds and low humidity in the Harmattan dry season combine to evaporate sweat rapidly and produce cold-induced sickle cell painful episodes. The non-Harmattan dry season produces the highest temperatures of the year and water loss, associated with dehydration, is a different plausible pathway to the triggering of vaso-occlusive crises in those with SCD. The third peak was at the height of the rainy season (Figure 2.1), where increased vegetation and stagnant water pools favour mosquito activity, and the transmission of malaria-induced sickle cell crises (Ahmed *et al.*, 2012).

The Harmattan also seemingly plays a role in another major SCD symptom, the acute chest syndrome: sickling in the blood vessels of the lungs, accompanied by cough, infection and pain. The role of the Harmattan is thought to be in producing low humidity, thence vulnerability to infection, with infection the trigger to acute chest syndrome (ibid.). A third SCD symptom in which weather in northern Nigeria is implicated is that of priapism: a painful persistent erection of the penis, unrelated to sexual thought, which if untreated may leave the sufferer impotent. The key weather condition is the extremely hot temperatures of the non-Harmattan dry season in northern Nigeria and lack of hydration, the key

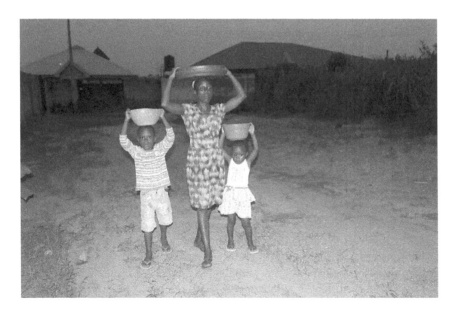

Figure 2.1 Cloudy weather portends rain, Lagos State, Nigeria, 2017.
Source: With permission of Funso Balogun and Ayoola Olajide.

trigger to priapism. Finally, ischaemic strokes (strokes caused by blockages, rather than bleeds), were raised in months of peak mosquito activity and malaria parasite transmission. The authors hypothesize that malaria is related to increased red cell adhesion to the lining of the blood vessels, and such increased adhesion may be related to raised levels of strokes in a small number of SCD patients (ibid.).

Air quality has also been studied for its possible effects on hospital admission with acute sickle cell pain. In one UK study, acute admissions were raised when ozone levels were higher, especially in the summer months (Yallop *et al.*, 2007). On the other hand, not all air pollutants operated in the same direction, that is, to worsen rates of sickle cell acute admissions. There was no association between sulphur dioxide, nitrogen dioxide or dust (particulate matter less than 10 microns). There was even an inverse relationship between carbon monoxide and acute sickle cell admissions. This may be because carbon monoxide and haemo-globin together form carboxyhaemoglobin, which cannot form the long, twisted rods of sickle haemoglobin, thus decreasing the amount of sickling. *In vivo* studies have also shown prolonged red blood cell survival when carbon mon-oxide has been administered, and carbon monoxide has even been investigated as a possible form of treatment for SCD. There was also a trend towards an inverse relation between levels of nitric oxide and admissions. People with SCD are usually depleted of nitric oxide, whose normal function would be to relax walls of blood vessels, and whose absence may lead to increased tendency of blood vessels to constrict. Presence of nitric oxide has been found to reduce levels of SCD pain (Yallop *et al.*, 2007).

Yet the possible effects of air quality depend on the particular symptoms of SCD and the pathways to those symptoms that one considers. Higher levels of dust (particulate matter less than 10 microns) were associated with increased blood velocity in patients with SCD (Mittal *et al.*, 2009). Such increased blood velocity in blood vessels in the neck is associated with risk of stroke in some patients (Deane *et al.*, 2010). This suggests a possible pathway between a particular form of environmental pollution and a particular symptom of SCD, stroke.

Quality of air in the home has also been implicated in possible routes to trig-gering SCD-related-illnesses. In low- and middle-income countries, many are compelled to prepare meals on inefficient cooking stoves or heat their homes using biomass fuel (wood or animal dung) leading to household air pollution. This can be associated directly with pulmonary hypertension or right heart failure but Bloomfield *et al.* (2012) suggest that a condition such as SCD may have a predisposing effect, producing a combined genetic and environmental pathway to severe symptoms. Young people with SCD have also been shown to exhibit increased frequency of respiratory symptoms when exposed to environ-mental tobacco smoke or passive smoking. The increased respiratory symptoms were found with current or past exposure to passive tobacco smoke, and even to exposure to smoke when in the womb (Cohen *et al.*, 2013).

The context-dependent nature of causality has also been reflected in medical debates: especially the issue as to whether treatments developed in non-malarial environments are transferable to malarial areas of the world where SCD is common. Thus, data from several African countries indicated that the main infection *streptococcus pneumoniae* found in non-malarial countries did not appear to be the leading cause of infections in children with SCD, and that, without further studies, the particular context may mean that pneumococcal prophylaxis was potentially inappropriate (Serjeant, 2005). However, Williams *et al.* (2009) found that the organisms causing bacteria in the blood in African children with sickle cell anaemia were the same as those in developed countries, and concluded that despite the difference in malarial context, introduction of vaccinations could substantially affect survival of African children with SCD.

Finally, as previously indicated, there can be no distinction between social and physical environment. For example, in the Middle Eastern country of Bahrain, ongoing tensions between the regime and its Shia population, tensions that are arguably a proxy for broader geo-political struggles between Iran (majority Shia Islam) and Saudi Arabia (majority Sunni Islam) have led to both historic and recent accusations of human rights abuses. In the 1990s, there were reports of the abuse of prisoners with SCD in Dry Dock Prison in Manama: sitting them in the direct flow of air conditioners, and presumably inducing the types of sickle cell crises when exposed skin is rapidly cooled (United Nations, 1997). Later tensions in Bahrain in the years following the failed "Arab Spring" of 2011 resulted in extensive use of tear gas on demonstrators, including those with SCD, which could result in lack of oxygen and exacerbate sickle cell symptoms, notably acute chest syndrome. Reports of deaths of people with SCD associated with use of tear gas by security forces were documented by the Bahraini Center for Human Rights (2013).

The collective environment

While the general principle that there are social determinants of health is well established (Marmot and Wilkinson, 2006), we need to disaggregate several factors in this broad relationship. The phrase social determinants includes *poverty*, and plausible pathways to worsening the lived experience of SCD caused by poverty include lack of access to good nutrition; exposure to infections and accidents through dangerous living environments, and lack of money to adequately heat housing. In the UK, Cronin de Chavez (2018) notes that sudden drops in home temperature are linked to the onset of sickle cell crises and argues that money to support adequate heating of homes in colder climates should be regarded as a form of preventive medicine. One US study suggested that individual socio-economic distress was associated with SCD pain-related disablement and with psychological and physical poor quality of life, but also that measures of neighbourhood-level socio-economic poverty were independently associated with poorer physical quality of life for young people living with SCD (Palermo *et al.*, 2008). A UK study notes that people with SCD from socio-economically deprived areas are at highest risk of both SCD readmissions and in-hospital mortality (Al Juburi *et al.*, 2013).

A related but distinct aspect of the social determinants of health is *inequality* (Wilkinson, 1996; Wilkinson and Pickett, 2009). Inequality in social standing means that those in subordinated positions, having to routinely defer to those in higher social standing (and this could be on the basis of class, gender, racism or disablement), are more prone to the damaging release of corticosteroids (adrenaline or "flight or fight" hormones) as they have to suppress legitimate anger in the face of injustice, and be faced either with accepting a toxic status quo or being positioned as a serial troublemaker. Since the chronic release of such corticosteroids is associated with heart disease and diabetes in all persons, it is easy to see recognizable pathways through which the health of a person living with SCD might also be compromised. The anger, frustration, disappointment of constantly deferring to someone of higher status damages health. But people with SCD in North America or Europe may have to defer to others as a low-paid employee, as a person from a racialized minority group to a racist state official (see Chapter 6) or to an unsympathetic health care provider (Haywood *et al.*, 2014). In the Global South, they may have to defer to others on the basis of disability discrimination (see Ola *et al.*, 2016). Of course people with SCD could choose the emotional stress and energy of fighting their positioning towards the bottom of several hierarchies, but we have seen that premature destruction of red blood cells, severe anaemia and chronic tiredness are characteristics that make ongoing struggle against this not impossible, but less likely.

A third dimension of the social determinants of health is the *neoliberal variant of capitalism*. Countries such as the USA and the UK, which adopted increasingly neoliberal policies after 1980, are associated with greater poverty and income inequalities, and greater health inequalities within nations (Coburn, 2004), and the disproportionate representation of African-Americans or Black British people living with SCD in lower socio-economic groups suggests that people with SCD will be over-represented as the victims of neoliberal policies. There are a number of plausible, but as yet unexplored, pathways to the relationships between neoliberalism and poor SCD health. Neoliberalism has been associated with an extreme intensification of the labour process (Braverman, 1974); requirements of emotional subordination in roles, with the individual as emotional shock-absorber of the structural injustices both of work (Hochschild, 1983), and of work-life balance (Hochschild and Machung, 1989); and increased requirements of what sociologists call performativity (Ball, 2003): having not only to do a good job but to be actively seen to be doing a good job, constantly self-auditing the quality of work through targets – all of which is about having an alienating lack of control over the flow and pace of work, and is strongly associated with poorer health (Wilkinson, 1996). For someone living with chronic tiredness and episodic periods of illness, without strong enabling disability laws, the work environment is likely to be hostile. In the UK, adults with SCD complain of discrimination by employers and by financial agencies, such as mortgage and insurance companies (Atkin and Ahmad, 2001).

To date, sickle cell and employment studies have tended to focus on the relationship between discrete SCD symptoms, such as leg ulcers and employment

(Okany and Akinyanju, 1993), or on the impact of treatment modalities on employment (Ballas *et al.*, 2010), and have implicitly individualized the problem by not looking at the constraints imposed by the overall structures of labour markets. The problem with a neoliberal context is also that the kind of research that gets funded may implicitly reflect those political biases, by treating the policy contexts as an unquestionable given. Clinical medicine and psychology tend to focus on individuals in ways that do not threaten neoliberal world-views. By contrast, research that framed the issue in terms of resource distribution in order to ensure young people with SCD had sufficient food to eat to underpin their nutritional status represents a challenge to the existing order of things. For example, the statement "children with sickle cell disease have worse health-related quality of life (HRQL) compared to children without sickle cell disease after adjusting for income level" (Panepinto *et al.*, 2009: 12) rather misses the point. The point is to see income level adjusted as a social policy to improve the health of those living with SCD (and their non-SCD peers), and (if necessary in the absence of immediate policy changes) strengthen more immediate pathways to mitigate effects of poverty on SCD (for example, supplementary feeding pro-grammes such as school breakfast clubs), *not* merely to treat poverty levels as an immutable variable to be adjusted for in research.

Although the low-income mothers of children with SCD studied by US sociolo-gist Shirley Hill (1994) were resource-poor by standards of the Global North, they at least had access to some social security monies to support the upbringing of children and, as we will see in Chapter 10, this is an important difference to those in the Global South, who have to frequently denude the household budget if they are to pay for basic medicines for young people living with SCD. The families in Hill's study were also facing racism. Racism damages health at a number of levels – not least by means of the link between reported experience of discrimination and hypertension (Krieger and Sydney, 1996). Moreover, studies in both the UK (Anionwu and Atkin, 2001) and in the USA (Rouse, 2009) have suggested that racism plays at least a part in negative encounters between those admitted to hos-pital with SCD and health care providers. Having SCD is usually associated with lower blood pressure, but, where blood pressure was raised in those with SCD, this was associated with strokes and premature deaths (Pegelow *et al.*, 1997).

There has been relatively little attention paid to the issue of gender and SCD. An exception is a study that notes different gendered child-rearing practices in low-income African-American families, in which boys are treated as especially vulnerable owing to their SCD, and deserving of protection and making excep-tions for, while young women with SCD are expected to be "valiant" and to exhibit resilience in their SCD experience, as in their wider life (Hill and Zim-merman, 1995). This may be in preparation for a context that the Global North and the Global South have in common: that it is women who disproportionately bear the double burden of work inside and outside the household (Hochschild and Machung, 1989). This extends to women caring for someone with SCD (Burnes *et al.*, 2008). Such double burdens of work probably also extend to women living with SCD, though at present we have no specific evidence of this.

Meanwhile, there are certainly gendered attitudes to the birth of a child with SCD, with fathers in a study in Kenya interpreting the birth of a child with SCD, in a context of education instructing them that both parents must be genetic carriers for them to have a child with SCD, as evidence that they cannot therefore be the father (Marsh *et al.*, 2011). We saw in Chapter 1 the putative role of polygamy as relevant to the sickle cell experience. In a context of lack of diagnosis of children with SCD, polygamous fathers who are carriers, experiencing serial deaths of children with SCD from one (carrier) wife, may, at least hypothetically, be more likely to take another wife, thereby creating a situation where sickle cell carrier fathers have greater fertility than non-carrier fathers (Konotey-Ahulu, 1980). There also gendered attitudes to prenatal screening for sickle cell trait reported in the UK (Reed, 2011; Atkin *et al.*, 2015; Dyson *et al.*, 2016b) and these form part of a longer discussion in Chapter 8.

Very little has been written that situates the experiences of SCD within a disability rights context (see Dyson *et al.*, 2007a; Abuateya *et al.*, 2008), and this is perhaps because those with SCD may not make SCD a central part of their identity in the first place (Atkin and Ahmad, 2001). The point about the environment, physical or collective, is that environments are changeable. This argument, concerning the alterability of the collective environment, especially within a framework of disability rights, is taken up further in Chapter 10, which considers possibilities for challenging stigma.

Service provision is itself an important determinant of the SCD experience and most evidence we have on this comes from the USA, where the encounter may often be between a white health care provider and an African-American client. Pain is experienced on most days for most people living with SCD in the USA (Smith *et al.*, 2008). Providers frequently complain of high users of emergency departments (with offensive epithets such as "frequent flyers"). Contradicting this negative labelling, high users of emergency departments with SCD are more severely ill, experience greater pain and distress, and have a reduced quality of life compared to those using emergency departments less frequently, suggesting their clinical need merits their greater use of services (Aisiku *et al.*, 2008). Negative stereotypes of people with SCD (as, for example, having lower pain thresholds, and being drug-seekers) are challenged by wider evidence that opiates are given to white hospital patients for pain at significantly higher rates than they are given to African-Americans (Pletcher *et al.*, 2008). This should also disabuse us from reaching for crude explanations that invoke "culture" as a reason behind such differences in experience. Different *social structures* of communities do indeed result in varying health care consultation behaviour for pain (Zborowski, 1952) but such an insight has become degraded into the caricature that, allegedly, different "cultures" have different pain thresholds. Discrimination is itself associated with pain in SCD (Mathur *et al.*, 2016). Haywood *et al.* (2014) suggest that SCD patients are accurately able to pick up on the attitudes exhibited by health care providers, thus validating patient reports of the problematic experiences and poor interpersonal interactions they tend to have with providers when seeking treatment for their pain, and that both racist discrimination and sickle cell-based discrimination were behind such provider attitudes. The disease-based discrimination was greater than even racist discrimination, and suggests that trust is a key component in securing good rapport necessary to pain relief in SCD (Elander *et al.*, 2011). The myriad ways SCD is marginalized: its symptoms difficult to objectively measure; its situation as an underserved disease, and its status as a disorder attached primarily to black people suggest that, in order for such trust to emerge, the sources and consequences of authority in biomedicine may need to be rethought (Ciribassi and Patil, 2016).

Conclusion

A generative, context-dependent notion of causality, typified by developmental biology and by realist sociology, could be a source of symbiosis between the biological and the social sciences. Through the specific example of sickle cell, this chapter has sought to explain why genes are not "for" anything. This is not because the social environment is able to act as a remedial adjustor to a given and fixed biology. As has been argued, we tend to conflate the concepts "inherited", "in-born" and "genetic" as if they are the same concept, and then to compound this mistake of a fixed "Nature" further in the notion that what comes from such a Nature is natural, in the sense of given, just, or fair. Attempts to challenge such circumstances are then considered unnatural or against Nature, the frequent last refuge in the arguments of regressive politics. In this respect, consider that "many elderly Europeans have small but noticeable amount of sickle-cell haemoglobin in their blood. This gene is normally found only in Africans but has, in their case, appeared as a new mutation within their ageing bodies" (Jones, 1994: 93).

In contrast to a view of biology that attempts to fix meanings, the chapter has argued that diversity, plasticity and the capacity to generate myriad experiences of SCD are to be found in genetics and genomes, because genes and genomes are not enacted outside of organisms and environments (Ingold, 2000). This has consequences for understanding why ultimately it makes no sense to delineate physical-biological and socio-cultural environments. If biological constitution is (wrongly) conceived of as a fixed genetic endowment, then challenging racism can only rest on asserting cultural differences overlaying biological similarities (ibid.: 389). Understanding that both the biological and the social entail capacities and constraints not only helps in our appreciation of sickle cell, but has wider ramifications in enabling us to challenge racist logics in which our destinies are "fixed" or "natural" or "just" simply because part of their genesis lies in our genome.

3   A long history of sickle cell
Sickle cell and malaria

Introduction

Most histories of sickle cell commence in 1904, the date of the first microscopic observation of sickle cell, or in 1910, the first publication of the scientific paper of that observation (Herrick, 1910). This small, twentieth-century fragment of the history of sickle cell, is deferred until Chapter 4. This chapter is concerned with a much longer time scale, and what may have occurred with respect to sickle cell before 1910. This has a number of benefits. It helps in moving our understanding beyond an anthropocentric view of sickle cell as an issue only of human provenance. It also aids our appreciation of the social implications of genetics. As discussed, part of the power of both conservative ideologies and racist logics depends on genetics providing a bedrock explanation that something is given, natural and "has always been with us". This pre-history of sickle cell undermines such assumptions. Finally, the pre-history of sickle cell provides useful lessons about social theory: the importance of animal, vegetable and mineral in analysing human societies; the limits of empiricism and the potential of absence of phenomena in explanations, and the benefits of distinguishing between the empirical, the actual and the real.

The genesis of sickle cell

The sickle cell gene most likely post-dates the movement of humans out of Africa around 50,000 years ago by several millennia. In fact, it seems likely to post-date the emergence of agriculture 10,000 years ago, and did not arise until the era of the Green Sahara (Shriner and Rotimi, 2018) or possibly even later when slash-and burn agriculture moved across West Africa around 4000 BCE. Agriculture first developed in the Middle East and provided an ecological niche for mosquitoes and their associated malarial parasites, but in that region animal husbandry meant that only a certain proportion of mammalian transmission of malaria was human transmission. By contrast, in Africa, the proportion of malaria transmission through human hosts was much higher, and it is malaria rather than race or ethnicity that holds the key to the association of sickle cell with Africa.

The US anthropologist Frank B. Livingstone is best known for elucidating one of the key insights underpinning theories of human evolution, namely, the role of sickle cell and malaria in explaining human genetic variation. His classic articles explored how the sickle cell gene was relatively absent in Liberia in the 1950s even though malaria was endemic (Livingstone, 1958a, 1958b). Livingstone tracked this apparent anomaly to the fact that, as relatively late adopters of agriculture (which meant clearing forests that previously had shaded and cooled flowing waters – conditions less favourable to mosquitoes, which require heated shallow pools of water for their larvae to breed), Liberians had only recently created the ecological niche suitable for the mosquitoes responsible for spreading falciparum malaria, against which sickle cell trait provides a strong survival advantage during early infancy. As the selective genetic advantage takes a number of generations to build up, this explained the relative lack of the sickle cell gene in a malarial environment.

Livingstone was a key opponent of the notion of distinct biological races (Livingstone, 1962) and it was his work on sickle cell, thalassaemia and other red blood cell adaptations to different forms of malaria that partly provided the basis for his beliefs. In a compendium of over 2,000 twentieth-century studies testing human bloods across the globe he outlined the notion of clines (gradients, as in the word "incline") of frequencies of particular genes across populations (Livingstone, 1985). His work carefully documents the date, place, type of sample (which might be a linguistic or ethnic group, an occupational group such as miners or students, or a group in relation to services, such as clinic attenders), and size of sample, as well as the results that included proportions carrying a gene associated with the various haemoglobin disorders. This is important. When conducting policy research in the UK on the viability of using socially constructed ethnic census categories as the basis for targeted prenatal screening for sickle cell and thalassaemia in the early 2000s (about which more in Chapter 7), a suggestion was made to me to make use of this classic work. It was as if the rates cited by Livingstone were thought to be somehow prevalence rates, preserved, as if in amber, that could be forever attributed to people whose ancestors came from particular parts of the world. This would be to miss important implications of Livingstone's work. The frequencies of genes associated with sickle cell may vary, even within ethnic groups, across quite short geographical distances. This may be to do with topography.

For example, in Kenya, in East Africa, rates of sickle cell were high on the coast and on inland lakes but low in the Kenyan highlands, whose altitude inhibited the survival of mosquitoes as the vector responsible for transmission of malarial parasites. One cannot therefore extrapolate from a small prevalence survey in one geographic area to a whole region or a whole nation state. The work of Livingstone ascribes prevalence rates for sickle cell to particular well-defined sub-populations, sampled at particular moments in time, in specific places and circumstances. It is precisely this level of mapping of the prevalence of genes associated with haemoglobin disorders that is required in order to have a solid evidence base to invest in public health measures (such as newborn screening for SCD, the subject of Chapter 9). Livingstone's work reminds us of the ongoing need to improve the quality of epidemiological data we have on sickle cell in order for countries currently less well-resourced to plan the response of their health systems to SCD.

Nonetheless, the work of Livingstone remains important as an historical record, and for its awareness that there is no primordial link, that is, no link dating back to the dawn of *Homo sapiens*, let alone to the dawn of hominids on Earth, that connects blood, geographical territory and the genes in human bodies (Carter and Dyson, 2011). This has not prevented what Carter (2007) has characterized as the return of scientific racism. Shiao *et al.* (2012) attempt to reassert genomics, against what they caricature as the "social construction" of race, advocating for the notion of clinal classes, which they claim closely reflect social perceptions of ancestry. This work has been extensively criticized by Fujimura *et al.* (2014), not only because the phrase "clinal classes" is itself an oxymoron, but because dividing clines into categories involves making arbitrary decisions about the placement of the dividing line on the continuum. The critique covers broadly three types of argument. First, in seeking to represent human populations, Shiao *et al.* (2012) misrepresent the nature of the groupings of people within genetics, namely, that neither African-Americans nor Africans represent a single branch (clade) on the human genetic tree of life. Second, apart from the methodological weakness in sampling, the argument is circular to the extent that genetic markers are used to differentiate *pre-defined* groups. Third, "human geneticists make decisions about which sub-set of individuals to use to 'represent' a 'race' or 'national group' in their sampling procedures and in their cluster analysis" (Fujimura *et al.*, 2014: 215). They conclude: "some African populations (the Kenyan Bantu, Mandenka and Yoruba) share more genetic variants with Europeans than other African populations such as the San or Mbuti" (ibid.: 215). For our purposes, I wish merely to note that the Mandenka and Yoruba groupings approximate to the respective regions where Senegal and Benin sickle cell haplotypes are found and that the Central African haplotype was formerly referred to as the Bantu haplotype. Sickle cell, as we have seen, was in European populations from at least Roman times, if not before. Let us leave the last word on this to Frank Livingstone, who, in the language of the time, and with racist concepts he himself disowned (Livingstone, 1962) concluded: "It thus seems that the sickle cell gene, although long considered a Negro characteristic, is absent in the 'purest' representatives of the Negro race" (Livingstone, 1958b: 40).

In order to understand more about the emergence of SCD as a disease of humans, we need to go back to what archaeologists call the Palaeolithic era, spanning approximately 2.5 million years of history, from the use of stone tools by *Homo habilis*, to a time just before the Neolithic transition to farming – dating around 10,000 BCE onwards, depending on the region of the world. At the time of writing, the consensus appears to be that modern humans were located in East Africa, that *Homo sapiens* migrated out of Africa around 50,000 years ago, and that *Plasmodium falciparum* may have moved at the same time (Tanabe *et al.*, 2010). There are several types of malaria in humans but the various types originated in different non-human organisms. While types of malaria can infect birds and reptiles, *Plasmodium vivax* and *Plasmodium malariae* appear related to a type common in chimpanzees. However, the type of malaria we are interested in with respect to sickle cell, *Plasmodium falciparum*, once thought to have arisen as a result of lateral transfer between avian and human hosts (Waters *et al.*, 1991) has more recently been thought to have transferred from gorillas (Loy *et al.*, 2017). The human red blood cell and its evolutionary adaptations, including sickle cell, are therefore intimately connected to the evolution of other species. The key *expansion* of malaria in human populations appears to date from around 10,000 years ago (Joy *et al.*, 2003), a process beginning with the transition to agriculture in the Middle East. However, it appears that the extant mosquito vectors there were zoophilic (preferred non-human mammalian blood sources).

The human adoption of agricultural practices over hunting and gathering reached West Africa by 4000 BCE. This took the form of slash-and-burn agricultural practices in which trees were felled and burned in order to clear spaces for human agriculture. Here the mosquito vectors for malaria, *Anopheles gambiae*, were predominantly human blood-preferring (anthropophilic) (Carter and Mendis, 2002), and conditions for the flourishing of *Plasmodium falciparum* malaria and the genetic mutations of sickle cell became possible.

At this point it is worth considering the various roles of non-human actors in the creation of sickle cell. The life cycle of the *Plasmodium falciparum* parasite that causes severe malaria interpenetrates both human and mosquito hosts. The infected bite of the female Anopheles mosquito injects materials through its salivary glands into the human. Inside the human there is a stage where sporozoites (literally, seeding organisms) invade the liver, and having undergone transformation and multiplication in the liver, parasite-filled sacs (merozoites) invade the red blood cells. Incubation can take 10–14 days before symptoms, but successive blood stages take 48 hours (hence the recurrent fevers of malaria). Some transformations later in the cycle involve production of female and male gametes, which are taken up by the mosquito in blood meals. These have a cycle of maturation in the gut of the mosquito before being injected into another human host through the mosquito bite. Meanwhile, the life cycle of the mosquito takes place. The mosquito lays eggs in still water, larvae and subsequently pupae develop from the eggs within the water, before the adult mosquito emerges from the water surface.

The ecological story underpinning the likely history of malaria and sickle cell has been outlined by Livingstone (1958a, 1958b). Prior to slash-and-burn agriculture, dense forests covered much of the ground, humans lived relatively dispersed existences, and the soil was subject to minimal impacting. This had a number of inhibiting roles with respect to the development of malaria. Fast-flowing streams would not have been slowed by irrigation, and remained too rapid for growth of Anopheles' mosquito larvae; canopy shade would have reduced the extent to which waters could be warmed by the sun; human population density would have inhibited the life cycle of the protozoan by virtue of being too dispersed to support reliable transmission through biting and taking up of human blood. With the particular form of agriculture – yam production in West Africa – different ecological conditions were created. These conditions included availability of slow or still waters created through irrigation, and the impacting of soil, favourable to the collection of water in puddles which could be heated in the sun, conditions favourable in turn to the larvae of Anopheles mosquitoes. Concentration of humans in settled communities made transmission from human to mosquito to another human more reliable, and in turn facilitated the reproductive cycle of *Plasmodium falciparum*. The wider ecological picture concerns the viability of the wider environment for the mosquito: as we saw in Chapter 1, mosquitos cannot survive as readily beyond certain latitudes, above a certain altitude and *Plasmodium falciparum* is less transmissible by mosquito vectors in the (non-oasis) desert context of relative human solitude.

An important consideration is the relative recent emergence of the sickle cell genetic mutation, perhaps as few as 40–75 generations ago in the case of one African haplotype (Currat *et al.*, 2002). The mutation, written in short form as [β6Glu → Val] involves a replacement of one amino acid at point six of the beta-globin chain. In the case of sickle haemoglobin, the usual glutamine (soluble in water) is replaced by valine, the latter notable for its insolubility. The recent nature of this mutation has two important implications for knowledge. First, we tend to talk about *the* Human Genome not only as if there were one standard ideal from which certain alleles represented an aberrant departure, when as we have suggested, in endemic malarial areas the sickle mutation may be the fittest (most fitting to an environment, not necessarily the strongest) of alleles. Second, the case of sickle cell represents an important principle of a philosophy of science termed critical realism. This principle is that things may be actual before they are empirical, and may be real before they are actualized.

The UK philosopher Roy Bhaskar (2008 [1975]) wrote of reality comprising three realms. The first is the realm of the *empirical*: things are observable and are known by humans. Second, the realm of the *actual*: things can be there (actual) before they are known (empirical). Although not credited with a philosophy that displaces humans from the centre of world events, Bhaskar's approach serves us well in the sense that the realm of the actual could help us to focus on the majority of global events beyond human encounters and knowledge (see Harman, 2018). Clearly much of what I am characterizing as the long history of sickle cell occurred in the absence of human knowledge about it. Furthermore, different forms of malaria affect many vertebrates – birds, reptiles and rodents, as well as other primates – and so things are happening beyond humans as well as beyond human knowledge. Third, Bhaskar writes of the realm of the *real*. This is a realm of mechanisms or causalities as yet not actualized. For realist philosophers, a mechanism is an emergent property of the interaction of parts of an entity, a process that depends on the structure and composition of that entity (Elder-Vass, 2015). As such, mechanisms or causal powers can be real but not actualized. For example, in the case of sickle cell, valine has a capacity to insolubility compared to the solubility of glutamine. The biochemical potential for a mutation to disable haemoglobin solubility, and to enable the formation of twisted rods of haemoglobin molecules, was real before it was actualized. Thus, it was always an immanent *potential* of a haemoglobin allele to develop partial resistance to malaria, but the mutation of glutamine to valine was not actualized until slash-and-burn agricultural practices were adopted in Africa. This created the specific ecological context that enabled the mechanism [β6Glu → Val], the replacement of glutamine by valine as the sixth amino acid in the beta-globin chain (Rees *et al.*, 2010) to be actualized. As we shall see, however, it is unlikely that sickle cell could have become known to humans had reproduction of two genetic carriers of sickle cell not subsequently resulted in embodied sickle cell disease. Actualized sickled cells in humans were not *empirically* observed under the microscope until the early twentieth century.

Sickle cell in the Palaeolithic era: a pre-history of sickle cell (pre-4000 BCE)

We have seen how the ecological conditions surrounding the introduction of yam cultivation helped establish conditions more favourable to the Anopheles mosquito and that the flourishing, if not the very existence, of sickle cell dates from this relatively recent period of history. But in the long period of time known as the Palaeolithic era, sickle cell was not embodied in humans, though the mechanism [β6Glu → Val] was an immanent potential, and the possibility for a genetic mutation offering partial protection against malaria therefore did exist. An important facet of the realm of the real is that in order to explore it, scientists have to be prepared to make use of counterfactual knowledge (Lukes, 1974). Thinking counterfactually literally means thinking counter to the apparent facts of a situation, and can be very productive. We had to think counter to the observed "fact" that the sun moves around the Earth in order to consider that the reverse is true and that the Earth, moon and sun might be related by gravitational pull. Only by thinking counterfactually in this way did humans understand the mechanisms of gravity, how to escape gravity in order to send a rocket into space, and were subsequently able to *empirically* observe the Earth move around the sun (Dyson and Brown, 2006). As we shall see in Chapters 5 and 6, it is the inability or unwillingness of state officials or policy-makers to think counterfactually that limits their understanding of sudden deaths associated with sickle cell trait. Or, to put it another way, racism depends on aggressive empiricist thinking. In Chapter 10, we further examine the importance of thinking counterfactually, thinking how current collective arrangements shape and limit our shared understanding of what is possible, and how, therefore, campaigning to change the organization of education, employment, housing, transport and health insurance could instantiate benefits for those living with SCD globally.

Thus, for a long period of time before the Neolithic revolution, the latent potential for the key sickle cell mechanism [β6Glu → Val] was not actualized. If, as I believe, one reason for developing human knowledge is to inform processes of policy formation, then anticipating unintended consequences is modelling in advance what something might be like, what Stenhouse (1974) called compensation. In this respect, thinking counterfactually is important. For example, another key haemoglobin variant, haemoglobin C [HbC: β6Glu → Lys] in which glutamine is replaced not by valine but by lysine (Rees *et al.*, 2010) is also thought to offer partial protection against malaria. Unlike sickle cell, however, both the carrier state (HbAC) and the homozygous condition (HbCC) are protective against malaria. Furthermore, haemoglobin CC disease is not nearly as severe a condition as SCD and may be asymptomatic in some individuals. This has led to the (counterfactual) suggestion that in the longer term, in the absence of human attempts to control malaria, haemoglobin C would eventually "out-compete" sickle haemoglobin as a protector against malaria and sickle cell would be replaced in malarial West and Central Africa (Modiano *et al.*, 2001).

Sickle cell in the Neolithic era (circa 4000 BCE onwards)

As we have seen, once the practices of slash-and-burn clearances making way for agriculture had reached West/Central Africa, ecology favourable to the Anopheles mosquito and to *Plasmodium falciparum* malaria was established. Medical science is frequently seeking the so-called "natural history" of a condition. The rationale of the public health researchers in the Tuskegee Syphilis Experiment (see Chapter 1) was to study the "natural" history of that disease (Reverby, 2000). Sociologists would no doubt point to the work of French philosopher Michel Foucault (1979), who documents the birth of the medical clinic as an institutional basis for making the idea of a disease, independent of its manifestation in any particular human body, thinkable. With the capacity to see continuities between different patients (now termed cases) the sick person, in which the disease and the person cannot be considered apart, disappeared from the medical cosmology in seventeenth-century Europe (Jewson, 1974).

It is this search for a basis on which to judge a natural history of sickle cell that has exercised a number of commentators. Data gathered as part of a World Health Organization study on controlling malaria in Northern Nigeria in the 1970s has been taken to be indicative of the deleterious effects of SCD in malarial conditions. The study, investigating the spraying of insecticide to control mosquitoes, and hence malaria, was based around Garki District, now in the Jigawa state of Northern Nigeria (Figure 3.1). The description of the area given in the WHO report was understandably concerned to carefully document current conditions (grasslands, agriculture, a poorly nourished population). This could be mistakenly read through Western eyes as an impoverished rural area without services, ridden with the unfamiliar disease of malaria. In fact, neither economic development level, nor disease ecology was primordial there. As we have seen, SCD was a relatively recent development of perhaps 40 generations. The context of rural poverty is perhaps better characterized as underdevelopment rather than lack of development. *Underdevelopment* is the term given by the German economic sociologist André Gunder Frank (1966) to a process where economic

Garki District

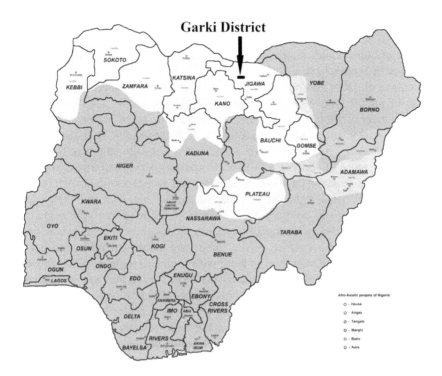

Figure 3.1 Garki District in Jigawa state in the Hausa area of Nigeria.
Source: Adapted from PANONIAN.

relations with a colonial power build up a network of expropriation of resources and establishment of economic dependencies. The subsequent withdrawal from such relationships leaves the area economically destitute: the area has been *under-developed* (verb transitive, something done to the area, not a naturally occurring state of affairs). The specific thesis of how Europe underdeveloped Africa is contained in the account of Rodney (1972). In this respect, the geographical location of Garki (then in the Kano kingdom) would once have been part of a powerful and wealthy Hausa trading empire in the eleventh to eighteenth centuries, before coming under British colonial rule by the early twentieth century. Although we may draw important inferences about the history of SCD from the Garki study, it is important to note that neither poverty nor sickle cell were natural or primordial in Northern Nigeria.

The Garki Malaria Project collected demographic data that included numbers with and without genes encoding sickle haemoglobin. Of particular interest was a comparison of cohorts at birth and at age five. By comparing the numbers with SCD soon after birth with the number in the population at age five, the study was able to show that the expected numbers of children with SCD in the older cohorts were not to be found. The implication was that nearly all children with

SCD, that is all but around 2 per cent of such infants, had already died before the age of five (Fleming *et al.*, 1979). This seems a powerful illustration of the impact of SCD on infant mortality in an area of endemic malaria, and as malaria is one of humankind's major global-historical killers, suggests that a very large number of infants have died historically of SCD and continue to do so today. Grosse *et al.* (2011) estimate that across Sub-Saharan Africa between 60–90 per cent of infants born with SCD died before the age of five, and that with the achievement of Millennium Development Goals, up to 16 per cent of all Sub-Saharan Africa under-fives deaths might be attributable to SCD. In the terminology of Bhaskar, introduced above, sickle cell is not fully empirical (at least in the narrow sense of accessible to Western science); sickle cell trait is embodied in the Garki population (at about 25 per cent) and even that embodiment may not have routinely been sufficient to make someone with sickle cell trait appear different to others in everyday life. However, SCD itself is barely actualized, with most dying before the age of five, even though there is a sickle cell mechanism – an ongoing balance of life, premature death and protection against malaria based on different fates of those with adult haemoglobin (HbAA), sickle cell trait (HbAS) and sickle cell anaemia (HbSS). As we shall see in Chapter 9, actualizing those born with SCD beyond infancy depends variously on identifying those infants with SCD, and providing them with protection against malaria and infections. Such figures inferred from the Garki Malaria Project do, however, suggest that, from the origins of sickle cell to the beginning of the twenty-first century, millions of infants with SCD may have died.

A theory that the Egyptian boy-king Tutankhamun, who lived around 1330 BCE, died of sickle cell has been advanced by Timmann and Meyer (2010). Their paper proposes eight reasons supportive of their argument. First, DNA analysis of his mummy suggested Tutankhamun had been exposed to several strains of *Plasmodium falciparum*: a killer, certainly, but more usually, as we have seen, in infancy rather than aged 18 when some immunity based on repeat exposures may have built up. Second, as we saw at the outset of this book, they note that populations around Egyptian oases are reported to have 9–22 per cent sickle cell trait (El-Beshlawy and Youssry, 2009). Third, other researchers had previously identified haemoglobin S in three out of six pre-dynastic Egyptian mummies dating from 3200 BCE (Marin *et al.*, 1999), ostensibly the earliest record of sickle cell. Fourth, they do not remark on their own observation that Tutankhamun had a shortened second toe, and dactylitis, or hand-foot syndrome, common in children with SCD, might explain that feature of his body. Next, they note the consanguineous nature of his parents' relationship, and in a family with sickle cell trait, consanguinity would increase the statistical chances of Tutankhamun inheriting a form of SCD. Sixth, they note his maxillary protrusion (overbite), a somatic feature also present, for example, in 21 per cent of SCD children in one Nigerian study (Oredugba and Savage, 2002). Then, they note the avascular necrosis of the femoral head. This is when the blood supply to the "ball" part of the ball-and-socket hip joint is compromised and the head of the femur bone begins to die off. This is a well-established feature of SCD, especially the haemoglobin SC disease type, and

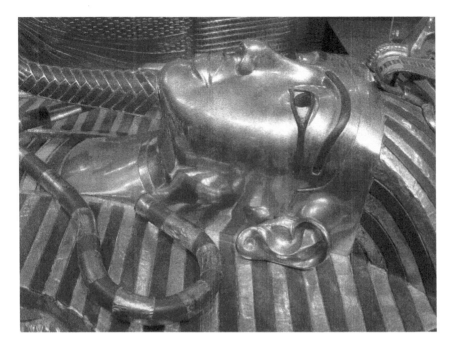

Figure 3.2 Mask of Tutankhamun.
Source: Lynn Greyling.

where health services organization, insurance or affordability permit, a hip replace-ment may be undertaken for people with SCD even before they leave teenage years behind. Finally, the authors note the enlarged penis is detached from the body, and make a highly speculative link to priapism in SCD: the persistent and painful erection that may result in scarring and thickening of the connective tissue within the penis, possibly ending in impotence if untreated.

Sickle cell in classical Roman times (circa 450 CE)

In the 1990s, archaeologists uncovered a remarkable burial site, dating from the late Roman period, in a villa outside the town of Lugnano, 100 km north of Rome (Soren and Soren, 1995). Dozens of infants were found to have been buried together in graves, indicating a wave of sudden and, to the local popu-lace, unexplained deaths. The deaths were accompanied by the burial of canine puppies, and evidence of plants such as honeysuckle associated with treatment of fevers was also found. The deaths were explained as the result of severe malaria, *Plasmodium falciparum* malaria having reached Southern Europe during the Roman Empire (Sallares *et al.*, 2004). Trans-Saharan trade routes flourished at this time, and transfer of malaria was possible either through the blood of human travellers themselves (as the incubation periods between infected bite and symptoms may be 10–14 days), and/or the transfer of mosquito larvae in water barrels, carried across the Mediterranean in trading boats.

We can see how mosquitoes and *Plasmodium falciparum* malaria may have been transmitted to Southern Europe, but this does not exhaust the explanation for genes associated with sickle cell. The Mediterranean island of Sicily has a relatively high prevalence of sickle cell genes, with up to 10 per cent of the population having sickle cell trait. However, analysis of alleles linked to African populations, alleles that are not malaria-linked alleles such as sickle cell, indicates that inter-ethnic unions, between those of African descent and Sicilians, only accounts for 1 per cent of the transfer of genetic material between the populations. The explanation for the high levels of sickle cell trait depends not on reproduction between African and Sicilian populations, but the expansion from an initially low rate of gene transfer. Given the high mortality of those without the protection in infancy afforded by sickle cell trait, it is the differential survival of those with sickle cell trait, in the face of successive waves of severe malaria, which may best explain the expansion of the prevalence of sickle cell trait in certain Southern European populations, such as Sicily. The initial 1 per cent prevalence was ostensibly amplified to nearer 10 per cent by malarial pressures on the population (Ragusa *et al.*, 1992).

Thus, a plausible account of the sudden deaths of the Lugnano infants was that it represented the mortalities of children without sickle cell trait in a population facing a challenge from *Plasmodium falciparum* malaria for the first time. However, what killed Lugnano infants is also likely to have amplified the sickle cell gene in this population, protecting greater proportions of any future generations in that area. In this instance, sickle haemoglobin exists in actuality, and is expanded as a proportion of the surviving population. Human empirical experience exists, but any specific causal explanation is confined to explanations of differential deaths of those we now believe died of malaria, and not those who survived. Even if the differential survival of those with sickle cell trait had been known, note that there remains a domain of knowledge beyond the reach of science. Those with sickle cell trait are more likely to survive, but why do some without sickle cell trait survive and others not? As we move to consider the human experience of sickle cell in parts of Africa, we come across explanations that do address this realm of knowledge.

Sickle cell in the golden ages of Africa

The Early Middle Ages in European history are sometimes pejoratively referred to as the Dark Ages, an era supposedly ended by the Enlightenment, and the rise of rationalist thinking and science. This Eurocentric terminology ignores what has been referred to as the Golden Ages of African societies in which Ghana, Mali, Songhai, Hausa and other empires and kingdoms rose and fell between the end of the Roman Empire and the advent of first, the chattel enslavement of Africans by Europeans, and later the colonial occupations by European powers.

Such broad cultural framings bias how Europeans approach the hidden history of sickle cell in Africa before the twentieth century. The title of a 1980s text, *From Myths to Molecules*, juxtaposes Igbo beliefs in *ogbanje* children (of the spirit world) and highly technical scientific explanations of the structure of haemoglobin (Edelstein, 1986). The title of the text strongly also implies progress.

However, even quite detailed scientific knowledge of the complexities of sickled red blood cells has not, as we have seen, resulted in reliable empathy for persons experiencing a sickle cell painful crisis from their (non-specialist) health care providers in the USA or the UK, nor in reliable levels of trust between patient and carers. Lack of such empathy, even for the most severe and enduring types of pain, stands in contrast to some reports of how some groups in Africa conceptualized the chronic illness. Konotey-Ahulu (1996: 115) reports a number of West African tribal languages describing what appears to be the sickle cell pain: the names given to the illness are onomatopoeic: *Chwechweechwe* (Gã language) *Ahotuto* (Twi) or *Nwiiwii* (Fante), with the repeated syllables mimicking reflecting cries of pain, and the meaning of the names (body-chewing, body biting) suggests empathetic recognition of the symptoms of those experiencing pain. In East Africa too, in the Chewa language of Malawi, the words for several types of pain *kupweta pweteka* (repeated or persistent pain); *kuwawa* (a biting pain) and *kulasa lasa* (stabbing pain) are noted to reflect the patterns of pain associated with SCD (Clendennen and Lwanda, 2003: 21). The intimate connection of the illness experience with the environment was also noted. Episodes of pain are more frequent in the rainy season, with its drop in temperature and the proliferation of water for breeding mosquitoes, producing symptoms described as rainy-season "rheumatism" (Konotey-Ahulu, 1996: 166). These conceptions of illness, attendant to the lived experience of the person in ecological context, are actually in stark opposition to modern conceptions of a "natural" history of a disease.

Moreover, in one Ghanaian tribe, the family-linked nature of sickle cell was observed: through oral family history, the Ghanaian Professor of Medicine Felix Konotey-Ahulu (1996) traces sickle cell in his own family back to 1670, reproducing a family tree going back over nine generations and three centuries. However, Edelstein (1986) has disputed that all the African language names listed by Konotey-Ahulu are necessarily coterminous with SCD, and proposed, for example, that the word listed under the Hausa language reflects a more generic word for chronic illness. This does suggest that, while there may be some overlap, it would be wise not to regard such tribal names as evidence of a one-to-one correspondence with people who had SCD. An illustration of this point comes from the work of Nzewi (2001). Among the Igbo peoples of South-East Nigeria, children regarded as *malevolent ogbanje* (spirit-children who die early and are believed to be reincarnated within the same family), overlap strongly with those children with a modern SCD diagnosis (ibid.). However, they do not correspond precisely, suggesting that childhood deaths from other causes may have been subject to *ogbanje* explanations. Spirit children were, and remain, a feature of many West African cultures, for instance, being referred to as *abiku* among the Yoruba of South-West Nigeria (Ogunjuyigbe, 2004). However, we need to remember that such spirit explanations are about *why* a particular child died, not *how* they died, the scientific cause of death (Denham *et al.*, 2010), and that spirit children are held to be living embodiments expressing relationships to kin, the environment and social norms (Schneider, 2017). As such, sickle cell disease and spirit children belong to different cosmologies, with different rules governing what it is that the cosmology is trying to resolve. *Why* a child dies, why that *particular* child, and why at that *time*, are explanations beyond science, which must content itself with mere causal explanation. This explains why a child with SCD may be taken to a medical doctor, but also to a spiritual healer. There are simply other issues at stake.

Sickle cell in the age of Maafa (1500–1888)

The advent of first genetic and subsequently genomic analyses has enabled a particularly disturbing phase of history to be mapped in news ways. The *Maafa* (African Holocaust) enslavement of some 11 million African peoples and forced transport to the USA, the Caribbean and Brazil has been documented by UK historian Basil Davidson (1996). Davidson also emphasizes that, though slavery existed before 1500 in Europe, Africa, the Middle East and India, the particular type of trans-Atlantic slavery prosecuted by Portugal, Britain, France and the Netherlands was chattel slavery: slavery that conceived the enslaved people as property, such that children of the enslaved became automatically considered the private property of the enslaver. This distinguished it from other forms of slavery, where the offspring were not only free but might rise to senior levels in the society they were born in.

The mapping of genes associated with sickle cell, and, in particular, reference to haplotypes, has enabled researchers to make estimates of which groups of peoples were kidnapped and transported to which areas of the Americas, and to triangulate such findings with documentary sources (Schroeder *et al.*, 1990). As will be discussed in the final chapters of the book, the use of sickle cell as a marker enabling, so it is claimed, the tracing of other academic interests, stands in stark contrast to the relative lack of applied social policy research aiming to improve the adverse experiences of those living with SCD. Schroeder *et al.* (ibid.: 175) suggest a breakdown of Senegal (10 per cent), Benin (60 per cent) and Central African (25 per cent) haplotypes in the US sickle cell population, and argue that these figures are consistent with information from documentary sources on the embarkation point of peoples enslaved, provided one adjusts for lower overall incidence of the sickle cell trait in Senegal compared to Benin and Central African areas. Gonçalves *et al.* (2003) indicate that the state of Bahia in Northern Brazil received more enslaved peoples from West Africa, compared to the rest of Brazil, who received more from Central Africa, and claim confirmation for this by dint of the greater proportion of those with the Benin haplotype in the contemporary Bahia population compared to those with the Central African haplotype.

Yet another study highlights the genetic diversity of the Guianese population and states that results are concordant with historical data on the slave trade. Such results show a West African origin for the *Noir Marron* population and a Central African origin for Haitians, while Guianese Creoles are highly admixed (Simonnet *et al.*, 2016). The interest in the *Noir Marron* population by researchers is noteworthy. This population represents the descendants of maroons: people who had escaped slavery and who subsisted in mountains or dense bush areas of the country where they had been enslaved. Genetics researchers have been highly interested in such groups, for the reason that they supposedly represent a less admixed (or allegedly more "pure") version of a claimed original African population. The *Noir Marron* fulfil just such a role for Simonnet *et al.* Such thinking has been extensively criticized, for reasons including problems, such as: (1) circular thinking, that starts not with the DNA but with taken-for-granted folk classifications of race or population; (2) failure to recognize that genetic recombination means that people may share genetic material who are not related; and (3) failure to recognize that Africa contains more genetic diversity than the rest of the world put together (Duster, 2009; Royal *et al.*, 2010; Fulwilley, 2011). We might add sickle cell-specific cautions to this list. One is that having a gene associated with sickle cell may tell us about our ancestors' exposure to falciparum malaria rather than our own degree of relatedness. The other is that the assumption that "European" and "African" populations have been continuously separated so that only "later" can they become admixed. There is ample evidence of the early presence of sickle cell in European populations (Lavinha *et al.*, 1992), and Fryer (1984) documents Black Africans among the Roman Army occupying Britain over two millennia ago.

Moreover, people do not always concur with the evidence thrown up by genomic studies: Arnaiz-Villena *et al.* (2001) suggest that Jews and Palestinians share common genetic ancestry, both being part of populations who have circulated around the Mediterranean basin for millennia. In Brazil, people overestimate the proportion of ancestry attributable to both African and indigenous Indian descent (Santos *et al.*, 2009). Genetic evidence has led to something of a three-way stand-off between Brazilian sickle cell activists, Brazilian social scientists and international social scientists. The Brazilian sickle cell activists foreground an identity as the descendants of Africans as a political mantle, framing their struggle in this way (Creary, 2018). They do this partly as a reaction to the fact that the (accurate) claims of genetic diversities in Brazil may be misused as political rhetoric to prevent black and brown communities gaining social advancement, pointing to biological admixture, while forestalling improved social equalities. Social science academics in Brazil point to the genetic evidence that distinct races do not exist, that the basis of disadvantage lies in the capitalist economic order, and that positive discrimination initiatives (quotas for universities) simply have a perverse result in recruiting wealthier black students from outside Brazil rather than poorer black students from inside Brazil (Fry, 2011). Meanwhile international social science commentators argue that Brazilian community activists, in acceding to a campaigning strategy that seeks to unite black and brown, have simply given in to the cultural imperialism of the USA by adopting the one-drop rule of hypodescent: that anyone with one black ancestor (in popular parlance, with one drop of black blood) is categorized as black (Bourdieu and Wacquant, 1999). This one-drop rule has also been employed in a US historical study to try to rehabilitate the US South (Sweet, 2005). This revisionist history correctly notes the lack of physical anthropology evidence for distinct biological races, and describes how social divisions were effected through operating a colour line (who may marry whom), further noting that it was the Union North that effectively imposed the one-drop rule in defining who is to be considered black onto the Confederate South. However, through amplifying the small number of white slaves, the existence of brown Hispanic enslavers, and the occasional fluidity of ethnic categorization in the ante-Bellum South (Sweet, 2005), the greater obscenity of the enslavement of millions of African descent people is downplayed when set alongside the triumph of a discriminatory conceptual framework imposed by the North on the South, a framework troubling African-Americans, and by association the population of people living with SCD, to this day.

An instructive caution to the implicit narrative of genes associated with sickle cell traversing the Atlantic for the first time in the bodies of enslaved peoples can be taken from studies of different haplotypes. As we have discussed, the Benin Haplotype was widespread across the Mediterranean by the end of the Roman Empire. Lavinha *et al.* (1992) studied the distribution of haplotypes of sickle cell across Portugal, the Portuguese being the first enslavers of Africans during the *Maafa*. In the port cities of Lisbon and Oporto, the haplotypes of Senegal and Central African were represented. Before colonizing Brazil, Portugal had enslaved Africans from Mauritania and Guinea (Senegal lies approximately between the two). However, the presence of the Benin haplotype was not solely focused around the two ports, but spread across the remainder of Portugal. Since the Benin haplotype moved into Mediterranean populations from the end of Roman times, it was in the Portuguese populations by the sixth century, a millennium before the transportation of enslaved Africans to Brazil in around 1530. It is at least theoretically possible that some Portuguese colonizers were sickle cell genetic carriers, and were possibly therefore the first transmitters of genes associated with sickle cell across the Atlantic. The subsequent transfer in the bodies of enslaved Africans was of course in far greater numbers.

Schroeder *et al.* (1990) dismiss the possibility that anyone with SCD could have survived enslavement and transportation to the Americas. They write:

> The severity of medical problems of sickle cell anaemia is so great that any individual with the disease who was unfortunate enough to have been forced on to a slave ship would almost certainly not have survived the trans-Atlantic voyage.

> (Ibid.: 169)

As perhaps two million people died in any case in the process of capture and transportation, survival prospects of those with sickle cell anaemia would indeed seem grim, though whether the transportation of those with other, perhaps less severe forms of SCD, such as haemoglobin SC disease, could ever be reconstructed from fragments in shipping logs or plantation records is not known.

The first point to note about the Americas was that *Plasmodium falciparum* malaria was not itself endemic until transferred by virtue of the transport of enslaved Africans (Yalcindag *et al.*, 2012). In this sense with respect to the Americas at least, the introduction of *both* malaria, and sickle cell as its co-evolutionary genetic adaptation, accompanied the forced migration of enslaved African peoples. However, the North of the US was not conducive to malaria and malaria declined in the US South from the 1930s onwards (Sledge and Mohler, 2013). Thus, at first, the North, and subsequently most of the South, did not provide the malarial environmental pressure to keep prevalence of sickle cell trait at the levels they were at the time of enslavement. These levels would have been as high as 25 per cent in some groups of enslaved West and Central Africans. Twentieth-century figures for African-Americans suggest a rate of around 8 per cent with sickle cell trait (Schroeder *et al.*, 1990). Part of this decline in prevalence will be the absence of the malarial pressure favourable to genes associated with sickle cell.

Sickle cell in the nineteenth century

US historians have noted that the very environmental and poverty-stricken conditions of enslaved peoples would make identification of any sickle cell very difficult (Savitt, 2002). On a trip to the USA the retired UK haematologist Roger Amos noted a particular poster in the exhibition, "Purchased Lives: New Orleans and the Domestic Slave Trade, 1808 to 1865". The poster is a newspaper advert offering a monetary reward for the return of Charles Jackson, an enslaved person who had run away from his captors. The complete inability to conceive the enslaved person as anything more than property led the enslavers to offer monetary rewards, in this case $25, for the return of their "property". One such advert, from the *Louisiana Gazette* of July 10, 1826, seemed to contain the hint that the person might have had SCD (Amos, 2015). The advert, for one Charles Jackson, described him as having "yellow skin, mild and suffering appearance. When it rains he feels in the reins (veins?) a great pain causing him to limp" (Figure 3.3). The reference to yellow skin may not be to jaundice (a common feature of SCD) but to the mixed heritage of Charles Jackson (ibid.). The other features mentioned do recall SCD strongly: the reference to suffering might index the bearing of frequent pain, and the specific reference to the cold, wet weather worsening symptoms recalls the rainy season rheumatism in the accounts of Konotey-Ahulu (1996), and the links between adverse weather conditions and SCD in the contemporary medical literature.

Generally, sickle cell disease would have been an invisible malady during the period of slavery in the USA (Savitt, 2002). In 1846, a paper entitled "Case of absence of the spleen" was published in the *Southern Journal of Medical Pharmacology*. It discussed an enslaved person, Jack, on whom a post-mortem had

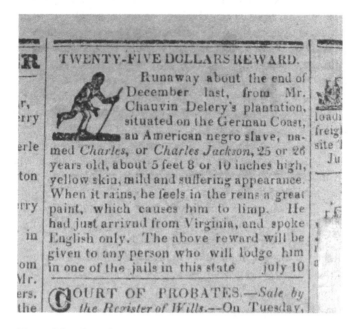

Figure 3.3 Advert in *Louisiana State Gazette*, 1826, offering reward for runaway enslaved man, Charles Jackson.

Source: Louisiana Division/City Archives, New Orleans Public Library.

been carried out in 1834. The autopsy had uncovered "the strange phenomenon of a man having lived without a spleen" (Lebby, 1846). Jack was described as of "very spare make" and suffered both the fevers and pleurisy typically associated with SCD. One possible consequence of having SCD is that the spleen, an organ that would usually remove damaged red blood cells from the circulation, is itself subject to repeated infarctions, so that by adulthood all splenic function, or indeed all the spleen, has been lost. The enslaved person may well have had SCD, but this would not have been known to medicine at the time. A similar case of a missing spleen is reported in a case by Hodenpyl (1898), where the 32-year-old African-American is also noted to have pains all over the body, jaundice and scars, possibly from sickle cell leg ulcers (Serjeant and Serjeant, 2001: 76). It should be noted, that especially in the case of those with haemoglobin SC disease, another possibility is progressive enlargement of the spleen as a result of repeated infarctions. Absence of spleen, absence of functionality of spleen, or chronic enlargement of the spleen may all therefore be indicators of SCD.

Another route by which sickle cell history might be constructed is through the written accounts of European missionaries in Africa. In 1863, an expedition led by David Livingstone was in the process of exploring an area around Lake Malawi in order to understand its relationship to the Arab-Swahili slave trade in East Africa. Livingstone employed a number of Africans from various ethnic groups. These included five Shupanga men; Kokolo from Botswana, Zambia and Zimbabwe, and Comoro Islanders. The Shupanga were from lowland areas of endemic malaria in south-east Mozambique, but on the arduous journey several became ill, and one died, in colder, windy conditions at altitude of over 1,000 metres above sea level (Clendennen and Lwanda, 2003). In favour of a sickle cell-related explanation are the accounts of pains suffered all over the body and limbs, throbbing pains that did not subside until many days later, and the fact that these were not malarial fevers (which would have been well recognized by the men themselves, as well as by Livingstone who instead described it as a new unexplained condition). Against this is the sheer implausibility of numbers, with Clendennen and Lwanda suggesting a 9 per cent prevalence for sickle cell trait. Even with their reference to consanguinity in the group, and the possibility of a milder form of SCD, the chances of one adult with SCD, as opposed to one with sickle cell trait, let alone more than one are slim. If we consider any of Livingstone's employees to have had sickle cell trait instead, then we move down a whole order of possibility of symptoms, although the altitude documented (1,049 metres) was approaching the level (1,100 metres) referred to in current US health education advice (CDC, 2018). The controversies as to whether sickle cell trait can be associated with symptoms are extensive (Carter and Dyson, 2015; Dyson *et al*., 2016a) and some of these debates are noted in Chapters 5 and 6.

A further possible account of what we now term sickle cell is found in the writings of James Africanus Beale Horton. Born in Sierra Leone of Igbo descent, he qualified as a doctor at Edinburgh University in 1859, where he took on the name *Africanus* as a demonstration of pride in his heritage. His early political texts refuted racist conceptions of Africa as undeveloped and its people as inferior to Europeans (Horton, 2011 [1868]). Later medical texts have been suggested to describe symptoms compatible with a sickle cell diagnosis. The difficulty in this interpretation is that in describing pains in the joints, enlarged spleens, decreased red blood cells and increased white blood cell counts, leg ulcers that fail to heal, irritability and weakness, jaundice, amenorrhea in women, and so on, we can only guess that some of the instances of some of the symptoms may have been one of the few adults with SCD who then lived to adulthood in endemic malarial environments, rather than other plausible reasons such as malaria itself.

For example, in one passage, Horton writes:

> When chronic enlargement of the spleen has lasted for any length of time in an active state, besides the results already described, the patient is very apt to suffer from dropsical effusions, which might terminate his life; also from sloughing ulcers from the most trivial injury; from pains, and not infrequently collection of matter in the extremities; and in females in amenorrhea.
>
> (1874: 482–483)

Again, though, since SCD is a multi-system disorder, symptoms of SCD extend to virtually every part of the anatomy and physiology, and this fact is reflected in comprehensive medical texts that document the effect of SCD in chapters corresponding to different systems of the body (Serjeant and Serjeant, 2001). It is this dispersed pattern of symptoms that has been suggested made it difficult to describe SCD as a discrete disease, at least before the advent of laboratory medicine (Wailoo, 1997). To the extent that anyone may be credited with a written account of *treatment* of the symptoms of what we now call sickle cell disease, then Africanus Horton is arguably the strongest contender, predating James Herrick by over 30 years. In this respect, I emphasize the focus on treatment. As we shall see at least some twentieth-century scholarship had as much to do with reinforcing colonial or racist prejudices (see Tapper, 1999) as it had to do with treatment, and the alleviation of suffering was not always the framing within which research was conducted.

Conclusion

The long history of sickle cell affords us important lessons in the production of knowledge (Dyson, 2018). First, it draws our attention to the importance of *absence* in explanations: for example, the absence of extensive animal husbandry in early African agriculture enabled mosquitoes preferring human blood to thrive, and the sickle mutation to be enacted (Hedrick, 2011), or the absence of malarial pressures leading to a decline in sickle cell gene prevalence in, say, African-Americans compared with West/Central Africans. Second, and developing this first point, it draws our attention to the importance of having a conceptual framework that performs the function of compensation (Stenhouse, 1974). What might things be like? What if things were like this? For instance, examples would include the realm of the real (Bhaskar, 2008 [1975]) or the notion of the virtual (Delanda, 2016).

The long history of sickle cell also confirms recent philosophical emphasis on non-humans, and the difficulty of sustaining a notion of distinct natural and social realms (Latour, 2013). As Morton (2017) has remarked, the human body is an historical record of the evolution of non-humans. In considering the gene encoding sickle haemoglobin in contemporary human bodies, we have a record of the evolution of animals, birds, insects, protozoans and of plants grown in the Neolithic Transition. Finally, and in a lesson with important consequences for challenging the association of genetic reductionism and regressive politics, genetic does not mean primordial (Carter and Dyson, 2011): the sickle cell gene has not always been with(in) us.

4 A short history of sickle cell

The twentieth century in the USA

Introduction

This chapter focuses on the history of SCD in twentieth-century USA, with occasional reference to other Anglophone contexts. It does so in order to de-centre those understandings of SCD derived from the US experience in the twentieth century. First, it moves us beyond a chronology of medical innovations, since people living with SCD are more than patients, and we need to consider the broader context of their lives. Second, slavery and its legacy stratified African-Americans into poverty. Racialized poverty made for very poor quality survival: SCD thus appeared empirically as a severe chronic illness with ostensibly "inevitable" debilitating symptoms. At other times, and in other places, SCD as an illness is, and could be, a very different experience than in the twentieth-century USA. Third, the experience of SCD is bound up with the history of racism in the USA. However, it is not just that the history of racism is different in, say, the UK or Brazil, and that this difference will alter the framing of SCD, but that other settings may link SCD to other forms of stratification not based on race (for example, to scheduled castes in India) or indeed may not frame SCD within concepts of blackness or racism at all. Finally, in this anthropocentric twentieth-century history, almost everything is a correlate of human experience, right down to the quest to find key celebrity figures who can be iconic representations of living with SCD. By contrast, Chapter 3 explained the importance of climate, ecology and the role of non-humans in SCD. The hope, paradoxically, is that by detailing racism, anthropocentrism and SCD in twentieth-century USA, something of the future possible of alternative understandings of SCD may be opened up.

Medicine and sickle cell

The historiography of sickle cell suggests that histories have tended to be reduced to accounts of early biomedical papers from the "discovery" of "peculiar elongated cells" under the microscope (Herrick, 1910) to subsequent case studies, such as Washburn (1911), Cook and Meyer (1915), and Emmel (1917), through to Mason (1922), who first named sickle cell anaemia as such. There is, though, a more hidden history, beyond a medical history narrowly conceived. In this chapter we look at some of the social and political features of the way in which sickle cell has become visible. The account is restricted in several important ways. First, sickle cell symptoms are very disparate, and sickle cell was once regarded as the "great masquerader" as its varied manifestations could equally well be the consequence of other diseases (Winsor and Burch, 1945). As Wailoo (1997) observes, it was not until laboratory medicine began to emerge that a connection between the generative mechanisms of the disease and the manifestation in symptoms could be noted. More generally, laboratory medicine consolidated the power and resources accorded to medical practitioners in the twentieth century. Second, the wealth and resourcing of medical technologies in North America mean that any twentieth-century account of sickle cell is liable to be US-focused. Moreover, such accounts are liable to follow key published articles, almost all of which are in US journals (Savitt, 2014); key individuals, such as Lemuel Diggs, who treated a cohort of US sickle cell patients in Memphis (Nollan, 2016), and key historical accounts written by US academics (Tapper, 1999; Wailoo, 2001). This means that the history of sickle cell is dominated by written medical accounts, produced in English, in the Global North, and that what was happening with regards to sickle cell throughout Africa, India and Brazil may require other resources to reconstruct other narratives. To give just a simple example of how this bias operates, the rare haemoglobin variant haemoglobin D was referred to initially by the term haemoglobin D-Los Angeles, reflecting the first geographical location of medical identification in the 1950s, but is now known as haemoglobin D-Punjab, reflecting the area of the world where it is common and where it is now presumed to have arisen. While this chapter can go some way to redressing an over-medicalized view of the history of sickle cell, it cannot redress imbalances in the production of knowledge. This history of sickle cell is, then, actually a social history of sickle cell in twentieth-century USA, with occasional references to other times and places.

Carib's Leap and Jump Jim Crow: how sickle cell became linked to colonialism and racism

Medical case reports are often, though not always, anonymous. It is thanks to the US historian Todd Savitt that some of the more personal aspects of sickle cell case reports have been developed, beginning with what is now regarded as the first documented case of sickle cell in Western medical science (Savitt and Goldberg, 1989).

Walter Clement Noel was the son of affluent plantation owners in the north of the small Caribbean island of Grenada. He had migrated to Chicago to study dentistry at the university medical school. He had become ill in the winter of 1904 and a smear of his blood, examined under a microscope, was noted to be characterized by strange-shaped red blood cells. It was the intern (a recently qualified junior doctor) Ernest Irons who produced the report dated 31 December 1904, but it was not until 1910 that the presiding physician, James Herrick, published a medical paper describing "peculiar elongated cells". Noel recovered, qualified in the class of 1907 (Savitt, 2010) and returned to his native Grenada. There he ran a dental clinic until his early death aged just 32, from a chill apparently caught when attending a horse-race meeting. He was buried in the Catholic cemetery in Sauteurs on the northern tip of Grenada (Savitt and Goldberg, 1989).

Although by the eighteenth century Grenada was a British colony, the earliest colonizers had been the French. In 1651, the French had cornered the last of the indigenous peoples of the island, the Caribs, at the top of a promontory overlooking the sea. The Carib peoples resisted capture by leaping from the cliffs to their deaths below. The place is now known as Carib's Leap, and the French for jumpers or leapers is, of course, *sauteurs* from the French *sauter* to leap. The Sauteurs cemetery now contains plaques commemorating, on the one hand, the deaths of the last First Peoples of the Caribbean and, on the other hand, the resting place of Walter Clement Noel, the first named person with SCD known to medical science in the Global North.

In another part of his historical work, Savitt (1997) notes that the very social conditions that led to the documented first case of sickle cell disease, also led to the relative lack of attention given to the person in the next case reported in the medical literature. The time in the USA in which sickle cell first became visible is known as the *Jim Crow* era. Between the end of formal slavery following the US Civil War in 1865, and civil rights legislation in 1964, a century of racist apartheid prevailed, characterized by failure to make any restitution for slavery (Kerr-Ritchie, 2003); a continuance of extreme poverty through the practice of sharecropping; continued exclusion from political voting rights; segregation of lives (which included separate blood banks for black and whites when these were first developed, a segregation sometimes ignored in practice by the SCD physician Lemuel Diggs, who recognized its basis in prejudice rather than science (Nollan, 2016)), and the violent murder of black people in mob lynchings.

The term *Jim Crow* was derived from the song *Jump, Jim Crow* sung by a white performer in blackface. The legend is that, around 1828, the white performer Thomas Dartmouth "Daddy" Rice appropriated the song and syncopated dance-style from a disabled, enslaved African-American stable-hand. With damaged shoulders and legs, and syncope (associated with low blood pressure), the reported symptoms of the stable hand are all redolent of possible SCD. However, the story itself is doubtful as: (1) the location of the encounter is undocumented, and inconsistently given as Ohio, Baltimore, Louisville, or Pittsburgh (Christgau, 2004); (2) the only documentary record is in *Atlantic Monthly* in 1867 (Christgau, 2004), nearly 40 years after the claimed encounter by Rice, by which time, in order to justify continued gross discrimination in the post-Bellum absence of slavery, the alleged "authenticity" of the black culture that was being used to justify discrimination was important to establish; and (3) Rice had himself followed several earlier performers, including a certain Charles Mathews, who performed imitations of African-Americans, including black actors, as early as 1822 (Burrows and Wallace, 1999). That is 45 years before the *Atlantic Monthly* account, by which time post-Bellum justifications of racist discrimination against emancipated slaves were being developed. Former slaves, now nominally free, were denied "forty acres and a mule" because Northern capitalist interests prioritized increased land values and recommencement of the Atlantic international cotton trade over following through with promises of land for freed slaves to grow their own non-cash crops (Kerr-Ritchie, 2003). Rice's stage-shows thus followed earlier imitations of African-Americans by Mathews: a white upper-class English actor. My interpretation is that, by 1867, it served a purpose, as part of a post-slavery reconfiguration of a racist ideational system, to explain the subjugated impoverishment of many freed slaves, to present the Jim Crow origins as based on a single actual event. This purported event anchored racist views in (alleged) *actual* enslaved people's culture, and not merely as following on from the earlier racist mimicries of Charles Mathews and others (Burrows and Wallace, 1999: 489). As such, the actual stable hand, about whom we might have speculated around sickle cell symptoms, possibly did not even exist. In this instance, *avoiding* reading back in time the stable-hand's reported symptoms as SCD is important in resisting the construction of the very caricature of black culture upon which *Jim Crow* rested.

In any event, *Jim Crow* law is now a phrase used to describe the racist segregationist laws that lasted well into the twentieth century. In such a *Jim Crow* context, white physicians in the US South would frequently refuse to treat black patients. Medical schools in the US North began to accept some black students and this formed the backdrop to the presence of Walter Clement Noel in Chicago in the early 1900s. As such, Noel was a *contrast* to what many US white peoples might have expected when interacting with a black person. He was male, educated, and from a family of sufficient means to pay for a US university education. He lived in the US North, and in an urban setting. In all of these ways, he was a noteworthy person to the doctors Herrick and Irons. This contrasted to the second case reported in the medical literature, Ellen Anthony. She was female, denied formal education, and located in an impoverished rural setting in the US South. By all such dimensions of disadvantage – gender, poverty, regionalism, rural location, and literacy – she was of little interest (Savitt, 1997).

In such *Jim Crow* times, Nollan (2016) notes that it only took three or four case reports for the notion that SCD was a racially specific disease to become established. Thereafter, papers had to address themselves to this racialized framing. A further (racialized) feature of early twentieth-century medical reports on what we now term SCD, was the reference to syphilis. The higher rate of syphilis in African-Americans was a standard trope of the racist cultural system at the time. It was associated with sickle cell from the very first (Herrick, 1910: 520 offers syphilis as a possible diagnosis) through until at least 1945 when sickle cell is compared to syphilis as a masquerader of symptoms (Winsor and Burch, 1945). Western medicine, having described sickle cell in "Negro" patients, was subsequently, in the 1920s, unable to accept the notion of sickle cell in a white person – instead the argument was advanced that the person could not really be a "proper" white person (Tapper, 1999). This view persisted late into the twentieth century, and the US sociologist Troy Duster recalls being cautioned, in his study of sickle cell in Greece (Duster, 2003), that, since sickle cell was confined to black people, he must have confused sickle cell with beta-thalassaemia.

Among the first 40 or so medical articles documenting sickle cell cases up until 1933, there are glimpses of the human nature of the suffering endured (Savitt, 2014). The reports include reference to severe pain, some noting (as did Memphis physician Lemuel Diggs (Nollan, 2016: 112)) that treatment with morphine had little or no effect. Patients or relatives recount that being sickly was a life-long experience for the person with SCD, undermining both attempts at schooling and work (Savitt, 2014). Of 54 patient histories, most were children or young adults, with an overall mean age of 15, and only four were over 30 years old. Case reports were sometimes also autopsy reports of the deceased person with SCD. Savitt notes that persistent leg ulcers affected many of the people with SCD, as they had Walter Clement Noel, as well as other signs, such as enlarged spleens, yellowed whites of the eyes associated with jaundice, respiratory infections, late onset of puberty, and an emaciated or undernourished condition. There is a hint at distrust of medicine with respect to blood tests, especially of members of the extended families, and of surgical procedures, a distrust of medicine later characteristic more widely among African-Americans (Reverby, 2000; Skloot, 2010; Benjamin, 2011).

Savitt *et al.* (2014) suggest that the term sickle cell crisis first appears in print in Sydenstricker (1924a) who refers both to abdominal crisis and to a crisis associated with the spleen; and subsequently to a haemolytic crisis (Sydenstricker, 1924b). The word crisis was familiar to physicians from a variety of fevers and conditions, but was at the time also applied to a variety of symptoms associated with syphilis, a condition especially associated with African-Americans in racist discourses and soon to be rendered more infamous by the Tuskegee Syphilis Study of the 1930s–1970s (Reverby, 2000). This does suggest a negative linking of the term crisis to sickle cell by virtue of both sickle cell and syphilis being associated (in the racist ideational system) with being black. A more positive possibility is suggested by Savitt *et al.* (2014) who propose that the term evokes a white physician's genuine sympathy for a black patient's extreme suffering in an era not noted for such empathy. The term does evoke empathy, and is favoured by some patients because it is held to communicate both the extreme nature of the sickle cell pain, and the urgency of the situation to health care providers (ibid.). However, "crisis" also possibly conflates three issues, namely, sickle cell pain, a vaso-occlusive episode, and the urgent need for health care (ibid.). However, sickle cell pain is chronic as well as acute: a pervasive everyday experience for people with SCD in the USA, not just an emergency (Smith *et al.*, 2008). Furthermore, a crisis implies sudden onset when vaso-occlusion may be a product of chronic factors, such as ongoing red blood cell destruction and ongoing adhesiveness of red blood cells and blood vessel walls, Finally, the majority of sickle cell pain is reportedly managed at home, not in the acute setting (Savitt *et al.*, 2014). Despite the ambiguity of the term and the manner in which it can unhelpfully conflate these distinct issues, people living with SCD express the hope that the term crisis can successfully convey to reluctant health care providers the seriousness and the urgency of their needs.

1930s: sickle cell emerges in the context of racialized poverty

Wailoo (2001) provides an account of how sickle cell emerged with specific reference to Memphis, Tennessee. He notes that sickle cell became visible to the medical profession in the US South under particular circumstances. The decline of the cotton industry in the US South displaced already impoverished African-American share-croppers into a deprived, urban environment in search of a living. At the same time, with many white physicians refusing to treat black patients, new medical schools were required. The declining cotton industry meant that attracting federal funds for new medical schools to cities such as Memphis became an important factor to the civic authorities in replacing income. Such revenues, lost to the local economy from the decline of cotton, could be replaced with the wages of doctors and other hospital staff. For the medical schools, impoverished African-Americans in poor health provided good "clinical material" on which medical staff in training might practise their skills.

If the notion of people as "clinical material" sounds a cynical interpretation, we might note that the 1930s also saw the commencement of the Tuskegee Syphilis study (Reverby, 2000) and the 1940s the beginning of the Henrietta Lacks controversy. The former involved permitting African-American men with syphilis to go blind or die, even when treatments became available, in order for generations of junior public health doctors to study the so-called "natural" history of the disease. The latter involved taking the cells of an African-American woman, Henrietta Lacks, who was dying of cancer. The biopsy was undertaken without the permission or knowledge of her and her family. The cells were exceptional in that they could be cultured and reproduced in the laboratory where other cells had failed. Subsequently the so-called *HeLa* cells were cultured for laboratories across the US and the world, all without explicit acknowledgement of their original source (Skloot, 2010). Even when the extended family received belated recognition of this fact, there were subsequent attempts to claim rights over the genomic sequence of the cells, attempts which the National Institutes for Health had to avert. In such circumstances, the view of people with SCD as good clinical material resonates with the social attitudes of mid-twentieth-century America.

African-Americans living in cities such as Memphis were already resource-poor, and faced a poor diet and an insanitary environment, even without specific consideration of those living with SCD. Those with SCD who became ill did so in a situation where "for someone earning very little, it would be easy for a visit to the doctor or hospital to amount to a week's or a month's income" (Nollan, 2016: 54). Sickle cell came into view for the first time as providing good clinical material for staff of new medical schools (though not for straightforward altruistic reasons, at least at the policy level), and the identity of sickle cell as a disease of black people was further cemented.

It is worth noting the ways in which the first *cohort* of SCD patients, as opposed to single cases, came to be brought together, offered treatment and made subject to medical study. First, Lemuel Diggs was a white physician willing to treat African-American patients. Second, "he never charged his sickle cell patients a fee" (ibid.: 45) – altruistic certainly, but this also encouraged people to return to him, making ongoing study a possibility. Third, teaching SCD patients about their condition in terms of management and prevention became important, but was carried out by Diggs in reported opposition to the dean of the medical faculty (ibid.: 96). Diggs is also credited with indirectly educating other medical practitioners. Through recognizing SCD as a multi-system disorder, cross-consulting with a wide range of other specialities regarding particular symptoms, he was able not only to build up his own knowledge of SCD but impart something of SCD to physicians in other specialities (ibid.: 97). Finally, by the 1950s, Diggs was lending his car to an African-American phlebotomist, James Childs, to transport SCD patients to hospital. This fulfilled three functions: (1) ensuring appointments were kept; (2) subsidizing transport costs, allaying chronic lack of funds; and (3) helping to overcome the suspicions and fears of African-Americans of going to hospital (ibid.: 124).

Nollan attributes to Diggs genuine sympathy for the suffering SCD patient, though this does not necessarily contradict the notion that building research required a series of cases forming clinical material (Wailoo, 2001). However, the work of Lemuel Diggs in Memphis had to be tempered with recognition of the racist political landscape within which he operated, such that some political battles, for instance, the desegregation of blood within the blood bank, had to be tackled indirectly rather than head-on. But the combination of racism and poverty meant that SCD became visible in a historically-specific, highly compromised population. The first accounts of what SCD was actually like would not therefore have been accounts of what the experience of SCD *could* be like. In different historical and social circumstances, cohorts of people with SCD in Jamaica exhibited better health outcomes (Lee *et al.*, 1995), even when per capita GDP in 1970–1980s Jamaica was at or lower than in the 1930s USA. What may have appeared as the "natural" state of SCD was in fact determined by the legacy of slavery and the historically-specific racialized poverty in which most of the cohort of SCD patients treated by Diggs then lived.

1940s: science prospers but not people with SCD

A particular feature of racist ideas at this time focused on the issue of miscegenation. The term came from an anonymous propaganda pamphlet in 1863 in the US Civil War in which Southern Democrats attributed to Republicans the policy of being in favour of mixed black-white unions to the point of races becoming indistinguishable, an idea apparently abhorrent, even to those opposing slavery (Hollinger, 2003). Anti-miscegenation laws subsequently remained in place in many southern states until ruled unconstitutional by the Supreme Court in 1967.

This notion of miscegenation, the suspicion and outlawing of marriages that crossed the colour line, framed the understanding of scientists when attempting to infer reasons for the better health outcomes of adult Africans with SCD compared to African-Americans. In a miscegenation world-view, the racist conclusion was that mixed relationships between black and white partners made SCD worse because such admixture was not natural in admixed African-Americans, whereas it purportedly sat "naturally" within the bodies of pure Africans (Tapper, 1999). We would now explain this phenomenon in different ways. As we have seen in Chapter 3, the majority of those born with SCD in malarial Africa would have died in infancy. The survivors would have been the hardiest and/or those born into families with sufficient resources to provide good nutrition to enable survival into adulthood. By contrast, African-American infants with SCD would not have been vulnerable to malarial deaths, since *Plasmodium falciparum* malaria either never was, or by the 1940s was no longer, endemic in most US states, and so they were not exposed to this principal threat of infant death. The lack of malaria may have left more infant survivors, but the extreme poverty, poor nutrition, and insanitary environment, which most would have been exposed to, would have left those survivors in very poor health. Moreover, at the time, the potential SCD infant prevalence in West Africa would have been as much as 1 in 50 compared to 1 in 400 in the USA, and this differential increased survival of African-Americans with SCD would have tended to equalize the apparent respective adult prevalence when comparing the USA and Africa.

A lack of flourishing characterized the lives of those with SCD, and contrasted with scientific advances. A paper by US biochemist Linus Pauling is frequently fêted as one of the key twentieth-century publications in the whole of science for identifying sickle cell as a molecular disease (Pauling *et al.*, 1949). However, Feldman and Tauber (1997) take issue with accounts of sickle cell research, with grandiose titles such as *The Eighth Day of Creation*, that credit Pauling's work as representing a radical disjuncture in science. Feldman and Tauber note that, over time in his written accounts, Pauling positions himself more and more as the central instigator of the insight. Furthermore, they note that several factors influenced the course of sickle cell research in the decades before. These factors included the privileging of laboratory blood pictures over patient symptoms in studies by Emmel (1917), Mason (1922) and Huck (1923), the latter even reducing clinical symptoms to an appendix of the published article. Even when Diggs brought the patient back into view by suggesting that the sickle-shaped cells might be responsible for blockages and hence for symptoms in those patients (Diggs and Ching, 1934), the sickle shape, as seen in laboratory slides, dominated and framed the view of sickle cell. As we will see in Chapter 6, this emphasis on sickled cells, rather than on the whole person with SCD, and on the sickle shape, rather than anaemia and other contributing factors in the SCD experience, continues to distort assessments of cause of death.

Feldman and Tauber (1997) also suggest that in addition to a patient-symptom/laboratory-slide spilt, there were broader scientific disputes yet to be resolved into a working consensus, rendering the scientific context fragmented and diverse. This fragmentation prevented the emergence of paradigms that might make it possible to think that SCD might have a molecular basis, and also ensured that dominant theories of inheritance prevailed, with both sickle cell anaemia and sickle cell trait conflated in the term *sicklemia*. However, as we saw in Chapter 1, the capacity of cells to sickle *in vitro* is a dominant characteristic. The mistake was to think that all phenotypic features must be inherited according to the same Mendelian principle: dominant or recessive. As we saw in Chapter 1, the capacity of red blood cells to sickle *in vitro* is dominant, but chronic anaemia and haemoglobin motility in an electrical field, for example, are not.

Finally, Pauling *et al.* were not the first to demonstrate that different haemoglobins move at different rates using electrophoresis techniques. A 1944 paper noted different mobility and rates of sedimentation between foetal and adult haemoglobin, and drew the conclusion that there were different molecular species of haemoglobin behind these observations (Andersch *et al.*, 1944). As the lead author of this paper was a woman, Marie Andersch, this perhaps also says much about the gendered nature of attribution of credit in the history of science.

One issue, hidden at the time of Pauling's work on the molecular basis of sickle cell, but of later significance in assessing the politics of sickle cell trait (about which more in Chapters 5 and 6), was the role of a group of African-American pilots during the Second World War. The Tuskegee airmen were a group of over 900 African-American trained aircraft pilots in a segregated unit who engaged in both combat roles and bomber escort roles. Most importantly a proportion would have had sickle cell trait, and no reports of any problems with sickle cell trait and altitude in unpressurized aircrafts were reported (Duster, 2003). As well as representing notable achievements in their own right as the first black US combat air pilots, the Tuskegee Airmen also stand as a testimony to counter the exaggerated accounts of the role of sickle cell trait in restricting aircraft travel. In the decades that followed, alleged susceptibility of those with sickle cell trait rested on molecular distinctions, and in one specific instance, discussed below, on Pauling's status as a great man of science, and not on such socio-historical evidence.

1950s: sickle cell and political blackness

In the 1950s, hundreds of studies of blood in Africa were undertaken, with sickle cell being marshalled as part of colonial medicine as a particular resource with which to examine questions of belonging and territory, a central concern to late colonial rule (Tapper, 1999). From the colonizers' perspective, Africa was characterized by non-tessellating constituencies: peoples, languages, and cultures did not exhibit a one-to-one correspondence with particular territories (Braun and Hammonds, 2008). The needs of colonial administrators demanded the imposition of order as a condition of effective colonial rule. The prevalence of sickle cell trait in different populations came to be seen as a deep marker – one that had the ostensible advantage of appearing objective and scientific – of who legitimately might belong in a particular territory as well as a marker of who was a "real" African (Tapper, 1999; Carter and Dyson, 2011). Sickle cell aided a particular colonial distinction between Sub-Saharan Africa and North African Arabs, with rates of sickle cell regarded as objective markers of otherwise indeterminate populations (Tapper, 1999). However, identifying frequencies of haemoglobin variants was not geared towards development of therapeutic interventions for those living with SCD.

While African nationalist leaders sought independence from colonization by Europeans, with the advent of the Cold War with the Soviet Union, the US government worried that such African nationalist movements were also attracted by Marxism and they supported decolonization as part of the strategy against communism (Watts, 2011). Such anti-communist concerns seem also to have had an impact on how sickle cell became incorporated into anthropocentric disputes.

The physician James Herrick, the author of the 1910 paper, became noted, over the course of his career, for his work on myocardial infarction (heart attacks). By the time an English researcher arrived in the USA to seek a conversation with the now elderly Herrick, in the early 1950s (Lehmann and Huntsman, 1974), another social prejudice was gripping the US: McCarthyism and the witch-hunt for anyone with left-leaning political views who might be labelled a communist. Three factors are worth citing in this regard. First, a number of prominent black people (such as the great singer, Paul Robeson) were implicated. Second, as we have seen, Marxist ideologies were influential among black African figures seeking independence from colonization by Europeans (Rodney, 1972). Third, African-American anti-colonial thought was well established in the inter-war period (Bergin, 2016). For these three reasons, the cultural system of the time, functioning "as if" a language, might conceivably have linked sickle cell to being black, and political blackness to anti-US communism. Perhaps this explains why Herrick did not foreground sickle cell in his life's achievements and seemed to shun someone who sought him out in 1950s USA on the subject of sickle cell, a topic rendered dangerous by political association:

> One of the authors visited Herrick some 40 years later, and as it turned out, shortly before his death. It might be worth recording that Herrick was by no means pleased to be specifically associated with the discovery of sickling, a 'minor peculiarity', because he wanted to be remembered for his work on coronary thrombosis. Perhaps the interview was altogether not fortunate. It was at the time when Senator McCarthy investigated the political past of University Professors retired or not retired. The enthusiastic visitor, straight from England in a black overcoat and black Eden hat was at first taken for a Federal Investigator!
>
> (Lehmann and Huntsman, 1974: 141–142)

Around 1953–1954, then, there is evidence that sickle cell was firmly attached to political blackness in the USA, and even the author of the first paper, James

Herrick, then in his nineties, apparently wanted to dissociate himself from such a dangerous topic. To their credit, others did not.

The association of sickle cell and black people brought white physicians such as Lemuel Diggs into the orbit of racialized politics. In the 1950s, he received a letter from a citizens group, aligned to the Ku Klux Klan, seeking support for the view that sickle cell indexed the "racial inferiority of the negro race" and that sought to use sickle cell as justification for segregation. In reply, Diggs noted that white populations had other inherited conditions (thalassaemia, hereditary spherocytosis) and that "One might, therefore, with equal accuracy, argue that intermarriage would degrade the Negro race" (cited in Nollan, 2016: 133).

1960s: disablement, racism and sickle cell

To the extent that Sylvia Plath's novel *The Bell Jar* is semi-autobiographical, the complaint of her protagonist Esther that she was taken to "a lecture on sickle-cell anemia and some other depressing diseases, where they wheeled sick people out onto the platform and asked them questions and then wheeled them off and showed colored slides" (Plath, 2005 [1963]: 60) might plausibly be taken to reflect actual attitudes: people with SCD were assumed to be chronically ill with a shortened life expectancy, but made interesting case studies for display to medical students.

By the 1960s, treatment for sickle cell in the USA was so still lacking that the Black Panthers described the situation as amounting to genocide. Those who might have comprised more enabling voices in the scientific establishment did not help matters. Linus Pauling remains the only person to win two (unshared) Nobel Prizes (for Chemistry, in 1954, and for Peace in 1962). As we saw above, Pauling was credited with being the first to identify that sickle cell anaemia was a molecular disease. More controversially, in one of his letters he later writes:

> I have suggested that the time might come in the future when information about heterozygosity in such serious genes as the sickle cell anaemia gene would be tattooed on the forehead of the carriers, so that young men and women would at once be warned not to fall in love with each other.
>
> (Pauling, 1967: 269)

Of course, Pauling was influenced by his own social location and the context of his era. Sickle cell was considered and referred to as a disease of childhood, with very high rates of under-fives mortality still reported in the late 1960s (Prabhakar *et al.*, 2010). Lemuel Diggs noted no overall improvement in life expectancy for sickle cell right through to the 1960s (Nollan, 2016: 136). Sickle cell was known to be inherited but the development of prenatal diagnosis through analysis of DNA (Kan and Dozy, 1978), and the possibility this opened up for diagnosis and selective termination of pregnancy was a decade away. As such, the rationalist scientific mind-set and the white male paternalistic world-view led Pauling to exhibit what we would now regard as disability discrimination. Furthermore, since historically, enslaved peoples were branded with the letter R on their fore-head, signifying that they had run away from their enslavers (Higginbotham, 1978: 182), to twenty-first-century eyes, Pauling's comments are problematic with respect to both disability discrimination and racism.

By the late 1960s in the USA, it has been argued that sickle cell became an important springboard to citizenship rights for African-Americans in the Civil Rights era (Tapper, 1999). For example, sickle cell community education and testing represented the contradiction in practice of the 1965 Moynihan Report, a report that had characterized African-American communities as allegedly dis-organized and uneducable (ibid.). A key part of this effort concerned the Black Panthers, who, through their sickle cell programmes, demonstrated precisely that black communities could organize for self-education. However, in securing the US 1972 Sickle Cell Control Act that ushered in the era of Sickle Cell Compre-hensive Care Centers, the cause of sickle cell became detached from the broader issues of equity in access to health services, based in the community and under community control that had been a feature of the services developed by the Black Panthers (Nelson, 2011). The work of US Professor of Pathology James Bowman implies that the Black Panthers did not have access to haemoglobin electrophoresis equipment and suggests therefore that use of the sickle solubility test may have been behind the confusion of sickle cell trait and sickle cell disease at that time (Bowman, 1977). This is disputed by Nelson (2011), who argues that the Black Panthers did indeed make use of such equipment. This dis-tinction between types of laboratory testing was to become crucial in struggles over the confusion between SCD and sickle cell trait, a confusion resonant to this day.

1970s: detaching sickle cell from broader causes

When the first legislation on sickle cell was enacted, it incorporated the basic confusion of sickle cell trait and SCD into law. The first line of the National Sickle Cell Anemia Control Act of 1972 refers to two million blacks having sickle cell anaemia, when this was the figure for sickle cell trait, not SCD (Draper, 1991: 224). In the period before 1972, sickle cell faced several chal-lenges in securing resources. First, grant-giving organizations considered that sickle cell only affected black people, and so was an unimportant disease, not worthy of funding (Nollan, 2016: 123–124). Second, "anything that could portray blacks as sickly or weak was also a potential threat" (ibid.: 125). Third, it was not possible for African-Americans to allow racist discrimination to become a non-issue, which "made it impossible to sentimentalize sickling in accordance with the model of disease representation required by the genre of the (charity fund-raising) telethon" (Tapper, 1999: 104).

The US National Sickle Cell Control Act was signed into force by Richard Nixon on 16 May 1972 (Nixon, 1972), but is notable for a number of problems. First, the monies released to support sickle cell were not always additional monies but were explicitly subtracted from research programmes for other disease conditions (Nollan, 2016: 138). Since Nixon erroneously stated that "the disease is especially pernicious because it strikes blacks and no-one else", African-American peoples were positioned not only as receiving special funding but as "taking away" the funding of others, when in fact funding was still way below parity for comparable diseases (Scott, 1970).

In part contradiction, then, of Tapper's claim that sickle cell was the bridge to civil rights for African-Americans at this time, the legacy of Nixon's cynical appropriation of sickle cell as an issue is that sickle cell funding became framed as taking away from whites, and explains the power of sickle cell to evoke the enduring misconception that black people are receiving special funding. Second, it is notable that the Act emphasizes control. Control implies that the priority is the prevention of births of children with SCD rather than the provision of comprehensive treatments, or as the Black Panthers wanted, policy action that improved social conditions (employment, education, housing, diet) for all African-Americans (Nelson, 2011). Such generic improvements would also have helped in the prevention of illness episodes for people living with SCD. Instead the focus was on screening and genetic counselling, with the unspoken rationalist assumption that a reduction in SCD births would inevitably follow. Community education was primarily community education on the genetic risks of having a child with SCD if both partners had sickle cell trait (Figure 4.1).

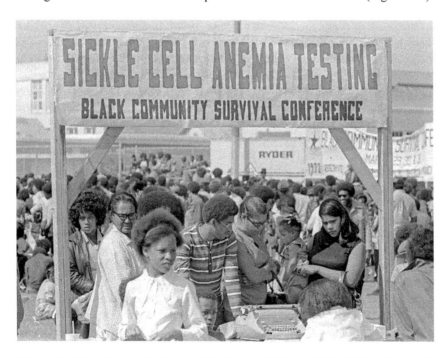

Figure 4.1 Black Community Survival Conference, 30 March 1972, sickle cell anaemia testing.

Source: Courtesy of the Department of Special Collections, Stanford University Library.

Finally, any care is subjugated to its role in supporting research into diagnosis, treatment and control.

Apart from making care of people living with SCD a mere adjunct of participation in medical research, the third aim repeats the emphasis on control. Thus, we have an ostensibly tripartite message that is effectively the same message three times. Aim 1: Screen and genetic counselling (for prevention of births). Aim 2: Community education on patterns of inheritance (for prevention of births). Aim 3: Research (at least partially) into how best to control (for prevention of births). Furthermore, to the extent that sickle cell research monies also benefitted white scientists and clinical researchers, and were directed at a condition affecting perhaps 1 in 400 US African-Americans, this meant that such sums could not be spent on broader social welfare projects in African-American neighbourhoods (Markel, 1997).

As is well documented, the 1970s sickle cell screening that ensued has been held up as an example of how not to introduce such screening, leading one New York activist to describe mandatory screening as "genocidal health practices of the white medical establishment" (cited in ibid.: 4). Discrimination against people with sickle cell trait followed in areas such as education, employment, insurance, marriage certification, and service in the armed forces (Bowman, 1977; Draper, 1991; Duster, 2003). Medical knowledge was lacking, with numerous case reports misunderstanding or misrepresenting the sickle cell trait as the cause of symptoms (Konotey-Ahulu, 1996). In one survey of physicians' knowledge about sickle cell in 1974, one in seven thought trait indicative of SCD; one in five could not distinguish clinically between trait and SCD, and one in two did not know of other types of SCD such as the combinations with haemoglobin C or beta-thalassaemia (Markel, 1997: 4). Later work reports a transition from physicians lacking any awareness of SCD, to subsequent over-compensation whereby any African-American presenting with any symptoms was regarded as a patient with SCD (Hill, 1994).

Furthermore, Witzig (1996) notes that such racialized assumptions about presumed identity of patients misled physicians into unduly narrowing their differential diagnosis, and cites two cases: one where a "phenotypically European" (of Indian, North European and Mediterranean ancestry) eight-year old boy was prepared for (unnecessary) surgery before establishing his symptoms were associated with sickle cell anaemia. A second case, assigned a black identity by physicians, and reporting that a previous doctor had told him he "had sickle cell", was mistakenly treated for sickle cell anaemia before bleeding to death from a peptic ulcer.

Hampton et al. (1974) note a further deleterious consequence of mass screening. Parents of those with sickle cell trait were found to have imposed a sick role onto their offspring. Hampton et al. refer to sickle cell "non-disease" (sickle cell carriers mistakenly thinking they have a chronic illness) as a potential public health issue arising from the hasty institution of ill-judged sickle cell screening programmes. The result of so much discrimination was to produce a very hard-and-fast public health message distinguishing between sickle cell trait as harmless and

SCD as a very serious health condition. The place of this distinction in the sub-sequent politics of sickle cell trait is the subject of Chapters 5 and 6.

1980s: the politics of susceptibility

Nollan (2016) notes that even Lemuel Diggs did not himself go out into the African-American community until near or after retirement. One study did examine the social context of African-American mothers facing up to racism while living in poverty in the inner city and raising a child with SCD (Hill, 1994). The study by US sociologist Shirley Hill stands as a counter to the white rationalist medical framework within which sickle cell had usually been con-sidered. Until that point, continuing to have children born with SCD in the knowledge that they were sickle cell genetic carriers was attributed to a combi-nation of ignorance and/or irrational behaviour. Hill's study examines the issue from the context of the mother. She notes that, historically, the African-American family was formed in the context of enslavement: quite apart from the raping of black women, enslavers deliberately broke up family relationships. In the 1980s, in inner city areas, this legacy was overlaid with social policies (briefly, employ-ment discrimination leading to small-time drug dealing to make a living, leading to criminalization within a skewed criminal justice system, leading to male absence in the family, placing dual demands of unpaid domestic labour and low paid employment onto women, and promoting a particular type of disharmony in gender relations). This led to a preponderance of African-American lone mothers. The legacy of enslavement and the immediate narcotization and criminalization of black men created a context in which white observers could compound their toxic historical and policy legacies by then blaming the African-American community for an alleged dysfunctional family structure. However, in a deprived urban environment, and facing racism and poverty, mothers regarded children with SCD not as a flawed child but as a child to be valued as symbolic of the survival of the race. The many policy confusions of the 1970s sickle cell screening lent the mothers' rejection of technically accurate estimates of genetic risk greater credibility.

One consequence of a growing economy and of civil rights legislation appears to have been an increase in the proportion of black workers employed in the chemical, rubber, steel, textile, motor and petroleum industries between 1960 and 1980 (Draper, 1991: 84). US sociologist Elaine Draper argues that genetic testing was associated with *susceptibility politics*. Such politics focuses risk onto the worker and disputed risks of genetic traits; draws attention away from scien-tifically robust evidence of environmental work hazards, and is used to exclude black workers, who constituted a minority with only recent and partial access to the types of higher-paying manual jobs in the industries listed above (ibid.: 84–85). Excluding workers with sickle cell trait effectively excludes 10 per cent of all blacks and few whites (ibid.: 83). The US conglomerate Dupont led the way in testing all black job applicants for sickle cell trait and SCD in 1972, but Draper points out the unequal power relationship when sickle cell testing becomes part of an industrial company's policy (ibid.: 130). Dupont's pro-grammes failed to match five principles for occupational genetic screening: (1) initiation (employees were not involved in setting up the programme); (2) informed consent (Dupont physicians did not routinely inform job applicants they were being tested for sickle cell); (3) no systematic counselling was arranged (those tested were simply referred to their own doctor); (4) job place-ment (Draper notes some evidence of work restrictions or job transfer for those identified with trait); and (5) confidentiality (which cannot exist where company management have access to files) (ibid.: 130–133).

Sickle cell testing can permit a situation where only African-Americans are tested, and where employers (especially in the chemical, airlines and military fields) have tested and excluded only African-Americans (ibid.: 92). Moreover, when industry test results were not kept confidential, this led to job discrimina-tion and raised insurance premiums (ibid.: 103). Half of 40 insurance companies surveyed raised rates for sickle cell trait when sickle cell trait had no significant effect on life expectancy rates (ibid.: 93, 224–225) and 9 out of 12 insurance companies raised rates for sickle cell trait even though not actuarially justified (ibid.: 228). Those with sickle cell trait were reportedly also denied employment when screened outside of their occupation as part of public screening pro-grammes (ibid.: 93).

1990s: visibility and priorities

The increased visibility of sickle cell in the USA in the 1970s had an impact in the UK, and two UK sickle cell pioneers, founders respectively of OSCAR (Organization for Sickle Cell Anaemia Research), in 1975, and the Sickle Cell Society, in 1979, report visits to the USA to learn more about sickle cell advo-cacy (Clare, 2007; Anionwu, 2016). Like the USA, the UK labour market was structured by the insertion of black (migrant) labour into low-paid, dangerous and hazardous occupations (Miles, 1982), often in declining industries, leaving a subsequent legacy of high levels of black unemployment. Following inner-city rebellions in the 1980s in the UK, some monies were found for the inner-city areas, in which the majority of black people then lived, and money for local sickle cell projects became part of this development (Dyson, 2005). Valuable as these sickle cell initiatives were, however, they substituted action on sickle cell for broader changes in health, education, employment and housing opportunities for black people. This is discussed further in Chapter 7.

At the time in the UK, however, public health doctors pointed out that the relative numbers of health education leaflets available on a subject did not reflect the epidemiological evidence of ethnic inequalities (Bhopal and Don-aldson, 1988). Sickle cell has a huge impact on those affected, but, in compari-son, small differences between black and white groups in terms of relative rates of heart disease, strokes and diabetes accounted for much greater ethnic health inequalities overall. The resulting concern led to an implication that specific disorders such as sickle cell were over-represented in health education materials, comprising 6 per cent of the leaflets listed by the Health Education Council in 1984 and 9 per cent by 1987 (ibid.). Since the research consisted of sending a junior public health doctor to the health promotion office where I then worked, the junior doctor merely consulting a national catalogue produced by the UK Health Education Council listing available leaflets, there was no apparent interest in *who produced* such leaflets. Many were actually produced either by self-help groups such as OSCAR (who had six guides covering sickle cell and employment, social services, and housing) or were local leaflets reflecting vociferous local community campaigns, for example, the Hackney Sickle Link Project. The research amounted to blaming sickle cell community activism for a skewing of national health promotion priorities, as judged by comparing leaflets with epidemiological data. Two leaflets discontinued by 1990 were the Health Education Council's own official leaflets on sickle cell, aimed at health workers and teachers respectively. These leaflets, focusing on *sickle cell anaemia*, were never replaced, merely supplanted in the 2000s by leaflets on *sickle cell screening*. Having effectively been dismissed as a totemic issue because it had been misused to stand for doing something for minority ethnic communities in the UK, sickle cell was downgraded in terms of policy development for another decade. Community concerns as reflected in the leaflets (education, employment, housing, insurance, and family care) were overtaken by the focus on prenatal sickle cell screening by the 2000s, when a new generation of leaflets emerged, reflecting screening concerns, rather than concerns for those living with SCD.

Sickle cell in popular culture

The US cultural sociologist JC Alexander has written of a situation where, in mass societies, cultural meanings, which might in other times have been performed in ritual by all members of a society, become condensed in the role of a few performers. Initially this involved a separation between performers on the stage and the audience. By the early twenty-first century, we have celebrities through whom many live their own lives vicariously, what Alexander (2010) names the celebrity-icon, who encapsulate a range of key cultural meanings in a condensed form. For example, somehow, malaria and sickle cell matter more as issues if we can say that Alexander the Great died of *Plasmodium falciparum* malaria in the mosquito-inhabited swamps south of Babylon (Chugg, 2012: 31–34) or that Tutankhamun may have had sickle cell disease (Timmann and Meyer, 2010) and put aside the many other competing theories about the causes of their respective deaths. Thus, to bemoan the fact that people care more about modern celebrities than people living with SCD may be good morality, but it is bad sociology (Alexander, 2010), because it fails to take account of how meanings operate within the cultural systems of complicated mass societies.

Moreover, combine this insight with the knowledge that iconic status is racialized and globally uneven, and we are left with two principal avenues whereby twentieth-century figures with sickle cell disease may have achieved widespread recognition: the culture and sports industries. As professional sports participation is unlikely for many with SCD (Waltz *et al.*, 2013) and US football stars sometimes listed as "having sickle cell" actually have sickle cell trait not SCD, we are left with participation in art, music and film.

Miles Davis (1926–1991), the famous jazz trumpeter (Figure 4.2), recounts the pain of his SCD and sickle cell-related problems with his hip in his auto-biography (Davis and Troupe, 1989). Georgeanna Tillman (1944–1980) was a singer with the Tamla Motown group, the Marvellettes (Figure 4.3), whose best-known record "Please Mr Postman", was the first number one hit for that iconic record label in 1961. Paul Williams (1939–1973) (Figure 4.4) was credited with

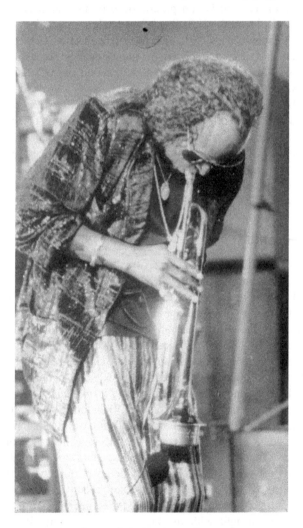

Figure 4.2 Miles Davis in Rio de Janeiro.

Source: Rui Brito www.flickr.com/photos/8018759@N04/483993302 (Subject deceased).

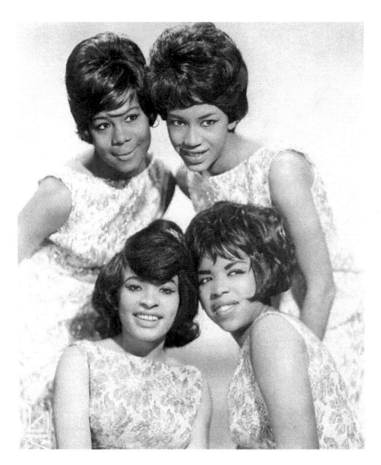

Figure 4.3 Georgeanna Tillman (bottom right) of The Marvellettes, 1963.

Source: Motown/Tamla Records Photographer: James Kriegsmann, New York.

the innovative choreography of another Motown group The Temptations, and his problem use of alcohol was attributed to attempts to deal with his sickle cell pain. Both Tillman and Williams are reported to have stopped touring because of the strain this imposed when combined with their SCD-related episodes of illness. Sean Oliver was bassist in the UK band Rip Rig and Panic (Figure 4.5), featuring Neneh Cherry, and Oliver later co-wrote "Wishing Well" for Terence Trent D'Arby, before dying of sickle cell complications in 1990. Tionne "T-Boz" Watkin (b. 1970) of the 1990s band TLC declared her sickle cell illness publicly and became a spokesperson for the Sickle Cell Disease Association of America. Albert Johnson, the rapper Prodigy (1974–2017) of the hip hop duo Mobb Deep, references his sickle cell anaemia in his song "Feel My Pain", and attracted one of the more infamous put-downs in rap music from his rival Tupac Shakur, who taunted him "Don't one of you niggas got sickle cell or

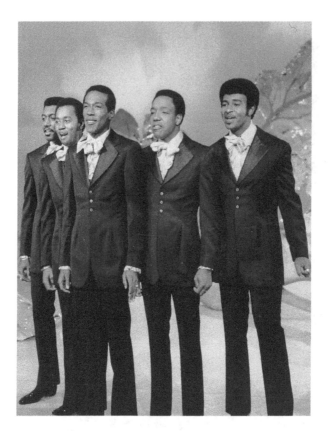

Figure 4.4 Paul Williams (fourth from right) of The Temptations, 1969.

Source: Bernie Ilson, Inc.

something?" Prodigy served time in a New York jail for firearms offences, wrote a cookery book on how to make prison food more palatable (Johnson and Iandoli, 2016), before being hospitalized with sickle cell complications and dying of accidental choking in 2017.

UK visual artist Donald Rodney (1961–1998) was part of the BLK Art movement that linked social issues, especially racism, to art. Rodney was born in an area of the West Midlands in the UK infamous for its racism in the 1960s, a racism so bad it drew a visit to the area by Malcolm X in 1965: "If You Want a Nigger for a Neighbour, Vote Labour" ran a racist slogan aiding the (successful) Conservative candidate at the time (Craig, 2007). Rodney sometimes made use of his SCD in his work, metaphorically linking the disease of sickle cell to the disease of racism. A long period of hospitalization with sickle cell in 1987 led Rodney to incorporate his own X-rays into his artistic work. The following year Rodney had a solo exhibition entitled *Crisis* (clearing referencing sickle cell crises) which brought together a variety of his X-ray-based works. In Book

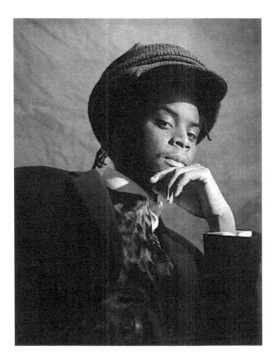

Figure 4.5 Sean Oliver of the band Rip, Rig and Panic.
Source: Alastair Thain.

Three of his notebooks in the Tate Modern, he sketches the pattern of inherit-
ance of sickle cell together with the name and address of the local sickle cell
NGO, the Birmingham branch of the Organization for Sickle Cell Anaemia
Research.

In film, one of the most iconic figures in cinematic history is *Alien*, the terroriz-
ing creature from the 1979 film of that name. Inside the alien costume was Bolaji
Badejo (*c.*1953–1992), a Nigerian studying in London, recruited specifically for
his skinny 6'10" tall frame, because the casting director apparently thought no-one
would quite believe that it could be a human inside the costume. Although it is
arguably a positive that someone living with SCD is a key cast member of an
iconic film of the twentieth century, the body image of people living with SCD is
framed in negative ways, and this is discussed further in Chapter 10.

Of course, and as will be emphasized in Chapter 10, many ordinary people
living with SCD have quietly registered important achievements. In particular,
achievements of people living with SCD outside the USA are less well documented. One exception was brought to my attention while attending the First
Global Sickle Cell Congress in Accra, Ghana, in 2010. Before the main congress, the Ghanaian Professor of Medicine, Felix Konotey-Ahulu convened the
Third International Conference on the Achievements of Sickle Cell Disease

Patients, a conference to celebrate Ghanaians living with SCD. Notable occupations of people living with SCD included bilingual secretary; consultant haematologist; head of a nursing agency; senior retail manager; university professor of ecology; banker; senior research fellow; epidemiologist; molecular biologist; children's educator; pharmacist and international pianist. Many speakers with SCD also had grown-up children of their own. While their biographies indicated relatively affluent origins and education and/or location outside Ghana itself, such achievements at least go beyond the Global North and the racialization that often frames black achievement as limited to excellence in sports or the arts.

Conclusion

If we take Chapters 3 and 4 together, we have two complementary types of reason for the contemporary framing of sickle cell as a black issue. Chapter 3 provides us with a longer time view than some histories of sickle cell: as part of the human genome it post-dates much of human history before the Neolithic Transition and, considered over even longer time-scales, the duration of hominids or non-human life on Earth, sickle cell is more like an event than an enduring condition. Chapter 4 provides us with a (mainly) US-focused account of sickle cell in the twentieth century, noting how the particular racialized politics of the USA have framed sickle cell in particular ways. The corollary of this is that other less well-known sickle cell studies are only just being written about, for example, in Senegal (Fulwilley, 2011); Ghana (Dennis-Antwi *et al.*, 2011); Mali (Lainé *et al.*, 2012); Oman (Beaudevin, 2013); India (Chattoo, 2018); Nigeria (Ola *et al.*, 2016); and Brazil (Creary, 2018).

In both time and space, we have the dimension of comparison that enables us to understand in what ways the twentieth-century African-American experience, which dominates understandings of sickle cell to date, may begin to be decentred in the current century. Sickle cell became visible partly through the rise of laboratory medicine, and molecular and genetic research has predominated over patient experience ever since. It also became visible in the context of twentieth-century racism and African-American poverty, and this racialization has arguably affected sickle cell experiences elsewhere (Dyson, 2005).

Finally, there is one more form of decentring likely to emerge, and that is a response to anthropocentrism. Herrick was not, in fact, the first person to see crescent-shaped red blood cells under the microscope, and nor even was Irons. This accolade goes to George Gulliver, Assistant Surgeon to the Royal Regiment of Horse Guards in London, who, in 1840, noted the peculiar shapes of red blood cells of particular species of deer (Gulliver, 1840; Conley, 1980). However, as the co-founder of the Sickle Cell Disease Association of America, Charles Whitten, pointed out, since these sickle-shaped cells do not represent SCD in deer, "These findings have relevance to the sickling phenomenon in humans in that they emphasize the importance of the physical properties of sickle cells, *exclusive of shape*, in the pathogenesis of sickle cell anemia" (Whitten, 1967: 650, my emphasis).

5 Sickle cell trait and athletics

Introduction

As we have seen in the early chapters of this book, many accounts of SCD place far too great an emphasis on the sickle shape as a key marker of SCD. This contrasts with early African accounts that situate sickle cell within the whole-person-in-pain-in-ecological-context. In the Global North, by approaching sickle cell via laboratory medicine, the sickle shape has been over-stressed in comparison to other key mechanisms in sickle cell disease, including inflammation, release of substances increasing risks of blood clotting, chronic damage to cell walls, and ongoing early destruction of red blood cells. Even within the vaso-occlusive sickle cell episode narrowly considered, the sickle shape is arguably as much a *consequence* of multiple interactive factors as its cause. However, because of the very name of sickle cell disease, and because the sickle shape represents a convenient point of entry into a beginner's explanation of SCD, the sickle shape has come to dominate in public, journalistic, legal and non-specialist accounts of sickle cell. This has had devastating effects for the politics of sickle cell, where the materiality of sickle cell trait has found itself misrepresented. The following two chapters address themselves to this concern. In Chapter 6, we look at the role that sickle cell trait has played in explaining away sudden deaths in state custody or state contact. In this chapter, we look at controversies surrounding sudden death in military or professional sports training and the politicization of sickle cell trait as a putative explanation.

Sickle cell trait and sudden death

A person jumps to their death from a great height. At autopsy they are found to have sickle cell trait. Would we say that sickle cell trait had contributed to their death? Hopefully, not. Worse still, would we conclude that people with sickle cell trait are more prone to deaths resulting from falling from heights than those without sickle cell trait? Again, hopefully, not. And yet this is precisely the flawed logic with which sickle cell advocates are faced in addressing the political fallout from sudden deaths in military training and elite sports. As we saw in Chapter 1, sickle cell trait is the genetic carrier state of sickle cell (HbAS) and not the actual chronic illness sickle cell anaemia (HbSS). People with sickle cell trait have around 40 per cent of their haemoglobin as haemoglobin S, compared to around 90 per cent in those with sickle cell anaemia (HbSS). Exercise physiologists can induce *in vivo* sickling in athletes with sickle cell trait through a combination of exercise and (simulated) altitude, but the sickling takes place outside the micro-circulation (in wider blood vessels, which sickled cells cannot block) and does not reduce the exercise performance in question (Martin *et al.*, 1989).

Following half a century of neglect, sickle cell became a prominent issue in the 1970s (Tapper, 1999). Numerous case reports linking sickle cell trait to various deleterious effects were produced, and many of these case reports were, in turn, debunked (Konotey-Ahulu, 1996: 358–371). One study involved a report of four deaths during training of armed forces personnel who, it transpired, also had sickle cell trait (Jones *et al.*, 1970). This was followed by a period of discrimination in admissions to armed forces, then by a reversal of this decision, with, initially, debarring decisions based on levels of haemoglobin S, before later developing a formula whereby those with "non-treatable anaemia" (Grant *et al.*, 2011) were debarred, thus focusing not on the sickle shape but on the destruction of red blood cells and consequent anaemia in someone with SCD, but not in sickle cell trait. At any rate, there are a number of problems with making deductions about sickle cell trait from such case reports.

First, sickled cells at post-mortem cannot legitimately be used to infer cause of death. In this respect, expert opinion combining sickle cell and pathology (Bowman, 1977), on the one hand, and sickle cell and exercise in the armed forces, on the other hand (Kark, 2000), make important points about deaths in the case of someone with sickle cell trait.

US Professor of Pathology James Bowman noted that:

> [T]he presence of widespread intravascular sickling in post-mortem or in surgical specimens has no relationship to the amount (if any) of intravascular sickling that may have been present while the tissue(s) were living, for intravascular sickling may arise as an agonal event or after death as a result of tissue hypoxia.
>
> (1977: 122–123; intravascular = inside the blood vessels; agonal = in the process of dying; hypoxia = lack of oxygen)

The importance of this testimony is that it emphasizes that sickled cells found at post-mortem in someone with sickle cell trait are only to be expected because the red blood cells are deprived of oxygen in the process of dying, in the throes of death or as a consequence of death.

US military physician John Kark wrote:

> Reversible sickling and unsickling of erythrocytes (reflecting the rapid formation and dissolution of deoxy-hemoglobin S polymers) take place in seconds. Hence, the presence or absence of intravascular sickled erythrocytes

in tissue specimens depends upon the degree of oxygenation of the sample just before fixation and only has clinical relevance if fixation occurred at oxygen tensions identical to those extant during generation of primary lesions. Agonal hypoxemia causes artefactual intravascular sickling.

(Kark, 2000; erythrocytes = red blood cells; polymers = chains made up of haemoglobin molecules, stuck together; intravascular = inside the blood vessels; lesion = region of an injury; agonal = in the process of dying; hypoxemia = lack of oxygen in arterial blood)

Kark therefore concludes that one cannot deduce the role that sickle haemoglobin may have played in clinical events while alive from the presence of sickled red blood cells in bodies after death, unless it were a medically supervised death in which the autopsy blood cells could be stabilized at exactly the level of oxygen present while still alive. In short, finding sickled cells in the body at post-mortem is more likely to represent a consequence of death and cannot legitimately be even considered to contribute at all without other substantial contextual evidence (see Lucas *et al.*, 2008).

Second, there are questions about the adequacy of the tests undertaken to identify sickle cell trait. This is more than simply the confusion between sickle cell trait and sickle cell anaemia, discussed in Chapter 4, where we noted the sickle solubility test cannot distinguish between (1) sickle cell trait, (2) sickle cell anaemia and (3) other compound heterozygous forms of SCD such as haemoglobin SC disease. Even haemoglobin electrophoresis may not suffice. For example, unless one has the test result before death, then one cannot measure the level of haemoglobin A_2. Hence, although someone may have bands of blood at the reference points for haemoglobin A and S (and the assumption made that they have sickle cell trait), one cannot exclude the possibility that the deceased person had one of the various forms of sickle beta-thalassaemia, in which the level of haemoglobin A_2 is raised above 3.5 per cent (Konotey-Ahulu, 1996). In many historical case reports of unexpected sudden deaths, the sickle cell status is inferred by the coroner and was not known before death.

Third, there is the possibility of interaction with another inherited factor, one where the X-chromosome-linked pattern of inheritance makes the condition far more common in men than women (and most deaths we are considering are in the gendered professions of the military and US Football). Glucose-6-phosphate-dehydrogenase deficiency (G6PD deficiency) is another adaptation to malarial pressures and is carried by a quarter of West African males (Ohene-Frempong and Nkrumah, 1994). G6PD deficiency entails the possibility of a serious rapid breakdown of red blood cells. This can be caused by foods (fava or broad beans, famously avoided by the Greek philosopher Pythagoras and his followers), by a wide range of pharmaceutical drugs, by stress or by a viral infection. Symptoms similar to SCD can be provoked in people with G6PD if exposed to unsuitable foodstuffs or drugs or *when someone with sickle cell trait also has G6PD* (Konotey-Ahulu, 1996: 365). G6PD deficiency does not appear to be part of any consideration in case reports in either military deaths or athletics deaths.

Finally, there is an inherent problem with case reports. In order to draw more generalizable conclusions, there should be a comparison of the respective frequencies of the incident between the population with sickle cell trait and populations without sickle cell trait. Case reports lack this perspective as well as other forms of methodological control essential to draw legitimate conclusions.

Exercise-related deaths and the military

A major work on sickle cell and deaths during US military training was published in the *New England Journal of Medicine* in 1987 (Kark *et al.*, 1987). This study had two major advantages over previous case reports. First, because military personnel were tested upon entry to the forces, reports of their sickle cell status were more reliable, having been obtained during life. Second, the study was able to make certain comparisons between populations of recruits, specifically those military recruits with and without sickle cell trait.

Kark's study is frequently misrepresented in the literature as evidencing sickle cell trait as a so-called risk-factor for exercise-related deaths. In this sense responses to Kark *et al.* (1987) mirror the problem that Draper (1991) finds with employment practices and sickle cell trait. Unscrupulous employers focus on so-called genetic risk factors, said to underpin the interaction of sickle cell trait and dangerous chemicals or environments, and so draw attention away from those very same dangerous environments. It is therefore worth considering what the key features of the Kark *et al.*'s (1987) study suggest. First, association is not cause (a prospective controlled study would be required with an intervention and a control group). Second, the relative risk ratios were very large. Black recruits with sickle cell trait were 28 times as likely to die of exertional heat illness as those without sickle cell trait. However, and crucially, while *relative* odds risk ratios were indeed very large, the *absolute* numbers were very small, there being 13 deaths among the 37,300 with sickle cell trait and 5 deaths in the 429,000 group without sickle cell trait respectively. In a point we will reiterate later, these numbers of deaths are infinitesimally tiny compared to (1) SCD deaths in the USA or worldwide; (2) deaths in the US armed forces (in combat or otherwise); and (3) deaths in sports. The relative numbers are also small in comparison to the total numbers going through military training or participating in sport. When actual numbers are very small, and very small in all kinds of ways, the fact that they become ontologically very large requires further scrutiny.

The reference in subsequent reviews of the literature to this odds risk ratio of 28 times the risk (Mitchell, 2007) betrays the weakness of empiricist thinking. If you point to a phenomenon as a given, and imply that it is inevitable and unchangeable, when in fact it is alterable, then this inertia is political. Quite what type of politics is stake is considered further as we move through this and the subsequent chapter.

In any case, the work of John Kark does not end there. As a US military physician, he was in the strategic position to undertake a form of research available to almost no-one else. He was able to undertake a prospective study of the effects of sickle cell trait in US military training with results in different controlled conditions. The ability of the armed forces to significantly direct those under their command in ways not possible with usual research participants was crucial here. Kark was able to instigate a study in which certain training policies were implemented in a set of army training centres. These measures were precautionary measures designed to minimize the risk of all recruits being exposed to exertional heat illness. Such measures included restricting training when the *wet-bulb globe temperature* (WBGT) was too high. The WBGT is a measure that takes account, not only of temperature, but also of humidity, wind speed and sunlight radiation. It is a measure that humans will become more aware of as the twenty-first century progresses and WGBT becomes known as a measure beyond which humans cannot work or even survive in areas adversely affected by climate change. In the work of Kark, where these environmental conditions exceeded certain WBGT levels, training was postponed to another time. In addition, recruits were trained with respect to building up conditioning slowly over time (as we shall see, some sudden deaths in athletics were during off-season periods when the condition of athletes had yet to be built up). Third, attention was paid to clothing to ensure that it dissipated heat appropriately. Next, there was not only close monitoring of the amount of water each recruit consumed to replace bodily fluids lost, but auditing of such fluid replacement. This contrasts strongly to a later statement made in 2007 by the US National Athletic Trainers Association (NATA, 2007: 3), which merely noted the need to "emphasize hydration", a vague reference without any specific requirement that water be available, nor that *auditing* of intake of the water be a feature of the process, a key feature of the Kark measures. Fifth, an episode of illness was an exclusion factor for participation in training. Finally, stationing of first aiders at the site of the exercises was an essential requirement. In those military training centres that implemented these specific precautionary measures, this entirely eliminated exertional heat illness deaths in recruits with sickle cell trait, and reduced deaths in those without sickle cell trait. By contrast, at army centres outside the intervention, the comparative death rates among those with sickle cell trait remained raised.

The inference that Kark himself drew from his own study was that it is possible to avert exercise-related deaths through altering the environmental parameters of the training:

> These data support the view that preventable unrecognized exertional heat illness is the predominant factor causing exercise-related deaths with sickle cell trait and may be a substantial factor contributing to such deaths in recruits without hemoglobin S. This approach appeared able to prevent excess mortality with sickle cell trait in recruit basic training.
>
> (Kark, 2000)

The important conclusion is that all deaths associated with exercise were eliminated in the study centres during the time of the study. The implication is clear: with proper attention to the parameters of training, there would be no exercise-related deaths from exertional heat illness. Challenges to this view seem flawed. Ferster and Eichner (2012) claim to identify ongoing deaths associated with sickle cell trait in the military, but can only achieve this claim by virtue of ignoring cardiac-related causes of death (which are sufficient cause in their own right without the need to refer to sickle cell trait). Moreover, cardiac-related sudden deaths are far more common than even the deaths misattributed to sickle cell trait (Harmon *et al.*, 2011). Ferster and Eichner also rely on the *assertion* of exertional sickling as a cause of death, with no demonstration of this mechanism as the initiating (as opposed to the accelerant) antecedent of death, an assertion given false concreteness by the circularity of references to the concept within the literature, often literature written by the same authors.

Further evidence that it is not sickle cell trait but rather environmental parameters that constitute the key issue, arrived in dramatic fashion in the UK in 2013. Corporal James Dunsby, Lance Corporal Edward Maher and Lance Corporal Craig Roberts were part-timers (which implies a lack of ultimate prior conditioning), training as part of the UK Special Armed Services (SAS) military. Specifically, they were undertaking a 16-mile hike across the Brecon Beacons on the hottest day of the year. All three died of exertional rhabdomyolysis, as a consequence of exertional heat illness, a form of exercise-related death involving the breakdown of muscles, release of resultant substances into the system, leading to compartment syndrome in which pressure from the increased fluid to the damaged tissues crushes the already traumatized area. None of these soldiers in training had sickle cell trait. Thus, it is important to note that exercise-related deaths (ERD) can and do occur in the general population.

To summarize: historically some military personnel have died an exercise-related death during military training. Some of these were found to have sickled cells at autopsy, which, as discussed above, is not even a definitive diagnosis of sickle cell trait, let alone an incontrovertible cause of death. A retrospective study found a strong association (not causation, remember) between having sickle cell trait and sudden death in training. A prospective study was able to demonstrate that precautionary measures were able to eliminate all exercise-related deaths, including in those with sickle cell trait. Where such precautions are not implemented (the 2013 UK SAS deaths), people without sickle cell trait continue to die.

Exercise-related deaths and US athletics

Devaughn Darling was an outstanding US football athlete at Florida State University. He participated in mat drills, training routines which emphasize high intensity, repetition and obedience to command, as part of student athlete off season football training in 2001. The ethos was that no-one was to quit, no-one was to have water, and trash-can-sized bins were available for athletes to throw up into (*SB Nation*, 2014). Coaches reassured student athletes that the body was resilient and that they would pass out before they died. Devaughn had passed out the previous week. This time, despite chest pain, complaining to fellow athletes of being unable to see or to stand, he was made to repeat failed drills with his group, then on his own, before collapsing and being carried out unconscious and labelled by a coach "F for failure". He was declared dead shortly after. A post-mortem revealed medication being taken for a cold virus (ibid.). It also noted the sickled cells. Despite Kark's evidence (2000), extreme drills had been instituted with an unconditioned athlete, specifically denied water, who had previously collapsed and who was recently unwell with a viral illness. Such (rare) student athlete deaths continued during the 2000s, with athletes both with and without sickle cell trait dying suddenly during exercises.

Over an 11-year period, nine US college student athletes died following exercise and were found to have sickled cells post-mortem. Leading sports science texts in the early 2000s noted that athletes with sickle cell trait show no differences in cardiac function, uptake of oxygen, peak exercise work rates and metabolic recovery (Bar-Or and Rowland, 2004), and indeed may excel in athletic achievements (Marlin *et al.*, 2005). Moreover, the authors took their lead from Kark's evidence and suggested student athletes should avoid precipitating conditions such as dehydration, poor fitness, inadequate heat acclimatization, and extremes of physical exertion after viral illness, but that such cautions should apply to all athletes not just those with sickle cell trait (Bar-Or and Rowland, 2004: 311).

A US Professor of Sports Medicine, E. Randy Eichner, became a key figure in the debate in the 2000s. He is cited by the same classic exercise physiology text as stating that "there is still no cogent evidence that sickle cell trait per se increases risk or consequences of exertional rhabdomyolysis or plays any role in exercise-related deaths" (Eichner, 1993, cited in Bar-Or and Rowland, 2004: 310), but subsequently directly reversed his views. Two factors in particular changed the context of the debate. First, the role of sickle cell was brought to bear in a different context: the death in 2006 of Martin Lee Anderson in a Florida youth prison "boot-camp", where exercise was being used as disciplinary punishment, one of numerous sudden deaths in state custody discussed in further detail in Dyson and Boswell (2009). Eichner's testimony successfully persuaded an all-white jury that sickle cell trait and exercise were more plausible explanations of Anderson's sudden death than the actions of the guards in forcing ammonia capsules up Anderson's nose and holding a hand across his nose and mouth (ibid.). Second, there was the case of student athlete Dale Lloyd whose sudden death following exercise in 2006, and discovery of sickle cells at autopsy, prompted a decade-long struggle over a financial settlement. Both cases were characterized by the potential for rich and powerful institutions to be sued for large sums of money.

The following year a statement on sickle cell trait was issued by the National Athletic Trainers Association (NATA, 2007). It was presented as a "consensus" statement, but sickle cell specialists had only two places on a panel membership of 40. Only some of the participants endorsed the overall statement, and the sickle cell experts were among the several notable exceptions to those endorsing the statement. The immediate antecedents of the meeting are also important.

Other accounts of this NATA statement move from noting the earliest-known sudden death of a student athlete found to have sickled cells at autopsy, Polie Poitier at the University of Colorado in 1974, to noting that in 2007 the issue "became" serious enough for the NATA to issue their statement (Gillham, 2011: 61). This critically interrogated neither the 33-year time gap, nor the flawed assertion of consensus, nor the very basis of the claim for the role of sickle cell trait.

The Polish sociologist Zygmunt Bauman has explained that we live in a death-denying society and that a sudden, premature, death offends modern sensibilities (Bauman, 1992). Moreover, in the litigious culture of the USA, a sudden death leads to legal action. This can either focus on the actions of the guards or athletics coaches as the environmental parameters of the deaths, or on the (alleged) role of sickle cell trait. As we shall see, it serves several interests to focus on the latter, however flawed the logic.

Chapter 4 outlined how the early 1970s was an era of enhanced attention to sickle cell, though an era frequently confusing SCD and sickle cell trait. Case reports linking sickle cell trait to medical symptoms and to alleged risk factors such as anaesthetics, altitude, air travel and sudden death in military or athletics training were criticized for failing even to establish that it was sickle cell trait and not a form of SCD that was implicated (Konotey-Ahulu, 1996: 349–371). Broader epidemiological studies of the period suggested sickle cell trait had no overall impact on overall mortality: hospital patients with sickle cell trait had no significant differences in death rates to those without sickle cell trait; African-American life expectancy was the same irrespective of sickle cell trait; and the prevalence of sickle cell trait did not diminish with advancing age cohorts (Bristow, 1974: 80).

The preponderance of case reports on sickle cell led one expert to propose a checklist to be used to appraise the validity of claims made (Konotey-Ahulu, 1996). Case reports, such as athletes whose sudden death following exercise were found to have sickle cells at post-mortem, should carry little or no weight unless these conditions are met:

1   *Certainty in the diagnosis of sickle cell trait.* As we have seen, sickle solubility tests cannot decisively identify sickle cell trait (HbAS). Nor can simple haemoglobin electrophoresis undertaken after death. Without identification during life, and/or other tests, we cannot even be sure it is sickle cell trait.
2   *A rigorous comparison is made with rates of morbidity/mortality in those who do not have sickle cell trait.* Only the second Kark study (Kark et al., 2008) and the later Nelson et al. (2016) study fulfil this condition.
3   *The environmental parameters do not result in deaths in those without sickle cell trait.* As is apparent, exercise-related sudden deaths in military or student athlete training can and do occur in the absence of sickle cell trait.
4   *The environmental parameters are not plausible causes of death in their own right.* There are also plausible causes of death without consideration of

sickle cell trait (which, we must recall, would result in sickled cells at autopsy as a consequence of death in any case).

In 2010, the National Collegiate Athletic Association (NCAA), who oversee US college sports, implemented mandatory screening of all student athletes in Division 1, around 144,000 students (Tarini *et al.*, 2012), subsequently expanding this screening to Divisions II and III. As well as the (unsubstantiated) assumption that sickle cell trait *initiates* exercise-related deaths, the further assumption of the NCAA programme appears to be that observation by trainers of known student athletes with sickle cell trait can prevent deaths (Eichner, 2010). History teaches otherwise. James "Buddy" Friend III collapsed when attempting a "freedom run" necessary to complete training as a naval recruit as long ago as 1986 (Friend, 1994). Many of what are now known to be the classic errors in training regimes were in evidence:

- training in unsuitable weather conditions;
- failure to provide water, let alone audit its intake;
- leaving Buddy on the ground after his collapse in the hot sun without being cooled;
- sending an ambulance away when it first arrived;
- lack of training of drill instructors;
- an absence of first-aiders when strenuous exercises were being undertaken;
- the macho attitude of drill instructors, compelling recruits who collapse to continue.

Most telling in rebutting the NCAA position is the fact that Buddy had not only been screened but wore a red metal identity tag warning that he had sickle cell trait. Here is a direct contradiction to the assumption of the NCCA policy that screening and observation will prevent deaths. The fact that a further defense of this policy has been to focus on the fact that it was the person who died who pushed themselves hard, rather than the trainers per se, misses a very basic sociological truth. Rules work best when internalized and operated by the people themselves without external discipline. Thus, a macho, no-limits exercise policy works even more effectively if the people concerned can be inculcated to internalize at a deep level the ethos and assumptions of the trainer, and to conduct themselves in accordance with those precepts, even in the absence of the trainers themselves. This is what happened with Buddy and, as we shall see, is also a feature of the context of sudden deaths of a number of student athletes.

As the author of the book outlining her son's last hours, Peggy Friend focuses on the lack of research into possible clinical aspects of sickle cell trait, and criticizes key black institutions, such as the Howard Center for Sickle Cell at Howard University, one of the leading historically black universities in the USA and the National Association for the Advancement of Colored Peoples (NAACP), arguing that, for political reasons (the perceived need to challenge the ban of sickle cell trait recruits in the armed forces), clinical research on sickle cell trait was limited (Friend, 1994). A bereaved family's anguish is a powerful rhetorical device in attempting to foreclose an argument about sickle cell trait, but, as we shall see by the close of this chapter, the moral high ground belongs neither to the bereaved families nor to the NCAA.

SCT and unexpected death in athletics

Between 2000 and 2010 when the NCCA mandated sickle cell testing for student athletes, nine college athletes died following exercise, and were noted during post-mortem to exhibit sickled cells. These deaths included Preston Birdsong (2000); Devaughn Darling (2001); Aaron Richardson (2004); Aaron O'Neal (2006); Dale Lloyd, (2006); Ereck Plancher (2008); Chad Wiley (2008); Ja'Quayvin Smalls (2009) and Bennie Abraham (2010).

There are sufficient explanations for all nine US college student athlete deaths between 2000 and 2010 without the need to attribute the deaths to sickle cell trait per se. There are either sufficient causes in their own right including heat illness (Preston Birdsong, Chad Wiley) or heart problems (Devaughn Darling, Ja'Quayvin Smalls). In the case of heart problems, a meta-analysis of evidence in 2017 found sickle cell trait is associated neither with an increased risk of heart failure nor with abnormalities of cardiac structure and function (Bello *et al.*, 2017). A further frequent context is the reported macho behaviour of the coach. Examples include Devaughn Darling (reportedly ordered to repeat a failed drill as a punishment); Aaron Richardson (coaches are said to have cursed him); Aaron O'Neal (made to repeat failed exercises, coupled with a failure to call emergency services); Dale Lloyd (coaches apparently ordered others to leave him alone); and Bennie Abram (reports suggest he was chastised to continue). In one case the same head coach who oversaw training in Florida in the case of the sudden death of Ereck Plancher in 2008, was later head coach at the time of the case of the sudden death of Ted Agu in California in 2014. In four cases (Bennie Abraham in 2010 and Ted Agu in 2014; but also two subsequent cases, Eric Goll in 2016 and Nick Blakely in 2017), a test result for sickle cell trait *was* available, suggesting, as in the case of James "Buddy" Friend III, that identification per se does not prevent deaths.

Even when expert sickle cell medical testimony specifically stated that the athlete had exertional rhabdomyolysis and that it was *not* medically appropriate at all to refer to a "sickle cell crisis" in the initiation of death, one judge managed to reiterate the dubious phrase "exertional sickling" in summing up and making judgment in the legal claim over the Aaron Richardson death (*Estate of Richardson v. Bowling Green State Univ*, 2010-Ohio-3475). Case studies of the type cited in Ferster and Eichner (2012) or Pretzlaff (2002, cited in Nelson *et al.*, 2016) carry no weight since, as case studies, they fail to include the sickle cell status of all the ambient population (soldiers, athletes) under consideration and they fail to capture data longitudinally. Case studies therefore lack key compara- tors across both time and space. More recent work on armed services popula- tions finds no difference in deaths between sickle cell trait and non-sickle cell trait armed services population practising exertional injury precautions (Nelson *et al.*, 2016). While disproving any *necessary* association between sickle cell trait and sudden death, the same study confirms the greater risk of developing exertional rhabdomyolysis, but not of dying from it in an exertional-injury-precautionary setting (ibid.).

During the 2000s, academic exercise physiology articles have debated the relative risks of sickle cell trait and exercise (Le Gallais *et al.*, 2007). It should be noted, however, that once the debate moves into nuanced technicalities such as whether or not just one section, run at altitude, of an elite marathon race in Africa affects the success of athletes with or without sickle cell trait, then we have in any case moved to an esoteric level not relevant to the purposes of generic public health advice about sickle cell trait. Meanwhile, the US student athlete deaths have attracted the attention of sports journalists, and led to a questioning of the view of sickle cell trait as benign. The popular media coverage was unashamedly sensationalist. Sickle cell trait was the "monster within" (NCAA, 2011) and "college football's serial murderer" (Bautista, 2010). Such popular coverage is misleading in several ways. First, media abhorrence of complexity means that the sickled-cells-cause-a-blockage view, criticized in earlier chapters, is uncritically adopted. Second, the assumption of exertional sickling, unproven as a concept as an initiator of sudden death, presupposes and forecloses the key debate, such as whether sickled cells at autopsy have any relevance at all (Kark, 2000). Third, it is debatable whether attribution to sickle cell is even legitimate at all, given other plausible sufficient causes. Finally, it is to be questioned whether the claim for a "series" of deaths even deserves such a description, given that it mixes several independently sufficient causes of death together, with the commonality constructed by virtue both of foregrounding sickle cell trait and of ignoring coaching practices.

There is, moreover, a wider perspective that may be brought to bear on this issue. Two sports played in US colleges and universities merit particular attention in particular: men's football and basketball, which have been referred to as "big-time" college sports (Clotfelter, 2011, *passim*). Such sports purport to be run on an amateur, non-wage, basis, a situation rigorously policed by the NCAA. However, these two college sports are very big businesses, to such an extent that their finances may dominate the finances of the host universities (Clotfelter, 2011).

The US student athletes are not paid professionals, but what they may receive are sports scholarships to colleges. The hope of star athletes, often from materially poor backgrounds, is that they may progress to elite professional football and basketball, where levels of pay are extremely high. The actual chances of successfully moving from a materially deprived background to the riches associated with professional sports have been calculated as seven-in-a-million (Dunning, 1999). Men's professional football and basketball are associated in the USA with what has been described as the "sports-media complex" (Jhally, 1984). This sports-media complex is also a financial complex, and involves huge sums of money paid by TV companies to secure coverage of the sport, together with extensive, lucrative commercial sponsorships and endorsements.

However, with few life chances, young African-American men, growing up facing poverty and racism, may see football and basketball as their sole chance of social mobility. The pressure to succeed is enormous, the rewards of success great, but the probability of failure statistically overwhelming. As noted above, the student athletes are unpaid, and represent a form of indentured labour, which partly explains the ethos that permits sport coaches to routinely refer to grown men as "boys". Top sports coaches are often the highest paid staff within universities, and indeed within the state public sector overall (Clotfelter, 2011). The sudden death of a student athlete is a problem for the sports-media complex. It threatens the complex financially, and some large financial settlements have been made (Jordan *et al.*, 2011) though other cases have spent a decade in litigation (suggesting the tenacity with which the sports-media complex will fight to keep even the tiniest fraction of its overall wealth). The sudden deaths (potentially) simultaneously threaten the autonomy of the sports team and in particular their coaches. In such a context, the NCAA policy may be better understood as a defensive reaction to the possibility of being regularly sued by its impoverished student athletes, or at least by their bereaved families. And so in 2010, "for financial, legal and reputational reasons, the NCAA moved to police the status of sickle cell, specifically how (sickle cell trait) was to be regarded" (Carter and Dyson, 2015: 68). The NCAA did so through mandatory testing for sickle cell trait for athletes in Divisions I of the NCAA structure. This provision was extended to Divisions II and III athletes by 2013, despite opposition from the American Society of Hematology (2012).

There were, and remain, a number of concerns. Many basic principles of genetic screening (Lappé *et al.*, 1972), principles developed in the wake of disastrous 1970s sickle cell screening (Markel, 1992; Duster, 2003), were systematically broken. The population concerned, student athletes, were neither consulted nor involved in the NCAA screening programme design nor its operation. There was no provision for the privacy of genetic information (Grant *et al.*, 2011). The implementation of the screening paid scant attention to the problems of discrimination (Bonham *et al.*, 2010) nor to the confusion inherent in terms such as "sickle cell athlete" (McDonald *et al.*, 2017). As pointed out by the Sickle Cell Disease Association of America, there was no provision for genetic counselling by a qualified genetic counsellor. Such provision was made neither prior to the test to explain the consequences, nor after the test in order to counsel those identified as being sickle cell genetic carriers (Ferrari *et al.*, 2015; McDonald *et al.*, 2017). The test was also mandatory (or the student athlete could sign away their legal rights) and so failed the test of ensuring autonomy in decision-making (McDonald *et al.*, 2017). The desperation engendered by the seven-in-a-million chance of social mobility helps explain why student athletes may sign away legal rights rather than take a sickle cell test that might place a doubt in their coach's mind about weakness; concur in a power relationship that infantilizes them as "boys", and internalize an erroneous belief that training until exhaustion/collapse/vomiting is the most effective training at improving performance. The culture of inappropriate exercise in student sports has a long history (Anderson, 2012).

There are some theoretical concerns in the social sciences, philosophy and the humanities that may be of help in clarifying the situation with respect to sickle cell trait. Contemporary philosophy has begun to take seriously the role of objects and materials in everyday life (Latour, 2013; Delanda and Harman, 2017; Morton, 2017). In conjunction with a re-thinking of objects within experiments, such theories offer a new way of thinking about the sickle cell trait controversy. The UK sociologist Ray Pawson recasts our understanding of experiments. In experiments, the scientist *already knows* the result they expect, and actively constructs the conditions to produce this outcome. In this way the scientist is able to confirm that their conceptual understanding of the causal mechanism at work is an adequate or robust concept (Pawson and Tilley, 1997). This is developed further by the French philosopher Bruno Latour. Latour (2000) counterintuitively suggests that good experiments depend not on control but the opposite, that is, on creating special circumstances under which the object or thing in question is given as much freedom as possible from context, what Latour terms the freedom of material things to "strike back".

As we have seen above, precautions can greatly reduce the risk of death from exertional heat illness on the part of all recruits, including those with sickle cell trait (Kark *et al.*, 2008). The Kark approach stands in stark opposition therefore to the NCAA approach. For Kark, by implementing precautions for *all* military recruits or student athletes, one aims to prevent anyone exercising entering a danger zone where exercise-induced illness is provoked, including those who are sickle cell genetic carriers. In this model, it is not sickling which initiates the problem, but the onset of exertional heat illness. If (unnecessarily) initiated, then the sickle cell genetic carriers are more prone to experience an intensification of the progress of exertional heat illness, but the initiating factor is not sickling and this explains why clinical sickle cell experts regard references to the process as a "sickle cell crisis" to be badly mistaken. Quite apart from the evidence that it does not prevent deaths, the enforcement of mass sickle cell screening, with the well-documented consequences of discrimination where principles of screening are not put in place, is not necessary. Public health reductions in mortality and morbidity are possible without resorting to screening, by avoiding a pool of those with exertional heat illness developing in the first place. By implementing public health-type precautions, audited and applied to all recruits or athletes, this reduces exercise-related mortality and morbidity for all personnel engaged in exercise (Kark *et al.*, 2010). Those who are sickle cell genetic carriers are protected by virtue of preventing them entering the pool of risk in the first instance. Deaths in those with and without sickle cell trait are thus prevented. To express this in the imagery of Latour introduced above:

> Kark's arrangements permit the sickle cell gene freedom from the culture of US sports coaches to exercise unpaid sports workers in a reckless manner liable to induce exertional heat illness. Where it is accorded this freedom SCT (sickle cell trait) remains benign.
>
> (Carter and Dyson, 2015: 71)

Of course, sickle cell trait may find itself in newly constituted assemblages in the future, with climate change producing extremes of Wet Bulb Globe Temperature that have an effect on the human body irrespective of exercise. In the absence of concerted collective efforts to minimize climate change, or to attenuate the consequences of such changes, the virtual capacities of sickle cell trait may alter, though again this may be a matter of relative ratios, with risk an absolute reality for all human life.

Within the limits of the current argument, in preferring the public health precaution model over the NCAA "exertional sickling" model, it is also necessary to be cognizant of structured social interests. It is not just a question of the participants in a social policy debate, but of who garners the power to set the agenda for the debate, who has the resources (finances, media contacts) to prevail in the debate, and which social groups have the motivation and means to side-line the views of others.

The sports-media network, within which US student athletes sit, includes many with vested financial interests (for example, wealthy business people who can claim relief on taxes for financial donations to "universities" while actually funding college sport and hence garnering tax breaks conducive to their own leisure activities). Businessmen, sports coaches and support staff, media executives, advertisers and sponsors all have vested interests in expropriating the unpaid indentured labour of student athletes. Equally all such parties will be concerned if families of student athletes are able to successfully sue for large sums of money, and will develop defensive actions to mitigate this possibility. Sickle cell screening may be conceived of as one such defensive action.

There are several interest groups excluded from influential roles in the debate. The student athletes may be unwilling to speak up (being both infantilized in their relations with sports coaches and fearful of revealing any perceived physical weakness). The voices of the whole sickle cell community of interest, including people living with SCD, their families and the non-governmental sickle cell organization who support them, gain little traction even though they are intimately affected by the consequences of NCAA sickle cell screening. As we have seen, the attempt to create the impression of a NATA "Consensus" statement in 2007 that initiated the move to screen student athletes, involved the exclusion of most clinical sickle cell experts. It also involved the impression management technique of listing the many stakeholders who attended, but not reflecting the fact that some attendees did not endorse the statement that initiated the move to screen student athletes (Dyson and Boswell, 2009: 21–24).

The potential to create networks of influence falls disproportionately to those with financial resources, social networks and strategic positions in the first place. Furthermore, it is not just a question of power. There are wider questions to ask about what shapes social preferences and choices in the first place (Lukes, 1974), and what the unintended wider societal consequences of a policy may be. As previously outlined, social mobility from inner-city racialized poverty to college football scholarship, to a lucrative career in professional sports is available to the fewest of the few, namely 0.0007 per cent (Dunning, 1999). What damage is done to the many who try unsuccessfully (and to their families) and what damage is done in terms of narrowing careers mind-sets of young black people from resource-poor backgrounds are not known. The unintended consequences of the policy include the amplification of the sickle cell trait as a danger, and this amplification has deleterious consequences beyond sport and the military when used to explain away sudden deaths of black people in state custody (Dyson and Boswell, 2009), as we will examine further in Chapter 6.

The student athlete debate also leaves out of account the manner in which student athletes are effectively exploited, not even as wage-labour but as non-waged labour. The athletes who undertake the work are not only expropriated in the classic Marxist sense of creating surplus value, but they create (sports enter-tainment) value for no immediate monetary recompense at all. The fact that they may have a college sports scholarship deepens their dependency still further, by creating a form of indentured labour. Wider issues and debates struggle to get on the agenda. Such wider issues include the vast material inequalities in the USA, a poverty that is also racialized. Attention is drawn away from inequities in educational provision, and away from the combination of poverty and comprom-ised educational opportunity that creates conditions conducive to recruiting African-Americans as unpaid labour in college football. Moreover, the roles of sports coaches, their degree of freedom in operating training regimes, however dangerous or counter-productive, is rarely examined. Furthermore, while atten-tion is focused on sickle cell trait, the more serious unmet needs of people with sickle cell disease itself are marginalized. In the USA, nearly 80,000 adults with SCD may struggle to find a provider of adult haematology services (Sobota *et al.*, 2011). And as we shall explore further in Chapter 9, there are hundreds of thousands of infants with SCD who die unnecessarily worldwide for the want of funding for comprehensive newborn screening (Dennis-Antwi *et al.*, 2011). The lives of infants with SCD globally could be saved for a fraction of the monies that circulate the sports-media complex.

One retort to criticism that the sport-media complex operates against the inter-ests of the racialized poor is to point to racial integration in sports. The protagonists, black or white, we are told, operate on the same playing field and share camaraderie in the locker rooms. Whether such integrated camaraderie is inculcated at the expense of hyper-sexism and homophobia is not discussed. St Louis (2003) argues that arenas such as college sports serve a particular purpose of tutoring us that we have moved beyond racism by implicitly appealing to the harmless and innocent nature of blacks and whites playing sports together, while simultaneously obscuring the power structures – the racism, poverty and educational disadvantage – that sustain the terms and conditions of such participation. This has the effect of making it seem that we have achieved a post-racial settlement, though one in which, per-versely, the categories of black and white athlete are reified and naturalized (Car-rington, 2011). The lack of any such settlement is amply evidenced in the hysterical reactions to any black athlete who takes a stand against racism.

Part of this process of reification and naturalization rests on the manner in which the issue of sickle cell trait is taken up within the sports-media complex.

The problem with basing analysis around networks is that it assumes that power is widely distributed across such networks when this may not be the case. Elam (1999) suggests that key personnel at strategic nodes of a network may be confident in their ability to exert sufficient control across the network, and that this may be achieved through the twin tactics of being hyper-sensitive to certain information, while censoring other information: what Elam calls sensors and censors. This is arguably the role of sports media in sickle cell trait. The notion that an athlete has sickle cell trait, or has died suddenly and been found post-mortem to have sickle cell trait, fulfils media requirements for immediacy and sensationalism/ revelationism in news production. Viewers or readers of news are positioned as passive consumers of a sensationalist tale, which has the additional advantages of detracting from wider sports policy (on dangerous training practices), or on wider social policy (on issues discussed above, such as poverty, racism and educational provision). At the same time that sickle cell trait is misleadingly attached to sudden deaths, as the primary and initiating cause, a form of censorship is being applied. Other features of sudden death or other relevant contextual information are censored. Heart problems or meningitis are potential causes of sudden death in athletes, but these alternatives, and arguably more plausible primary causes, are downplayed. The fact that in some sudden deaths it is a form of SCD and not sickle cell trait at all is ignored (Carter and Dyson, 2015), as is the fact that identification in and of itself does not prevent deaths. Also ignored are other causes of athlete deaths and illness, associated, for example, with alcohol, a key commodity in the sports-media complex, both for its role in binge-drinking sports cultures and for its central role in sports sponsorship and purchase of media advertising platforms. Meanwhile the unintended consequences of framing sickle cell trait as a health issue now reach far beyond the sports context. For example, misusing sickle cell trait has detracted from appropriate scrutiny of possible non-accidental injury (Konotey-Ahulu, 2011) from environmental disasters (*Truth About Zane*, 2018), and as we shall see in Chapter 6, from deaths while in contact with state authorities (Dyson and Boswell, 2009).

The continued amplification of the purported dangers of sickle cell trait as an initiating cause of sudden death contains at least two possible types of interest for sports scientists and the NCAA: to continue to garner consultancy work around the issue (see Spracklen, 2008) and to exert some organizational control over fiercely independent sports coaches, teams and colleges. The interests of those involved in the sports-media complex are, however, "against the unpaid student athletes, against the poverty and educational disadvantage of African-Americans more generally, against the interests of those with either SCT (sickle cell trait) or those with SCD, and in favour of a white, rich, sport-business elite" (Carter and Dyson, 2015: 74).

Conclusion

This chapter has looked at the manner in which sickle cell trait, the genetic carrier status for sickle cell, has become a subject of political controversy in the case of sudden deaths in army or athletics training. It has been argued that the evidence supports a view that sickle cell trait may function as an accelerant of exercise-induced heat illness, but is not the initiator of such processes, and that references to a "sickle cell crisis" are inaccurate in such contexts. Changes to training practices on the part of army drill instructors and athletic coaches, not sickle cell screening, are therefore the key to reducing such deaths.

Much misunderstanding stems from the obsession with the morphology of sickle-shaped cells, whose presence at autopsy may simply be an artefact of death not a cause. Another way of putting this is that, because 1 in 12 African-Americans (or 1 in 4 West Africans) are sickle cell carriers, 1 in 12 of all such deaths of armed services recruits or athletes, and 1 in 12 deaths of African-American doctors, lawyers or CEOs would show sickled cells at autopsy. Most sickle cell carriers who die do not, of course, become the subject of post-mortems. The tiny minority of sickle cell carriers who do become subject to autopsy could display sickled cells throughout their body and throughout their organs. In terms of morphology, this must seem quite a dramatic finding, especially where the coroner has no other obvious signs to provide a credible explanation of death. But the dramatic nature of the morphology does not prove the cause of death. This leads to serious socio-political consequences in military or college contexts, but perhaps even more grave consequences when the notion of sickle cell trait as a cause of sudden death leaks out into the realm of criminal justice. This will be the subject of Chapter 6.

6 Sickle cell and deaths in state contact

Introduction

This chapter considers the relationship between sickle cell, racism and the criminal justice system. It commences with a brief review of a prevailing concern of criminal justice researchers in Europe and North America, namely, that both indirectly by criminalizing the poor (where racialized minorities are over-represented) and directly by racist practices, that discrimination and racism are central challenges in criminal justice systems. The chapter then provides an overview of how sickle cell disease (SCD) and its genetic carrier state, sickle cell trait (SCT). are implicated in criminal justice issues. The autopsy finding, that a person died following contact with officers of the state has SCT, has been used to deflect attention from instances of sudden unexplained deaths in African-Americans, Black British and other deaths in other situations where SCT is associated with a politically less powerful group within the broader society. There follows a critical appraisal of approaches to analysis that cite institutional racism as a driving cause of the outcomes of the criminal justice systems. The chapter proposes that we look to the theory of critical realism for an approach that distinguishes in time frames between, on the one hand, the historical origins of contextual resources and the structural antecedents of institutional arrangements, and, on the other hand, the historically produced, collective and relational agency of individuals in situated activity in the present (Layder, 1993). This, it will be argued, permits both a more adequate assessment of the relation between sickle cell and unexplained deaths while in contact with officers of the state.

The concept of institutional racism in criminal justice

In the UK, following the publication of the Macpherson Report into the racist murder of a black teenager Stephen Lawrence, the phrase "institutional racism", a term originally associated with Stokely Carmichael (Carmichael and Hamilton, 1968), came into policy and popular usage. The term was defined as:

> The collective failure of an organization to provide an appropriate and professional service to people because of their colour, culture or ethnic

origin. It can be seen or detected in processes, attitudes and behaviour which amount to discrimination through unwitting prejudice, ignorance, thought-lessness and racist stereotyping which disadvantage minority ethnic people.

(Macpherson, 1999: 28)

The report defines a racist incident as one which the victim themselves perceives as racist in character. Mason (1982) was an early commentator who drew atten-tion to the analytical problems inherent in the term. Others have elided an argu-ably important difference between *institutionalized racism* and *institutional racism* by ostensibly treating the terms as equivalent within the same passage of text (Bourne, 2001). While it is plausible that individual racist attitudes may become part of the ongoing culture within an organization and that these prac-tices become accepted because they are unchallenged, that is, that racism is insti-tutionalized within an organization, the meanings associated with institutional racism seem to go beyond this initial formulation. The problem with the concept institutional racism is threefold. First, institutions do not have intentions: indi-viduals within those organizations act and their position in that institution accords them certain agency. Second, there appears to be a slippage between the concept that actions with discriminatory outcomes may be practised unwittingly, without cognition of if and how they might be distantly connected to outcomes – not least because human actions frequently result in unintended consequences (Carter, 2000) – and the notion that racism may be practised unwittingly, that, as Macpherson stated, there may be "unwitting prejudice". This is simply commit-ting a logical fallacy of treating the consequence as a cause. In such circum-stances racism may follow to the extent that, faced with convincing evidence of a linkage between past actions and current inequalities structured along racial-ized lines, a person either demonstrates bad faith in not recognizing this and/or does not agree to actions designed to address the situation. Third, there appears to be an implicit assumption that institutional racism is a sophisticated concept that is to be contrasted to naïve concepts of racism, for example, concepts that reduce racism to the sum of acts of individual racist behaviours. Indeed, an explanation of social relations that reduced explanation to the sum of social rela-tionships would indeed be a weak sociological explanation. There is a way of returning to a structural analysis, through the sociological approach of critical realism, without reducing our analysis to individual actions. However, it is an explanation that requires us to recognize that not all social processes are identity-sensitive (Sayer, 2005).

Carter (2000) has made two important points in this regard. First, drawing on Layder (1993), he argues that the analytical scale of contextual resources (for example, socio-economic position) and institutional arrangements (for example, in the police, or prison service) constitute a different scale of analysis to situated activity (the interactions of individual officers and those with SCT on the streets, in police stations or in prison). The former are *social relations*, pertain to social structure, and are necessarily opaque to individual people. This is very different from the *social relationships* observable at the scale of situated activity. Second, the rigour required of concepts of everyday language is not the same as the pre-cision demanded of social scientific concepts when deployed in analysis. For example, by adopting the everyday practical category of "race", the American Sociological Association embeds into analytical practice a subjective concept and treats it as an objective one. In such an analysis, the term institutional racism conflates two processes, one at the scale of historically reproduced social struc-ture, and one at the scale of contemporary interpersonal interactions.

In this respect, the work of the British sociologist Margaret Archer (1995) is apposite. Her approach distinguishes between, on the one hand, structure (the historically given socio-economic and institutional arrangements of society which are the products of interactions in the past), and culture (idea-tional resources, again made available to current generations by actions in the past), and, on the other hand, agency (what individual actors and groups of actors make of these material and cultural resources bequeathed from histor-ical struggles). In adopting this approach to racism, Carter (2000) argues that concepts such as institutional racism conflate two distinct time frames. Past historical interactions may leave structures that have discriminatory outcomes in effect. This is important as it taps into a growing body of sociological work that argues that we have over-emphasized ethnicity-based explanations as driving *causes* of social phenomena (Todd and Ruane, 2004; Carter and Fenton, 2010; Carter and Dyson, 2011).

Sayer (2005) usefully distinguishes between mechanisms that are identity-neutral (the macro-economic workings of capitalism, for example, where cur-rency weakening renders companies insolvent and workers redundant, operate irrespective of the identities of the workers) and mechanisms such as sexism and racism that are identity-sensitive. In practice situations may entail both identity-neutral and identity-sensitive mechanisms. Workers may be laid off, but employ-ers may discriminate in identity-sensitive ways by targeting women or black workers for redundancy first. Indeed, as we saw in Chapter 4, in the case of workers with SCT (the genesis of the sickle cell gene being an identity-neutral mechanism), employers used SCT as an ostensibly identity-neutral mechanism in order to effect an identity-sensitive outcome of laying off black workers (Draper, 1991; Duster, 2003). However, this took the actions of key individuals in thinking about, and acting upon, racist ideas.

Sickle cell and deaths in custody

In earlier chapters I have suggested that popular accounts of sickle cell are mis-guided in over-focusing on two things: (1) the sickle shape of the cell (rather than the myriad other physiological processes involved in SCD illnesses); and (2) the blockage of sickled cells (when usually even in SCD, let alone SCT, most sickling occurs in blood vessels much greater than the width of a red blood cell, vessels which the sickle cells cannot therefore block). Moreover, popular accounts of sickle cell misuse the notion of sickle cell crisis, partly because, as we saw in Chapter 4, this term conflates pain (which may be chronic as well as acute); a vaso-occlusive episode (when haemolysis, splenic sequestration aplastic events are other potential crises in SCD, but not SCT), and the demand for urgency in treatment. As discussed in Chapter 5, there is widespread agreement that when someone with SCT dies, their red blood cells will sickle as an artefact of death (Bowman, 1977; Kark, 2000; Lucas *et al.*, 2008; Jordan *et al.*, 2011) and that therefore no casual effect can be inferred merely from the presence of sickled cells in the autopsy of someone with SCT. Sickle cell experts dispute the use of "sickle cell crisis" as appropriate to use at all in describing events that may occur in someone with SCT.

Dyson and Boswell (2006) drew attention to the work in the 1970s of the late African-American pathologist, James Bowman, the father of Valerie Jarrett, a former senior advisor to Barack Obama. Bowman recounted a case in 1974 where, merely because sickled cells were found at autopsy, a defence lawyer succeeded in averting charges against guards who had forcibly subdued a prisoner. Bowman commented bitterly that the judgment effectively gave guards the possibility of committing "legalized murder" without fear of prosecution should sickled cells then be found at autopsy (Bowman, 1997). Between writing the article in 2004–2005 and publication (Dyson and Boswell, 2006), the Martin Lee Anderson case arose in Florida in January 2006. Here a 14-year-old boy, in his first day at boot camp, was compelled to run punishment laps of the compound before entering a prolonged altercation with nine guards who, over a 30-minute period, were seen on video to strike him and repeatedly haul him forcibly to his feet despite his apparent collapse. The first medical examiner attributed the death to "natural causes" of SCT. After exhumation of the body, and a NASA-enhanced examination of the surveillance tapes, the second examiner concluded that the death was attributable to the forcing of several ammonia capsules up the boy's nose while the guards held his mouth closed, a conclusion the first examiner did not challenge while witnessing the second autopsy. As we saw in Chapter 5, the key sports scientist behind the flawed "exertional sickling" hypothesis gave evidence, and the all-white jury acquitted all nine guards of several charges, including lesser charges of child neglect (see Dyson and Boswell, 2009: 106–111, for a fuller account).

Dyson and Boswell (ibid.) further documented 28 cases where the discovery of SCT at autopsy effectively led to a form of premature closure, in which the actions or inactions of officers of the state (police, prison guards or army personnel) were not fully scrutinized. Since sickling of cells in an SCT death occurs anyway, it has been pointed out that no logical attribution can be made implicating SCT in the death, unless the following conditions are met:

- the relevant laboratory tests have been undertaken to exclude forms of sickle cell disease;
- an appropriate comparison to rates of the phenomenon in those *without* sickle cell trait has been made;
- assurances that other environmental circumstances present produce no deaths in those without sickle cell trait;

- other conditions in their own right are not responsible for the death (Konotey-Ahulu, 1996).

All the 28 deaths were in close time proximity to one or more of: application of a conductive electrical device; use of pepper spray; physical assault; placing in a chokehold; placing into a prone position relevant to positional asphyxia; extreme restraint consistent with production of muscle breakdown, or a combination of two or more of these factors. The conclusion was that SCT was being misused to explain away sudden deaths in contact with officers of the state, deaths that could potentially be explicable in other terms without resort to SCT. What has been termed the "state talk" of officials of the criminal justice system (Sim, 2004) surrounding sudden death in custody has been found to follow a distinct pattern: dehumanizing the victim, exaggerating the degree of threat posed, if any, and minimizing the lethal actions of officers of the state (Pemberton, 2008). Unexpected deaths with SCT at autopsy comprise an important sub-set of this overall pattern. Sometimes the person killed comes into state contact because they are experiencing mental health issues. Just one such death that has been the subject of ongoing protests was the death in 2003 of Mikey Powell in Birmingham, UK.

In a typical series of events, such sudden deaths are not immediately announced, or grossly inaccurate information (ostensibly from sources close to the investigation) appears in the press. Accurate details of the deaths are subtlely changed in first reports appearing in the media (for example, undercounting the number of times a conductive electrical device was used or the numbers of officers involved in the restraint). CCTV equipment malfunctions or tapes are missing or wiped. It is then announced that the dead person had a "sickle cell crisis". The more precise fact that they have sickled cells at autopsy (an artefact of the fact they carry SCT) is lost, as the disorientated relatives of the deceased complain that their loved one did not have SCD. Indeed, SCD and SCT are used inaccurately and interchangeably in media accounts. The state officials affect surprise that the person had this "undiagnosed condition", both words rhetorically cementing the image of SCT as a medical condition rather than as a genetic carrier state. As such, the state officials present themselves as shocked bystanders who could not be blamed for a death by "natural causes" (Dyson and Boswell, 2009).

There are further ways that such finessing of events through state talk and through the reportage of journalists can be accomplished. If state officials *were* concerned about SCT, then logically their care of those with the clearly more serious SCD would be exemplary. It is not. Dyson and Boswell (ibid.) further documented 21 cases where the death of someone living with SCD takes place in custody where cries for help are serially ignored, where treatment is denied (for example, to keep costs down in order to boost medical incentive payments) or delayed, resulting in death, or where treatment is grossly incompetent (killing someone with an overdose of painkillers by titrating the dosage at the level of a heroin addict because of the assumption that a black-skinned person in jail must therefore be a drug addict) or where jail staff actively obstruct the emergency paramedics. One woman with SCD, Charisse Shumate, imprisoned for defending herself against serial domestic violence, led a class action lawsuit against the governor of California to press for improved medical treatment for prisoners. Complaining also leads to specific retribution: in the case of Charisse, this was to be denied parole even unto death. In other cases, the prisoner was allowed to go blind for want of treatment, and in yet another the person was deliberately placed in a cell to be raped by a serial violent sex offender (ibid.).

Since the publication of Dyson and Boswell (2009), a book which, based on English-language sources, mainly documented cases in the USA and the UK, but cited individual cases in Canada, Australia and New Zealand, a number of developments have taken place. First, such sudden deaths in contact with officers of the state, where it later transpires that the deceased person is an SCT carrier have continued unabated in the USA. In 2008, Baron Pikes had a conductive electrical device applied multiple times while handcuffed and lying on the ground, but the officer responsible was found not guilty (*Final Call*, 2010) despite apparent claims from the American Civil Liberties Union of Louisiana that:

> [the] State of Louisiana Death Certificate states that his death occurred when he was "electro shocked x 9 while in police custody and restraint". The certified document goes on to state the cause of Mr. Pikes' death to be "Cardiac Arrest following nine 50,000-volt electroshock applications from a conductive electrical weapon."
>
> (ACLU, 2008)

In 2011, Derek Williams died despite exhibiting signs of obvious distress while handcuffed in the back of a police car in Milwaukee. In 2011, Darrin Hanna died after being beaten by Chicago police and suffering internal bleeding (*Chicago Tribune*, 2012). Also in 2011, David Campbell (Leigh Valley, Pennsylvania) was stripped naked, restrained by up to eight guards (who allegedly turned off the CCTV), was pepper sprayed in the face, and placed in a restraint chair, as a result of guards trying to place him on suicide watch for failing to respond to questions and saying he heard voices (*Morning Call*, 2013). Sergeant James Brown (El Paso, Texas) died in 2012 after being injected with a sedative during a two-day jail sentence for drink-driving (*Huffington Post*, 2015). In each of the four cases, the death was attributed wholly or in part to sickle cell trait. Moreover, since the initial work on sickle cell and deaths in custody, an additional evasive tactic has emerged. This tactic is one in which state officials deny a person was "in custody" and therefore cannot be counted in such sudden deaths in custody. This is the reason the title of this chapter differs from the title of Dyson and Boswell (2009).

Second, it is now clear that in other socio-political contexts where a socially less powerful group also has a prevalence of SCT, the appearance of SCT at autopsy can potentially be misused to detract from unexplained sudden death that requires further scrutiny. In Spring 2011, in Bahrain (where 18 per cent of the population carry SCT), protests against the regime ended with doctors who treated protestors themselves being tortured and/or facing criminal charges. The deaths of two protestors, Hassan Jassim Mohammed Makki on 3 April 2011 and Zakaria Rashid Hassan al-Asherri on 9 April 2011, were attributed to "sickle cell anaemia" even though the men were only SCT carriers. Photos of the dead men posted on Facebook suggested extensive bruising consistent with being beaten (*Human Rights Watch*, 2011). Even in cases where the state is prepared to charge and convict police, the misuse of SCT still helps others evade conviction (BBC, 2013a). The death of Mohammed Ibrahim Yacoub in 2012 in Bahrain was attributed to "sickle cell disease" and little scrutiny has taken place concerning accusations that he was injured by being trapped between two moving police cars and later tortured (ABNA News, 2012). However, this illustrates that even with SCD (that is, the disease not the carrier state, which appears to have been the situation in this case), this does not mean a death does not deserve independent scrutiny. It is clear that in any country with extensive numbers with SCT (most of Africa, the Middle East, India and Brazil), and in minority ethnic groups in North America, Europe and Australasia, there is global potential for SCT to become a standard deflector of scrutiny of sudden unexplained deaths while in contact with state officials, and that sickle cell is not merely a global public health issue (Dyson and Atkin, 2011) but a criminal justice issue of global importance.

Third, the specific role of SCT is explaining away sudden death in contact with state officials appears to have expanded. A particular case of the unexpected death of a five-year-old child has been ascribed to SCT (Kepron *et al.*, 2009), but commentators have raised numerous concerns about the quality of the analysis, with the implication that the attribution to SCT is seriously flawed (Konotey-Ahulu, 2011). In 2009, Ashley Jewell, the partner of a high profile reality TV star, was killed during a brawl outside a night club in which he was hit over the head. An initial murder charge was dropped when Jewell was found to have SCT at autopsy. Thus, it seems that the dubious use of SCT in explaining sudden death has moved beyond the immediate realm of contact with state officials.

Fourth, there are ongoing developments in other spheres that have a reciprocal effect on the criminal justice debates. As we saw in Chapter 5, SCT has been mobilized to explain away sudden deaths in military training or elite sports training, and to support near-compulsory sickle cell screening of athletes. Since the evidence that compulsory screening without counselling leads to discrimination is overwhelming (Duster, 2003), and since the alternative approach claimed by the NCCA is based on unaudited cases that have not been subject to clinical review (Jordan *et al.*, 2011), the question then becomes which social interests are at stake in pursuing a flawed policy of mandatory screening? As outlined above, the reciprocal link between the spheres of college athletics and criminal justice was made when Professor E. Randy Eichner, a professor of sports medicine, and a leading advocate of screening for athletes, gave evidence in support of the guards in the Martin Lee Anderson case.

Finally, a series of events including the acquittal of George Zimmerman of the 2012 killing of black teenager Trayvon Martin, and the 2014 death of Eric Garner who was placed in a chokehold by police and died after repeatedly stating that he could not breathe, led to the formation of the international activist movement Black Lives Matter. What is instructive about many cases around which Black Lives Matter opposition has formed is that, even where the black person is unarmed or in their own home, or where evidence from mobile phone cameras documents the death, the police officers are rarely indicted and, if charged, rarely found guilty. To this extent sickle cell trait has been a canary in a coal mine. For 40 years, sickle cell trait has functioned as a key resource in deflecting blame and responsibility from police actions. The incidents to which Black Lives Matter is now responding now polarize opinion so dramatically, between state officials and anti-racists, that one suspects authorities might not even need to invoke the smokescreen of sickle cell trait in the future, should a person who dies suddenly in state contact prove to have sickled cells at autopsy.

Having established sickle cell as a major public health issue, and misattribution of sudden deaths in state contact to SCT as a major issue for criminal justice systems worldwide, I now turn to consider potential responses to this emerging situation, driven by concerns of the lack of any impact of the publications on sickle cell trait and sudden deaths in custody on practice. In doing so, I begin to question a mainstay of recent analysis in criminal justice work, the concept of institutional racism.

The analytical limitations of "institutional racism"

The tendency in controversies surrounding SCT and sudden death has been for observers to see what they wish in these events. For some, such as the Reverend Al Sharpton and the Reverend Jesse Jackson, active in protesting the Martin Lee Anderson and Darrin Hannah cases, among others, this is a clear example of racism at work. For others, such as the National Association of Medical Examiners, this is a case of politics at work interfering with science (*News Herald*, 2007). Is it possible that the officers of the state have no individual racist intents but that, by following custom and practice, they are engaged in reproducing what has been called "institutional racism"?

Street (2003: 30) exemplifies the imprecise use of racism "understood in institutional terms" as an analytical concept. In decrying the obscene numbers of African-Americans incarcerated in the USA, he notes the colour-blind approach to, say, local politicians welcoming building of new prison complexes as an economic replacement for closed industrial plants. He evades consideration of non-racialized explanations for this by his extensive and pejorative use of the use of the term "it just happens" (as in, it just happens that a process disproportionately affects African-Americans) thereby positioning critics of this view as on the wrong side of arguments to those in favour of racial justice. However, in a long list of reasons for over-representation of African-Americans in the resource-poor and criminalized sections of US communities, only some are legitimately categorized as racism, such as racist discrimination in employment practices. Most of the reasons proposed cannot be definitively assigned to racism. This becomes clear when he moves to suggested remedies: most are non-racialized in character, including a moratorium on building prisons, emphasis on rehabilitation for non-violent offenders, reclassifying the laws on drugs, and a re-focus on "suite crime" not street crime. If implemented, they would, to use his phrase, "just happen" to disproportionately benefit African-Americans (and would, in my view, constitute entirely appropriate policy suggestions). The analysis fails to separate the non-racialized *social relations* that generate the discriminatory outcomes in the first instance from the racist *social relationships* that characterize stages of the criminal justice process (for example, stop and search where skin colour is used as a racist resource in stereotyping where crime is anticipated to occur, or arrest, to the extent that officers operate with racist stereotypes of alleged black male aggression). The problem with the failure to operate with such a distinction is that it limits the likelihood for change that might enable black people to prosper.

By separating the structures and cultures at the scale of broader societal resources and institutional arrangements from the activities of individuals in situated activity and then considering the relationship between the two, we can perhaps move to a more effective challenging of inappropriate actions by state officials.

For instance, there may be occasions in sudden death where SCT is referred to but this does not in itself constitute racism. Thogmartin (1998) notes a case where, following police pursuit on foot, a person collapses and dies and is found to have SCT at autopsy. There may well be contextual factors to the death that comprise discriminatory outcomes (post-slavery social relations have left African-American disproportionately trapped in low-income situations and officers may focus disproportionately on street crime rather than white-collar crimes of the wealthy) but such discriminatory outcomes of policing do not require that the individual officers are racists. However, if they engaged in racist profiling in focusing on certain neighbourhoods where people with black rather than white skin predominate because they held that that is where crimes are committed, this would constitute racism, in addition to committing the ecological fallacy (*ecological fallacy*: a false assignment of presumed characteristics to individuals based on their membership of a group, such as being residents of an area. For example, individuals living in an area of high crime might be victims rather than perpetrators of crime). However, we do not have details in the Thogmartin incident. To the extent that there are no accounts of use of conductive electrical devices, pepper sprays, chokeholds, positional asphyxia, assault or restraint, the cause of death may remain a puzzle, or be contested, but the individual officers appear to have no case to answer.

On the other hand, in the cases of a series of chokehold deaths in the 1970s in Los Angeles, the Chief of Police Darryl Gates was challenged by the *Los Angeles Times* to explain why a disproportionate number of chokehold victims

(12 of the 16) were black. Gates was reported as saying that this "might be because their veins did not reopen *like normal people*" (my emphasis) (Dyson and Boswell, 2009: 68). This can clearly be labelled as racism since Gates was using ideational cultural resources (the idea that there are, biologically, beneath the skin, black people and white people; the notion that the black body is qualitatively different from white bodies, and that the black body has inherent flaws compared to the white body).

Furthermore, if one examines the case of Alton Manning and Denis Stephens in the UK who both died in UK custody in 1995, we can see that the reactions, in 1998, of the Director of Prisons, Richard Tilt, clearly draw on similar racist assumptions, namely, sharply distinct racialized categories and the attribution of flawed bodies compared to white bodies (ibid.: 76–77). Moreover, Tilt did so, not merely in response to an individual death, but as a putative attempt to explain different *rates* of deaths between black and white prisoners. With regard to deaths of those with SCD as opposed to SCT, in the case of Damien Henderson, killed by an overdose of morphine because officials presumed that, since he was a black man in jail he must therefore be a heroin addict and gave him the dose for an addict, the officials concerned were clearly equally operating with racist ideational resources (ibid.: 156–157).

On the other hand, it is more difficult to find that a concept such as institutional racism is helpful in analysing a case such as the Martin Lee Anderson one, however "obvious" it may seem. We cannot "read off" racist intent from discriminatory outcomes, however real those discriminatory outcomes are. That is because, first, we need to distinguish between intended and unintended consequences of purposive human actions (Merton, 1936). Second, the structures of society are relatively opaque to social actors in situated activity. Unless actors in situated activity use racist ideational resources, as did Gates and Tilt, attribution of racism (as opposed to identification of discriminatory outcomes) becomes problematic: a matter for difficult judgements on the basis of empirical research (Carter, 2000).

The context of a low-income African-American (with or without SCT) facing an officer of the state in a criminal justice encounter is a product of historical developments ranging from centuries to decades in time span. Such socio-historical antecedents include:

- enslavement of African peoples by Europeans and forced transportation to the Americas (Davidson, 1996);
- the development of a racist ideational cultural system to justify slavery, exemplified by the so-called illness of *drapetomania*, the alleged pathological tendency of enslaved people to run away, an illness to be cured by whipping, (Cartwright, 1851);
- the failure to change social relations in the post-bellum South by redistribution of land (Kerr-Ritchie, 2003);
- as we saw in Chapter 4, the reinvigoration of racism post-slavery by Jim Crow representations, as based on actual black culture, rather than on the racist caricatures of an English aristocrat;

- the social processes by which, also discussed in Chapter 4, a cohort of sickle cell patients first became visible in the urban poverty of Memphis, making it appear as if it were both a black disease and (because it affected African-Americans in extreme poverty) as if it were "naturally" an illness associated with premature death before adulthood (Wailoo, 2001);
- the later incorporation of sickle cell within broader Black Panther campaigns for social justice (Nelson, 2011).

Such historical antecedents also include the particular combination of:

- urban poverty;
- contemporary problematic gender relations in some African-American families (problems traceable to the rape and deliberate family dislocation that were integral parts of slavery);
- unemployment and criminalization of young African-American men;
- the systematic confusions of early screening programmes discussed in Chapter 4.

All these rendered low-income African-American communities intensely suspicious of any official pronouncements on matters concerned with sickle cell (Hill, 1994).

Challenging the place of SCT in criminal justice systems requires different types of strategy at different scales of analysis. At the scale of contextual resources, this requires sustainable paid employment to be made available for resource-poor communities both within countries, and, because of uneven capitalist development that generates global migration from post-colonial to higher-income countries (Carter and Virdee, 2008), between countries as well. At the scale of institutional arrangements, the suggestions of Street (2003) for criminal justice systems are apposite: a moratorium on building prisons, emphasis on rehabilitation for non-violent offenders, reclassifying the laws on drugs, and a re-focus on white-collar crime rather than street crime. At both these scales we are faced not with racism per se but with long-standing identity-neutral mechanisms. At the scale of situated activity, there is more scope for immediate response to "state talk", which deflects attention away from controversial actions of individual officers by reference to SCT. At this scale of situated activity, it is at least possible to raise awareness of the issue with sickle cell, criminal justice and human rights NGOs, by contacting journalists where new cases arise to point out the patterns in events, and by suggesting that there are experts in SCT autopsies who accept that, in some rare instances, deaths can be complicated by SCT (Lucas *et al.*, 2008) but who also challenge attributions of sudden deaths to SCT in many instances documented by Dyson and Boswell (2009) and whose expertise in sickle cell trait autopsies (Lucas, 2004) could be a valuable global resource.

Conclusion

In this chapter I have demonstrated the importance of an analytical distinction between discriminatory outcomes, the societal availability of racist ideational resources, and the specific activation of those resources towards a desired discriminatory ending. I have chosen to do this in order to illuminate the politics of SCT, where a combination of longer-term and shorter-term historical trajectories has made SCT available as a key resource in effecting racism, especially in state talk deflecting accusations of racism. The argument is that state officials, in an increasingly wide range of countries, engage in state talk that uses SCT to deflect attention from circumstances surrounding sudden unexplained deaths within particular criminal justice systems. However, caution is required against a straight-forward attribution of racism as a *driving force* behind these events. Racism does exist, but consists in these instances of state talk using SCT to deflect attention from the very real patterns of disproportionate detentions, and deaths during state contact, among black men. However, the roots of discriminatory outcomes that people describe as racist may not all in fact be racism. What is defined as a crime (and who gets to encode their definitions in law); what types of crime are then prioritized (street as opposed to corporate or white-collar crime); neighbourhoods where resources are targeted: all such concerns could also affect white low-income communities. The general shift to replacing social services and welfare payments (what used to be termed social security) with processing through criminal justice systems – what has been termed warehousing the poor (Herivel and Wright, 2003) – will evidently also over-represent black communities to the extent that they have been historically rendered resource-poor.

The problem with an analysis of "institutional racism" is that where a discriminatory outcome has non-ethnic structural antecedents, the argument collapses when such non-ethnic social origins are shown. The arguments of anti-racist protagonists can then be side-lined. It has been argued that there is a political as well as a sociological purpose to distinguishing between social relations and social relationships. Politically, white low-income groups can currently be co-opted against anti-racist strategies, whereas they would themselves benefit from changes at the scale of contextual resources or institutional arrangements. What can more readily be challenged, within the type of resources available to the academy, are instances of state talk, where vigilance is necessary to help ensure journalists, sickle cell communities of interest and human rights organizations recognize the dubious nature of attribution of sudden death in state contact to sickle cell trait.

7 Ethnicity, migration and sickle cell

Introduction

The status of ethnicity as an objective variable is increasingly contested in health research (Carter and Dyson, 2011; Bradby, 2012). Where research centres upon human genetics, there is the danger that, in a racist society, genetic information will be used to reinforce existing prejudices (Atkin and Ahmad, 1998). In this chapter, I assess the processes by which SCD became an ethnicized condition, one described by European physicians as pertaining to "immigration haematology" (Roberts and de Montalembert, 2007: 865). The chapter considers how ethnicity became the lens to bring sickle cell into view in particular ways at particular times, and how ethnicity was mobilized both in advocating, and in resisting, the development of services for sickle cell, especially in the UK. In part, the account becomes semi-autobiographical, noting how the author has had a role in amplifying the relationships between ethnicity and sickle cell and thalassaemia, and in assessing the degree of association between socially constructed ethnicity categories and prevalence of genetic carriers (Dyson et al., 2006). Finally, in line with contentions that sociological analysis has itself become over-ethnicized (Carter and Fenton, 2010), and with the inspiration of anthropological works past and present, the chapter concludes with an assessment of the prospects that ethnicity will disappear from the sickle cell cosmology.

Migration and sickle cell

It has been argued from the outset of this book that the power that the attribution to sickle cell represents lies in its relationship to the concept of race in overall systems of meaning. For example, in the UK at the end of the twentieth century, a majority of both health professionals (Dyson et al., 1996) and the African-Caribbean community (Dyson, 1997) wrongly believed that sickle cell was exclusively a "black" condition. Numerous authors have convincingly argued against the notion of distinct biological races (Montagu, (1998 [1942]); UNESCO, 1950; Livingstone, 1962; Miles, 1982; Lewontin et al., 1984; Cavalli-Sforza et al., 1996; American Anthropological Association, 1998; Carter, 2000; Sykes, 2001; Royal and Dunston, 2004; Fujimura et al., 2014; Duster, 2015;

Yudell *et al.*, 2016). The case of sickle cell above all illustrates the fallacy of race (see Dyson, 2005). The US philosopher Timothy Morton (2017) notes that the racist is someone who believes that race is something that can be pointed to in "ontic time-space", a philosopher's phrase that almost, but not quite, equates to the fascist notion of "blood and soil" (a slogan chanted at a white nationalist rally in Shelbyville, Tennessee, in October 2017).

The case of sickle cell disturbs many assumptions about the relationship between blood and belonging, and disturbs them for several reasons. First, in terms of timescale, as we saw in Chapter 3, the sickle cell gene is but a brief event in the timescale of hominids on Earth, and is a record of co-evolution of *Plasmodium falciparum* malaria in relation to birds, reptiles, mammals, and hominids, as well as, subsequently, humans. As we also saw, sickle cell reflects the fact that the sickle cell human body is a record of the evolution of *other* species (Dyson, 2018). Speciesism (anthropocentric discrimination against non-humans) is what permits racism (Morton, 2017), as, for example, when a columnist of a UK right-wing tabloid newspaper labelled cross-Mediterranean migrants as "cockroaches" Labelling humans as non-humans – racism – works because of speciesism.

Second, let us consider Figure 7.1, which is taken from a World Health Organization publication. It is of one of a series of maps describing prevalence of genes associated with haemoglobin disorders (beta-thalassaemia, as well as sickle cell and other variant haemoglobins). The WHO report includes a map entitled "Original Endemic Distribution of Haemoglobinopathies in Europe"; several maps showing migration to the UK, France, the Netherlands and Portugal, from their former colonies, as well a map of "internal" migration within Europe. Against this, examine the following quotation from the French philosopher Bruno Latour.

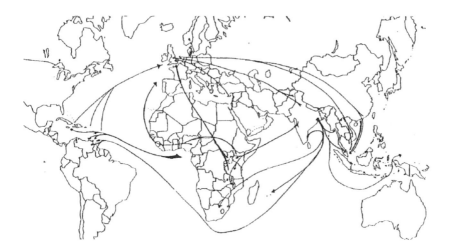

Figure 7.1 Colonial population movements; immigration; and re-immigration: UK.
Source: World Health Organization (1988: 13).

My enemy is arrows. I want to get rid of arrows. Because arrows is [sic] the proof that you have drawn things as if they were distant. In fact, they are not. So the more arrows in a drawing … every time there is something that doesn't fit inside a border you have to add an arrow. But the problem with the arrow just means that things which are actually very distant should in fact be close … So you are trying to characterize overlapping entities by projecting on a base map, which actually makes them distant … and then you add the arrows. But the problem is: can we make a geopolitical map without arrows, where we respect the overlapping (territories)? Territories are overlapped. Doesn't mean sovereignty is out. It means that the idea of sovereignty *on* a boundary means nothing now. This is why the old German empire metaphor [overlapping maps] is not that far-fetched. But then it means you have to be able to paint – to make the overlap visible.

(Latour, 2015; author's transcription)

Arrows on the map indicate that the map has been incorrectly drawn in the first place. Where bodies are in contemporary space *is where they are* and should be reflected in the map, but the map fails because it cannot handle overlapping constituencies (such as the dyads British resident/sickle cell carrier and African/ non-sickle cell carrier, or the more complex conjunction of white-skinned, British-born, British resident, sickle cell genetic carrier) without resorting to the use of arrows.

Third, genes associated with skin colour and genes encoding sickle haemoglobin are inherited independently from one another. This explains why someone may be a sickle cell genetic carrier or have SCD but also have white skin and fair hair. Where these territories of features – inside the body (haemoglobin type) and on body surface (hair and skin) – overlap in one person, advocates of biological race are faced with a dilemma. This dilemma is whether to privilege genes associated with skin colour or the genes associated with sickle haemoglobin in constructing the ideational construct of race. Such a choice is in essence a political decision, not a biological one.

Finally, let us return to examine the slogan "blood and soil". This slogan originated in nineteenth-century Germany before being taken up by the Nazis. It denotes an idealized view of a natural linkage between a national body, defined in racialized terms (blood), and an area of settlement (soil). The concept favours the rural, sedentary farmer over the urban nomad, and specifically in the case of European fascism, over the Jewish migrant. However, as we saw in Chapter 3, it was not the Palaeolithic era that produced sickle cell and other human genetic adaptations to malaria but the Neolithic transition to farming, with relatively more settled populations permitting the development of ecologies favourable to mosquitoes and malaria. It was sedentary, settled, farming populations that generated the sickle cell gene, not nomadic ones. Furthermore, what the WHO maps (WHO, 1988: 12–16) also fail to show is the *decline* of sickle cell gene prevalence over time in the migrants themselves. For example, at the time of forced movements from Africa to the Americas during the *Maafa* enslavements, the movement was from malarial to either non-malarial or less intense malarial environments in the Caribbean and the USA, and the prevalence of sickle cell trait fell from around 20 per cent to around 10 per cent, but varied according to the incidence of malaria in the receiving area (Allison, 1964: 141).

Notwithstanding the above, Anglophone literature has repeated the migration trope as a context for sickle cell every decade. In the 1960s "the haemoglobin-opathies [are] a new problem in Britain" (Lehmann, 1963: 571); in the 1970s, screening was undertaken for "abnormal haemoglobins in immigrant schoolchildren"(Stuart *et al*., 1973: 284) when, 11 years after the 1962 Common-wealth Immigrants Act ended primary migration from the Caribbean to the UK, most such children would not have been immigrants at all; in the late 1980s, a generation after Lehmann (1963), haemoglobinopathies were still a "recent arrival" (WHO, 1988: 1); in the 1990s, "haemoglobin disorders have been imported by immigrants" (Angastiniotis and Modell, 1998); in the 2000s, now two generations after Lehmann, service provision was still characterized as "immigration haematology" (Roberts and de Montalembert, 2007) and in the 2010s, "migration from different parts of the world to several European coun-tries leads to the *introduction* of haemoglobinopathy genes into the population" (Angastiniotis *et al*., 2013: 1, my emphasis). When sickle cell and other haemo-globinopathies are repeatedly constructed as alien, other, from outside, it is little wonder that some white English sickle cell genetic carriers reverted to notions of pollution, tainted blood lines and the Aryan race in reacting negatively to information they were genetic carriers of a haemoglobin variant such as sickle cell (Dyson, 2005, 2007).

Race, ethnicity and genes associated with sickle cell

Classic texts on medical screening suggest that targeting screening for sickle cell would be unproblematic. An early editorial at the time of the US Sickle Cell Control Act referred to "sickle cell disease, which for all practical purposes will be found among 22 million black Americans" (Nalbandian, 1972: 221) and Lappé *et al*. (1972: 1130) wrote: "To make testing more useful for certain conditions, pri-ority should be given to informing certain well defined populations in which the condition occurs with definitely greater frequency such as haemoglobin S in blacks." Carrier frequency of the sickle cell gene is up to 30 per cent in areas of West and Central Africa, but is nearly as high in parts of northern Greece, eastern Saudi Arabia and India (Serjeant, 1997), illustrating that sickle cell is not neces-sarily associated with recent African ancestry. As we saw at the outset of the book, the multi-centric theory of the origin of the sickle cell gene proposes five haplo-types (variations in the chromosomal context of the sickle cell gene), and one arose in either Arabia or India (Gabriel and Przybylski, 2010), again destabilizing the assumed link between African ancestry and the sickle cell mutation. Moreover, Parra *et al*. (2003) note that in Brazil, for example, there is no necessary associ-ation between phenotypic features associated in the popular imagination with race, such as skin colour, and genetic markers of African ancestry. They write:

Let us take as an example the historically common Brazilian mating of a white European male with a black African slave woman: the children with more physical African features would be considered black, whereas the more European features would be considered white, *even though they would have the same proportion of African and European alleles.* In the next generation, the light-skinned individual would assortatively tend to marry other whites and conversely the darker individuals would marry blacks. The long-term tendency would then be for this pattern to produce a white group and a black group, which would, nonetheless, have a similar proportion of African ancestry.

(Parra *et al.*, 2003: 181, emphasis added)

Even if sickle cell were of exclusively African derivation, it is a somatically invisible trait and is inherited independently of genes encoding presence or absence of melanin. The sickle haemoglobin variant would be one allele shared among both black-skinned and white-skinned. Furthermore, Lavinha *et al.* (1992) suggest that the Benin haplotype of sickle cell had spread into the Mediterranean population well before 1400 CE. Thus, Portuguese colonizers may have taken the gene to Brazil *before* those kidnapped from Africa were enslaved there. It is therefore not axiomatic that sickle cell indexes black skin or African ancestry. It is to the *social* processes underpinning this linkage of ethnicity and sickle cell that we turn in the next section.

The emergence of sickle cell as an ethnicized disease

The history of sickle cell is intimately tied up with medical power, colonialism and racism (Dyson and Atkin, 2011). As we saw in Chapter 4, the very term "sickle cell" is one of biomedical reduction to the cells seen under a microscope by white US physicians and not to the centuries-old onomatopoeic descriptions, in African languages, of the whole person in pain (Konotey-Ahulu, 1996). Ironically, even a post-colonial rendering of history, in which original knowledge of sickle cell symptomatology, and in particular of its inherited nature, is relocated in Africa (Konotey-Ahulu, 1974) risks deepening the assumed primordial association of sickle cell and black skin. However, since it was in the USA in the early twentieth century that the technology of laboratory medicine rendered sickled cells visible (Wailoo, 1997), the social context of the USA at that period becomes crucial.

We saw in Chapter 4 how the history of SCD in the USA ensured that cultural understandings of sickle cell would routinely associate it with black skin. From the fascination with the exceptional Walter Noel in Chicago (Savitt and Goldberg, 1989), to the racialized poverty that characterized the sickle cell patient cohorts of Lemuel Diggs in Memphis (Wailoo, 2001; Nollan, 2016), through to the use of sickle cell as a bridging issue attempting to secure citizenship rights for African-Americans (Tapper, 1999; Nelson, 2011), sickle cell became considered on all sides a black issue.

By the 1980s, SCD had become stabilized as a purported black disease to the point where sickle cell community pioneers in the UK, facing societal ignorance of SCD, and a marked reluctance of statutory services to engage with the issue, sought advice from African-American colleagues (Clare, 2007; Anionwu, 2016). The added impetus to the racialization of SCD in the UK came through the politics of Britain in the 1980s. The 1980s in Britain saw the beginnings of neoliberal politics, the attack on trades unions, and an economy of mass unemployment, with black youth unemployment running at 50 per cent for women, and 46 per cent for men (Brown, 1984: 190). Rather than see this unemployment as a combination of the UK's historical-material legacy and a racist ideational system, such unemployment was attributed by right-wing politicians to poor character, culture or even genes.

The historical-material legacy must be traced first of all to the enslavement of Africans and the triangular trade between Britain, Africa and the Caribbean (Davidson, 1996), a material history that later produced a cultural history of racist ideology to justify the brutal treatment of African peoples. According to Polanyi (2001 [1944]), the Great Depression in 1873–1886, and social dislocation attendant upon liberal international markets, led to nineteenth-century trade protectionism among the powerful nations. From 1881 onwards, this prompted the "scramble for Africa" by European nations, which, in turn, led to decades of economic imperialism. "Economic imperialism was mainly a struggle between the Powers for the privilege of extending their trade into unprotected markets" (ibid.: 226).

The legacy of the involvement of Britain in the slave trade, the scramble for Africa, and the role of the East India Company, was a series of British colonies in Africa, the Caribbean and the Indian sub-continent. After the Second World War, the British Empire became the Commonwealth: a reconfiguration, perhaps to render it more distinguishable from the war-time German propaganda that made the case for the legitimacy of Nazi *Lebensraum* on the basis of drawing explicit parallels with the British Empire. British social policy post-war entailed a struggle. On the one hand, there was the need for migrant labour from the Commonwealth (whose citizenship rights were at first encoded in the 1948 British Nationality Act) to fill acute labour shortages in the UK post-war economy (Carter, 2000). Politicians of both Labour and Conservative parties drew, or at least anticipated that the general UK population would draw, on the racist ideational system, fearing a problem of "assimilation" of (black) Commonwealth immigrants based on alleged incommensurability of different cultures. The consequences were several, exemplified by the development of the notion of the "British Isles": a fictional entity comprising the United Kingdom of Great Britain and Northern Ireland *and* Eire, the Republic of Ireland, which enabled white immigration to fill labour vacancies and for such processes to be invisible in policy terms. White Irish peoples were basically the same race as White British whether they liked it or not, remarked one Conservative Minister (Carter, 2000). Despite racist violence in the period 1948–1962 being directed by whites against black people (as in the 1958 Notting Hill riots, for example), concerns about assimilation prevailed over labour market needs and the 1962 Common-wealth Immigrants Act restricted primary migration to the UK. It was followed by a succession of immigration acts. These were a key factor in the rise of Margaret Thatcher in 1979. The previous year she had claimed in a speech that white communities were being "swamped". The Thatcher government passed the British Nationality Act in 1981, which abolished *jus soli*, the legal principle of being born in the country automatically according citizenship of that country.

A further impetus for the popular association of black and sickle cell in the UK derives from policy initiatives developed in the wake of the 1981 urban rebellions. These disturbances took place in Brixton (London), Handsworth (Birmingham), Toxteth (Liverpool), Moss Side (Manchester) and St Paul's (Bristol), centred on urban areas settled by post-war migrants to the UK from the Caribbean and subsequent generations, areas suffering material deprivation, youth unemployment and racist policing. It was living though times such as these that led the artist living with SCD, Donald Rodney, referred to in Chapter 4, to link his experience of SCD and his experience of racism by framing racism as a societal disease (Hylton, 2003).

The specific police operation in London that sparked the rebellions echoed the earlier offensive epithet of Margaret Thatcher: *Operation Swamp*. The reaction of a nervous government was to create special monies – Inner Area Programme monies – that supported inner-city regeneration. In some instances, sickle cell services, especially community-based sickle cell counselling centres, were funded following community demands (Valier and Bivins, 2002). This institutionalized the piecemeal nature of sickle cell provision in the UK from the outset (Prashar *et al.*, 1985), and, even as service provision for sickle cell became a site of struggle for black communities (Ahmad and Atkin, 1996), effectively misused sickle cell to stand for "doing something" for the health of minority ethnic groups. The further consequence was to cement, for a generation, the link in UK popular imagination of sickle cell and Black Caribbean populations. This may explain why health service letters inviting white people, who had been identified as carriers by genetic screening, to attend inner-city health centres, often in those very same inner-city areas listed above as the sites of rebellions, provoked negative racist reactions (Dyson, 2005). These reactions were possibly because of the strong association of certain inner-city neighbourhoods as "black" in ways that stigmatized whole areas (Howarth, 2002).

In the 1980s and 1990s, the association developed further in the USA. The ethical, legal and social mistakes incurred when attempting to introduce sickle cell screening in the USA (Hill, 1994; Duster, 2003) fed into African-American antipathy to medical research interventions in their lives (Reverby, 2000; Skloot, 2010) especially when African-Americans felt wanted as research subjects but not as patients deserving of treatment (Benjamin, 2011). In a context of material poverty, experience of racism, distortions of family structure and gender relations derived from slavery, unemployment, and of criminalization and narcotization of young African-American men, children with SCD were not stigmatized as allegedly flawed children but valued because they were symbolic of the survival of a group (Hill, 1994). This deepened further the association of sickle cell with African-Americans, despite 3–10 per cent of those with SCD in the USA being from ethnic groups other than African-American (Brousseau *et al.*, 2009).

The power of ethnicity in creating genetic knowledge of populations

Since the advent of Foucauldian perspectives on the development of medical knowledge (Foucault, 1979), it has become a truism that particular forms of power are associated with making visible certain forms of knowledge. The very concept of ethnicity is implicated in "making up" new bodies (Carter and Fenton, 2010) and the insertion of these new bodies, carriers of sickle cell and thalassaemia genes, into the nexus of genetic screening technologies in the UK. To be sure, this was already underway in terms of the historically established associations outlined above (Tapper, 1999; Wailoo, 2001; Wailoo and Pemberton, 2006).

The racialization of SCD in the UK was further intensified through the politics of the UK in the 1980s. The UK government attempted to include a question on ethnic origins in their 1981 census, but the extent of societal racism meant that pilot tests of such a question showed that it would not be answered in the extant conditions of racist policing and youth unemployment, those same conditions conducive to the 1981 urban rebellions in major UK cities. The racism awareness courses that subsequently pervaded public sector training, though fundamentally flawed (see Gurnah, 1984; Sivanandan, 1985), marked a change in public consciousness and in 1991 the UK Census asked an ethnicity (as opposed to country of birth, language or religion) question (Coleman and Salt, 1996). By contrast, Jans *et al.* (2012) note that, in the Netherlands, the legacy of Jewish deportations in the Second World War meant that selective screening, targeted by asking an ethnicity question, could not politically be considered. Meanwhile, in the UK, the 1991 Census results enabled a linkage to be made between census output areas and administrative districts of the UK health service. This link was first undertaken in a series of reports of community members' knowledge of sickle cell and thalassaemia (for example, Dyson, 1994). The reports tabulated the 1991 UK Census figures for different ethnic groups against estimates of prevalence of the sickle cell or beta-thalassaemia gene, and an estimate of the numbers of sickle cell/thalassaemia carriers in the health districts was made. Thus ethnicity was being explicitly used as a tool to make visible to policy-makers the likely number of carriers of haemoglobin disorders in a given area, and, by implication, the level of unmet need of services for sickle cell/thalassaemia screening and counselling. These reports were shared with medical researchers who then used the same principles in more systematic ways to produce guidelines for commissioners on likely numbers of carriers, at-risk pregnancies and expected foetal prevalence for different health districts (Modell and Anionwu, 1996; Hogg and Modell, 1998). This was furthered by the production of estimates of carrier rates, based on evidence of local screening results, for different ethnic groups in the UK (Hickman *et al.*, 1998; Kadkhodaei Elyaderani *et al.*, 1998).

At the same time, having used the concept of ethnicity to reveal the nature of the gap in service provision for sickle cell/thalassaemia counselling services, I myself was becoming uneasy at the readiness to naturalize ethnicity as a category, and to essentialize the relationship between ethnicity and the sickle cell/thalassaemia genes. Dyson (1998) noted how neither conceptions of distinct biological races, nor various social science frameworks for ethnic categorization, were adequate in mapping risks of carrying genes associated with sickle cell or thalassaemia, and that targeted screening risked processing people on the basis of assumed ethnicity rather than consulting them about whether or not they wished to be tested for sickle cell/thalassaemia trait. Dyson (1999) subsequently proposed a working solution to the problem. This suggested using the extant UK Census categories (in order to be able to contextualize the findings and possibly reduce the need for duplication of information requests for the client), but using an expanded set of categories, principally to capture Mediterranean, Arab and mixed ethnic groups who would be missed by the main UK 1991 Census ethnicity categories (ibid.). This approach was subsequently confirmed as feasible by a review of secondary evidence (Aspinall *et al.*, 2003).

Contesting sickle cell/thalassaemia services through ethnicity

Meanwhile the association of sickle cell and black/minority populations in Europe and North America continued in popular and professional minds, with haemoglobinopathy provision a site of struggles of minority ethnic groups for health and welfare provision (Ahmad and Atkin, 1996). Atkin *et al.* (1998a) note that various aspects of poor service provision for sickle cell/thalassaemia flowed from ethnic stereotypes about which groups should have which disease. Examples included health professionals not offering antenatal screening because of assumptions that a mother is from an ethnic group not traditionally associated as being at risk of carrying genes associated with sickle cell, and/or effecting screening without consent on the basis of observed skin colour or name. Over a decade later, Reed (2011) continued to note that White respondents to her study on men's participation in sickle cell screening tended to minimize its importance, assuming their white ethnicity placed them at low risk.

Commissioners of services were not knowledgeable about sickle cell/thalassaemia services or about the conditions (Atkin *et al.*, 1998b); there were problems with GPs neither understanding nor communicating test results (Dyson, 1997); and white health professionals were felt to marginalize the haemoglobin disorders because of their association with minority ethnic groups (Atkin *et al.*, 1998a). Clients had highest regard for the specialist sickle cell/thalassaemia workers (Dyson, 2005), sometimes appreciating common cultural background of specialist workers but responding positively to good services whatever the ethnic background of the service provider (Anionwu, 1996). A lack of health professional knowledge was attributed to the fact that sickle cell and thalassaemia were perceived by professionals to be associated solely with black and minority ethnic communities (Dyson *et al.*, 1996; Atkin *et al.*, 1998a). This lack of secure knowledge on the part of health professionals was confirmed by a subsequent audit (Lucas *et al.*, 2008). In particular, racist stereotypes associating black people with drug misuse dogged sickle cell services on both sides of the Atlantic as sickle cell patients in extreme pain were accused of being drug addicts when seeking treatment for the excruciating pain of a sickle cell crisis (Anionwu and Atkin, 2001; Rouse, 2009). Vulnerability to becoming over-whelmed by the challenges of living with sickle cell was, in the view of people living with SCD themselves, more related to life transitions and racism rather than to their medical condition or their individual psychology (Atkin and Ahmad, 2001).

Attempts to introduce universal newborn screening for SCD in England were met with criticism that it privileged ethnic equality issues over economic effi-ciency, and that it misconceived notions of equity (Sassi *et al.*, 2001a). In par-ticular, economists drew attention to ethnicity as the key dimension of equity in screening (ibid. : 61), ignoring, in their own conception of equity, the fact that those who do not readily identify with an ethnic group are effectively denied ser-vices (Hinton *et al.*, 2011: 379).

> Sickle cell disease disproportionately affects certain ethnic minority groups. The UK Standing Medical Advisory Committee recommended the use of universal, rather than selective, neonatal screening policies when ethnic minorities with a high risk comprise more than 15% of the population. At this threshold the cost of universal screening is as high as £430,000 to £1m per life year saved (depending on the ethnic minority mix) compared with selective screening. The adoption of universal screening does not appear to be justified by concerns for equity across ethnic groups, as the benefits to the white northern European majority would still be very small. Rather, it aims at reducing the number of cases missed because of inaccuracies in the selection. This NHS policy may reflect an aspiration to equal access for equal need, but one pursued at a very high cost. Significant efficiency gains may be sacrificed for what seems to be an inappropriate conception of equity in this context.
>
> (Sassi *et al.*, 2001b: 763)

At a broad level, this analysis missed the nuance that the Standing Medical Advisory Committee had referred to a threshold of 15 per cent of the *antenatal population*, an important distinction, given the much younger age structure of the UK minority ethnic populations at the time. More specifically, there are questions as to whether such analyses factor in effects of *all* preventive meas-ures, in addition to penicillin prophylaxis, associated with newborn screening, such as raising parental awareness of fever and of splenic sequestration (Grosse *et al.*, 2012) and whether all the costs of not screening are factored in. The latter include personnel costs and quality assurance costs of ethnic ascertainment, legal liabilities of missed cases, and possible costs in education of nursery personnel (Lane, 2001) as well as increased lifetime treatment costs for a disease, cumulative in nature, incurred by virtue of unnecessary morbidity endured in early life. Furthermore, economic analyses would need to model costs of lack of coverage of targeted programmes – as low as 70 per cent in one targeted programme in Georgia, USA (Lane, 2001) – *and* demand for screening by low-risk white European populations: as high as 51 per cent in that same programme (Harris and Eckman, 1989).

However, the work of economists appears to regard ethnicity an essentialist concept, treating it as an equivalent objective factor to socio-economic condition (Sasssi *et al.*, 2001a: 61). Their concern, that targeted screening was discriminatory against white North Europeans (ibid.: 64), ignored the more pertinent problem that services are effectively withheld from those who do not know their ancestry, or do not wish to acknowledge it or see it as significant (Hinton *et al.*, 2011: 379). Inequity was indeed there, but not in the manner proposed by Sassi and colleagues.

Crucially, *there was no awareness that it would more likely be black rather than white communities*, who would have perceived discrimination on the basis of selective screening by ethnicity. Wailoo and Pemberton (2006) note that screening in the USA was experienced by African-Americans as part of a wider undermining of their self-determination. Resistance to screening was not only for long-standing socio-historical reasons, but because newborn screening was first instituted to identify sickle cell trait, not the disease, with legislation in some US states confusing the two (Duster, 2003). As such, newborn screening (now presented as saving lives of infants) would originally have been received as an intervention contrary to Black fertility (ultimately preventing births by identifying carriers) in much the same way as antenatal screening might continue to be seen. This probably explains why, historically, uptake of screening by African-Americans in the Georgia newborn screening programme was as low as 70 per cent.

The manner in which the argument is set up – ethnic equity is transgressed, because wealthier, healthier white Europeans (Sassi *et al.*, 2001a: 64) disproportionately bear the costs of universal newborn screening to the benefit of poorer less healthy Black populations – seems to me perverse. First, Sassi *et al.*'s apparent use of the term equity is directly contrary to common usage in which equity refers to equality of outcome by means of unequal treatment, precisely what they accuse the policy-makers of. Second, they criticize economic analyses for comparing universal with no screening, and insist the comparison should be between selective and universal screening. However, there is no reason why a three-way comparison (selective and universal and no screening) should not be made. Indeed, third, when such three-way comparisons *are* made, selective screening (compared to universal screening) may be expressed as monies saved (largely for the rich, white North European low-risk populations) per year of lives lost (largely of the poor, Black populations) (Lane, 2001). Ultimately it has been argued that, in approving universal newborn screening in the USA and England, policy-makers did not favour equity over economic efficiency, so much as reck-oning with potential stigmatization, missed cases, and the perceived difficulty and discomfort in ascertaining ethnicity in giving greater weight to expert screening opinion than to economic analyses per se (Grosse *et al.*, 2005).

Selective antenatal screening for sickle cell and thalassaemia

In 2002, the NHS Sickle Cell and Thalassaemia Screening Programme covering England commissioned work on the development, piloting and evaluation of ethnic questions in relation to antenatal screening for SCD in an attempt to inform policy on the approach to screening in different areas of the country. The research investigated the validity, reliability, practicalities and displacement effects of attempting to target antenatal screening for people at risk of carrying genes associated with sickle cell or thalassaemia by means of an ethnic/family origins screening question (Dyson *et al.*, 2006). In a randomized controlled trial of two candidate ethnicity screening questions, a category-based question was significantly more reliable (i.e. produced the same reply to the ethnic/family origins screening question when asked a second time, several weeks later by a different health professional) than a binary plus open-ended ethnicity question (ibid.). This research programme also provided policy-makers with a measure of the degree of association between social constructs of ethnicity and genetic status at a particular historical point in time.

At the same time, qualitative research with mothers and midwives revealed problems on the ground with targeted screening. Some midwives used intuition to select/exclude clients from the screening questions rather than implement formal policy (Dyson and Dyson, 2014). The persistence of erroneous beliefs in "racial" groups displaced correct understandings of the relation between ethnicity and risk of carrying genes associated with sickle cell/thalassaemia (Dyson *et al.*, 2007c). In the low prevalence area studied as part of this policy research, an area that operated with a selective antenatal screening programme, the proportion identi-fied as at-risk of carrying genes associated with sickle cell/thalassaemia, when using specifically-designed ethnicity screening questions, as opposed to locally-devised "common-sense" categories, increased from 2.2 per cent to 13.0 per cent (Dyson *et al.*, 2007b). Moreover, only 10 per cent of those identified as at-risk by the ethnicity screening questions were actually subsequently offered a laboratory haemoglobinopathy screen: identifying those statistically more likely to carry genes associated with sickle cell through conceptual screening, by means of a questionnaire, but then failing to implement the laboratory screening.

By 2005, the NHS in England was using a Family Origins Questionnaire (FOQ), in connection with sickle cell/thalassaemia antenatal screening (Aspinall, 2013). The FOQ employed the term "family origins"; permitted respondents to tick multiple categories if this reflected their mixed ancestry; preserved the struc-ture of UK Census ethnic questions with broad groups followed by discrete sub-divisions; and highlighted the categories that implied further action to be taken by the midwife in terms of offering screening. Moreover, the question recognized that this screening information could help target laboratory tests for alpha-thalassaemia, and it permitted low-risk clients to request a test. The term "family origins" permitted an emphasis on (more stable) ancestry rather than (more fluid) ethnic identity (ibid.) but the FOQ differed from the original trialled question in important ways. These included the omission of the explanatory rubric which outlined the sickle cell-specific reason for which ethnic/family origins were being requested, and the expectation that the mother, not the midwife, would lead the completion of the instrument, with the attendant problem that midwives reportedly reverted to ticking one box rather than permitting self-location in relation to several family members by ticking multiple categories (ibid.).

As noted in Chapter 3, Frank B. Livingstone was the anthropologist who identified the historically changing relations of ecologies to human red cell mutations. By the time of the research programme in England into ethnicity and sickle cell screening, a classic resource – Livingstone's *Frequencies of Haemoglobin Variants* (Livingstone, 1985) – was out of print. Livingstone constructed a worldwide compendium of 2,220 references on the frequencies of alleles associated with resistance to malaria, including genes associated with sickle cell and the thalassaemias. As subsequent anthropologists have noted, Livingstone was baffled by why respected population geneticists such as Cavalli-Sforza *et al.* (1996) should implicitly assume, in their construction of phylogenetic trees, that shared genes necessarily indexed shared ancestry, when it might rather imply shared exposure to environment, notably malarial conditions (Vitzhum *et al.*, 2006). This suggests the need to reflect on the possible misuses that the compendium (Livingstone, 1985) might lend itself to. One potential misuse would be to assume that the compendium could be used uncritically as a resource to estimate carrier rates for sickle cell/thalassaemia amongst groups migrated, say, to Northern Europe. Livingstone's work implicitly refutes such an uncritical usage as it makes clear the study is "relating this certain segment of human genetic variation to human demographic, cultural and epidemiological history" (ibid.: 9). Thus the gene frequencies are seen as specific to time and place and a product of changing practices of humans and changing epidemiological pressures of malaria. Only by systematically ignoring the malarial context of place at particular times can such work be reduced to notions of ahistorical, distinct population groups, with assumed autochthonous ties to particular territories, which then somehow have a "natural" rate at which they carry genes associated with sickle cell/thalassaemia, a rate that remains constant as they migrate around the globe. This also undermines what was previously held to be a core aspect of a sociological definition of ethnicity: that peoples could be defined by ancestry and territorial affiliation to which other, subjective aspects, such as customs and culture might then be attached (Carter and Dyson, 2011). The Livingstone work also makes it clear that carrier rates differ markedly over short geographical differences and it should be no surprise, therefore, that a crude aggregations of ethnic categories such as "Indian" in multi-ethnic states such as the USA should show few sickle cell carriers (Lorey *et al.*, 1996) since the Indian sub-continent is covered by diverse groups with carrier rates ranging from 0 to 50 per cent.

Early medical expert working definitions in the UK proposed that ethnic groups should be defined as at higher risk of being genetic carriers of haemo-globin disorders if their ancestors originated in countries with a rate of greater than 1 sickle cell/thalassaemia carrier in 1,000. However, actual screening results in England later showed 1 in 540 "White British" babies carried a gene associ-ated with sickle cell (Streetly *et al.*, 2010), meaning that, in terms of original working definitions, *all* UK Census ethnic groups have a carrier rate for genes associated with sickle cell of greater than 1 in 1,000. Since this does not include thalassaemia carriers, the figure covering at-risk prevalence for sickle cell, other clinically relevant haemoglobin variants such as haemoglobin C, D-Punjab and E, and beta-thalassaemia carriers will be greater still, plausibly around 3 in 1,000. This suggests that even in a society such as England, where people are *made up* into ethnic groups, there are no constituent groups that can be legiti-mately regarded as without risk of carrying genes associated with sickle cell or thalassaemia.

Recent analyses have examined the impact of population movements within Europe (Angastiniotis *et al.*, 2013) or globally (Piel *et al.*, 2014) on the sickle cell gene in Northern European countries, such as the UK. However, extensive use of the term "immigrant" in the UK context reinscribes sickle cell with its racialized identity: it is not part of "us", it derives from outside. In analyses that do not subscribe to race or ethnicity as categories of essence, but that see race as a floating signifier in a system of meaning (Hall, 1997), the term immigrant in the cultural system of ideas in the UK (as drawn upon in right-wing tabloid UK newspapers in particular) itself connotes an ethnicized identity. This is a system of meaning into which SCD cell also fits, with deleterious consequences for what is associated with sickle cell (Bediako and Moffitt, 2011).

Conclusion

This chapter has charted the rise and decline of ethnicity as a key component of how sickle cell has been understood, particularly in the UK context. Sickle cell is originally associated not with ethnicity or ancestry but with the agricultural practices that created the ecological niche favourable to malaria. The particular socio-economic conditions of slavery, the subsequent ideational resource of race-thinking, post-bellum economic disenfranchisement in the USA, post-colonial labour shortages in the UK, the convergence of living with SCD in the context of material poverty and racism in the inner cities of both the USA and the UK created the conditions for the cultural association of sickle cell and being black. Subsequently ethnic categorization was used to reveal a lack of service provision to commissioners, to campaign for sickle cell and thalassaemia ser-vices, but also, conversely, to contest the (alleged) inequities in developing sickle cell/thalassaemia screening as universal services. Concern emerged that the UK Censuses of 1991, 2001 and 2011, which made people up into ethnic groups, naturalized such categories, and could be misused as quasi-racial cat-egories in targeting screening services for sickle cell/thalassaemia. Challenging misconceived arguments of inequity and developing universal screening services has produced a different domain of truth. In England, newborns categorized by their parents as "White British" carry genes associated with sickle cell/thalassaemia at rates around double the prevalence previously considered as a threshold for high risk. In conclusion, sickle cell and thalassaemia deserve appropriate health services because they are health issues, not because they are immigrant or ethnic minority issues, characterizations that socially exclude sickle cell in the very same processes they appear to acknowledge it. Meanwhile, for some comment-ators, the notion of ethnicity as an *objective* variable in research is itself in decline in sociological analysis, partly because its limitations have been exposed in addressing the issues of sickle cell and thalassaemia.

8 Genetic carriers and antenatal screening

Introduction

Chapter 7 examined the role played by the concept of ethnicity in rendering sickle cell (in)visible at different times and in particular ways, notably with regard to sickle cell screening. In this chapter, I examine the issue of prenatal or antenatal genetic screening, aimed at identifying genetic sickle cell carriers, more broadly. One characteristic of prenatal screening for sickle cell is the manner in which screening for a related condition, beta-thalassaemia major (hereafter, thalassaemia), in a specific historical and cultural context of Mediterranean countries in the 1970s, has come to be seen as a prevention-and-control model for reducing the "burden" of other inherited conditions, including sickle cell, in other times and places (Dyson, 1999). Such prenatal screening programmes raise issues of gender, racism and disablement. While some programmes have been relatively directive, others programmes, such as the ones in the UK, have claimed to be based on liberal concepts such as "informed choice". This claim is examined in relation to the notion that medicine is not merely a technical enterprise but a moral one, and one that will tend to reflect the dominant values of the society in which the screening is located. Meanwhile, as we shall see, those identified as genetic carriers of sickle cell or thalassaemia make sense of their trait in ways that do not conform to views of the world centred on notions of a rational choice. I begin this chapter with a consideration of a classic case of genetic screening for haemoglobin disorders: that of thalassaemia screening in Cyprus.

Screening for beta-thalassaemia in twentieth-century Cyprus

The genetic screening, prenatal diagnosis and selective termination of affected foetuses developed with respect to beta-thalassaemia has been regarded by some as a model haemoglobinopathies control programme (Angastiniotis et al., 1986), eventually reducing births of children with beta-thalassaemia major in Cyprus to near zero towards the end of the twentieth century (Angastiniotis and Modell, 1998). This programme has been positively referenced with regard to screening for sickle cell and screening in African contexts (WHO/TIF, 2008). However, as this section will seek to show, this "model" programme was a product of particular circumstances: historical, socio-economic, cultural and political as well as medical (Beck and Niewöhner, 2009).

Cyprus had one of the highest rates of beta-thalassaemia genetic carriers in the world, at around 1 in 7 of the population, and one in every 160 newborn children had beta-thalassaemia major. In such children barely any usual adult haemoglobin is produced, and by a few months old, when adult haemoglobin would usually have replaced foetal haemoglobin, the infants are noticeably pale and fail to thrive. By the 1950s, the treatment of monthly exchange blood transfusions (removing and replacing all existing blood) was being developed. This permitted survival until around 20 years by which time excess iron, introduced by serial blood transfusions, overloaded the heart and liver, often leading to organ failure. By the 1960s, drugs were developed that helped remove excess iron from the body (iron-chelating drugs) though the optimal treatment mode that eventually developed by the turn of the century, that of 10–12-hourly injections into the abdomen, 5–7 times a week, represented an extremely challenging treatment regime (Atkin and Ahmad, 2000a).

Cyprus, an island in the Eastern Mediterranean, was controlled by the British until independence in 1960. The British actively created ethnic conflict between Greek and Turkish Cypriot communities as a divide-and-rule strategy of colonial administration (Anderson, 2008). After a long and violent struggle Cyprus gained independence in 1960, though the legacy of colonialism bequeathed Cyprus its intercommunal tensions, which saw the island divided between Turkish and Greek communities in 1974 (Beck and Niewöhner, 2009). The largely agrarian society was centred on marriages, marriages arranged to ensure combined rural properties were sufficient to support the new family. In a context of economic hardship and communal division, a new custom developed of permitting co-residence before marriage. In this context, a screening result identifying thalassaemia genetic carriers, in a situation where thalassaemia was heavily stigmatized, was ruinous for the prospective bride, reducing or eliminating chances of an alternative marriage partner (ibid.: 80).

An assemblage of interests was enrolled to change this situation. Beck (2016) recounts how one doctor, Minas Hadjiminas, used his UK medical education, his preparedness to work within colonial administrative structures, his willingness to face down the Orthodox Church, who accused him at first of murder, and his capacity to talk in informal community groups across the island, to promote a type of community genetic education that framed thalassaemia as a collective cultural identifier, rather than as an individualizing problem stigmatizing discrete families. Given that parents had to find two pints of blood every month for their child living with thalassaemia, and that iron-chelating drugs were very expensive, WHO experts predicted demand for blood and treatment costs would outstrip the financial and human capacities of the island (Beck and Niewöhner, 2009). For example, iron-chelating drugs accounted for 44 per cent of the costs of all medicines purchased by the Ministry of Health in 1983 (Kalokairinou, 2007). Community education was linked with a requirement for genetic screening for couples if they were to receive the blessing for the church for marriage, a near-compulsory impetus to screening. In the Turkish part of Cyprus, the screening was compulsory, being imposed by law (Kalokairinou, 2007). When from the late 1970s onwards prenatal diagnosis and selective termination of affected pregnancies became technologically possible, this combined to produce a dramatic decline in births of children with beta-thalassaemia major (Angastiniotis *et al.*, 1986).

The near compulsory element of the screening was criticized by international genetic ethicists for breaching notions of autonomy (Hoedemaekers and ten Have, 1998), but in contrast stand accounts of suffering from international thalassaemia experts (Weatherall, 2010), Cypriot philosophers (Kalokairinou, 2007) or from Dr Hadjiminas in Cyprus himself:

> In the early 1960s there were mothers who suffocated their thalassaemic children with pillows, parents committed suicide and many marriages split after the birth of children; because of stigmatization, families avoided contacts with neighbours, fathers found it difficult to go to the village *kafenion*. We had to fight poverty, ignorance, prejudice and superstition – not only in patients but in physicians and nurses as well.
>
> (Cited in Beck and Niewöhner, 2009: 79)

Moreover, international concern over ethics has not prevented near unanimity of support for the thalassaemia screening policy, consistent over decades, on the part of the people of Cyprus themselves (ibid.). Comparable thalassaemia screening programmes have been adopted in conservative Islamic states where arranged marriages are the norm (Iran, Saudi Arabia). In the UK, the lack of such marriage customs in ethnic majority communities means that prenatal screening (rather than premarital screening) is the main route of entry into people's lives for a genetic screening programme (Christianson *et al.*, 2004).

The World Health Organization asserts that sickle cell can be prevented, but cites thalassaemia control programmes and either premarital screening and/or prenatal diagnosis and selective termination as the basis for this assertion (WHO, 2006). A joint meeting of the World Health Organization and Thalassaemia International Federation noted differences between the conditions but still cautioned that: "Prevention must also be considered for SCD since the burden it bears is considerable for both families and the health system" (WHO/TIF, 2008: 8). Such documents signify a possible tension between communities of interests representing the respective conditions.

In this respect, there is a danger of transferring a model devised in a particular historical context (Cyprus, in which couples had become informally engaged, had sex and developed pregnancies, before finding that they were in a carrier couple), and proselytizing on this basis to other genetic conditions, at other times and in other places. Other contexts where thalassaemia births have been greatly reduced, such as Iran or Saudi Arabia, have done so in the context of states, captured by conservative-religious norms, and able to base screening interventions around community matchmakers, arranged marriages and premarital screening, without the need to invoke prenatal screening, prenatal diagnosis and selective termination. A model developed in such Middle Eastern countries enabled socially viable interventions before conception. In countries without such social norms, the only known intervention that reduces births is prenatal diagnosis and selective termination (Christianson *et al.*, 2004). In England, this has been associated with genetic screening programmes offering women "informed reproductive choice". In liberal democracies, this is presented as more ethical on the basis of providing greater respect for Western ethical principles, such as autonomy and the right to know, though this equally involves subtle pressures of free choice in a directive educational environment (Hoedemaekers and ten Have, 1998). The section that follows traces the legacy of the Cyprus model of thalassaemia prevention for prenatal screening within the UK.

Screening for thalassaemia in the UK

Hoedemaekers and ten Have (1998) note that the Cyprus model of thalassaemia prevention implicitly drew upon three arguments about "burdens" (sic): (1) a burden of disease costs upon the community; (2) a burden of care for the family members raising a child with thalassaemia; and (3) the burden of disease management of the person with thalassaemia. Proponents of thalassaemia screening (Modell *et al.*, 1984) linked economic arguments in a subtle way with the pressures on patients and families (Hoedemaekers and ten Have, 1998: 278). Constructing a person with a long-term condition as representing a burden is of course the height of disabling discourse and open to criticism from a disability rights perspective. Such disability rights commentaries included criticisms that: (1) extant health education materials clearly presented people with thalassaemia in negative and pejorative ways; (2) analyses failed to account for much lower numbers likely to be born in a country like England, where (unlike Cyprus, Saudi Arabia or Iran) high thalassaemia carrier rates are in those ethnic groups in the numerical minority; and (3) false health economics analogies were being made because a wealthy country like England had greater capacity to absorb treatment costs and because decisions about such treatment costs depend in any case upon political priorities (Dyson, 1999). More broadly, disability rights authors noted that having a screening programme that resulted in reduced births itself undermined the potential future solidarity of disabled peoples; that the vested interests of condition-specific charities were not necessarily congruent with those of disabled peoples themselves, and that the voices of those living with the condition were often absent from policy debates (Shakespeare, 1995).

More importantly, with respect to the extension of thalassaemia screening to multi-ethnic societies, such as the UK, there is the question of the extent to which the overall framing of a genetic health care and screening programme, through a process of "sensitization" (Hoedemaekers and ten Have, 1998: 280), and bombardment with multimedia sources of information on screening, results in subtle pressures of social control persuading people to the choice not to have a child with thalassaemia. At the end of the twentieth century, Modell *et al.*

(1997) found that over 90 per cent of UK Cypriot parents used prenatal diagnosis and termination of pregnancy, but that rates were much lower and regionally variable (0–60 per cent) in British Pakistani couples. A few years later an audit of "informed choice" in thalassaemia screening in the UK was conducted (Modell *et al.*, 2000). A demonstrable service failure to provide informed choice was defined as failure to detect thalassaemia carriers, detection after 24 weeks (the then-standard limit for medical termination), failure to offer genetic counselling or failure to offer prenatal diagnosis. At the same time two Health Technology Assessment Reports included health economics cost analyses of the viability of offering universal or selective antenatal screening by ethnicity for both thalassaemia and sickle cell (Zeuner *et al.*, 1999; Davies *et al.*, 2000), before both newborn sickle cell screening and antenatal screening for sickle cell and thalassaemia were formalized into a national screening programme for England by 2004. This programme was based on the neoliberal notion of "informed reproductive choice".

Time, manner, place

We have seen how the type of screening that emerged in Cyprus for thalassaemia was intimately linked to economic deprivation, post-colonial tensions, subtle changes in marriage norms, rhetorical declarations of suffering, and changes in technologies and social relations over time. By the end of the twentieth century, practically no new infants were being born with thalassaemia in Cyprus itself and were greatly declined in the Cypriot diaspora in the UK (Gill and Modell, 1998). The contextual nuances of the Cypriot example are, however, precisely what render it less than wholly suitable as a model for other times, other places and other genetic conditions.

First, in the mid-twentieth century, experience of thalassaemia consisted of premature death, lack of any treatment, lack of affordable treatment, lack of affordable health sector costs, and demonstrable suffering (Weatherall, 2010). In many cultures, including Cyprus, to be an infant with thalassaemia was to break many social norms: that a newborn might thrive as a child and grow to adulthood; that such a person would carry on family lineage and traditions, and that the child would meet expectations of a normative body: expectations challenged when lack of haemoglobin led the bone marrow of someone living with thalassaemia to increase production of red blood cells, expand the bone marrow, affecting bone growth, and thereby creating somatic features marking out children with thalassaemia as physically recognizable from their peers (Kalokairinou, 2007: 293). However, with biomedical treatments, life expectancy has increased beyond 60 years of age, people with thalassaemia have become parents and grandparents, and treatment regimens have reduced the degree of changes in bone structure. In one respect, the past 50 years have seen the emergence of the social model of disability, which has challenged notions of a "normal" body (against which deviations are stigmatized). In another respect, a hyperconsumerist, hyper-sexualized culture has rendered body shape and image central to consumer identity and has been a powerful reinforcer of bodily norms, such norms being at once disabling, racist, ageist and (hetero)sexist.

Second, the particular location of Cyprus, as a site for the increased visibility of thalassaemia, is significant in a number of ways. As Beck and Niewöhner (2009) argue, strivings for post-colonial independence, and enhancement of communal identities through conflict, created a cultural space in which group identity could be attached to issues. Beck (2016) credits Dr Hadjiminas with skilful enrolment of the church to people, religious blessings to genetic screening, and in communicating with people locally in their own informal meeting spaces, such that an agrarian society came to embrace modernist technologies of prenatal diagnosis. However, what genetic screening, prenatal diagnosis and the potential for selective termination of pregnancy mean to people may be very different in other socio-historical contexts. At the Second World Congress on Sickle Cell in Rio de Janeiro in 2014, a speaker advocating such an approach of prevention was ill-received by the Brazilian audience. With a growing emphasis on an African-Brazilian identity as one framing the SCD experience in Brazil, an approach supported at that time by the Brazilian Ministry of Health through funding of sickle cell NGOs and initiatives, and an emphasis on non-hierarchical decision-making (rather than a genetic "control" programme) as a legacy of having only recently thrown off rule by military dictatorship, a Catholic Church opposed to termination, and with sickle cell presenting fewer acute pressures on blood bank services than thalassaemia, this meant that expectation of the Brazilian activist community was more focused on newborn screening to save the lives of infants born with SCD, and the human rights of those living with SCD, rather than on preventing births of people with SCD.

Third, beta-thalassaemia major is a very different condition from SCD in several respects. Although survival is compromised in the case of SCD, even in the harshest malarial conditions there are some adults surviving with SCD (Grosse *et al.*, 2011). They may survive partly on the basis of making use of traditional herbal medicines (Okpuzor *et al.*, 2008; Fulwilley, 2011) or through mutual aid strategies of sickle cell support groups (Dennis-Antwi *et al.*, 2011; Ola *et al.*, 2016), as well as by purchasing biomedical treatments. In contrast, beta-thalassaemia major remains fatal in the absence of biomedical treatments. Neither, with thalassaemia, is there an equivalent set of precautionary public health measures comparable to the benefits of newborn screening for sickle cell disease: identification of infants with SCD at birth and a range of measures (prophylactic penicillin, anti-malarial measures, vaccinations, health education of parents to identify key symptoms such as enlargement of the spleen or fever) with demonstrable benefits to the healthy survival of infants born with SCD. Newborn SCD screening is taken up further in Chapter 9.

Finally, the original rationale suggested as a reason for prenatal screening of women for sickle cell in the UK was to identify women with SCD in order to best care for the mother living with SCD during the pregnancy, *not* to identify sickle cell genetic carriers (Buckle *et al.*, 1964).

What is very clear is that, whatever the social context, in order to gain acceptance, a mass genetic screening programme needs to link to a strong social narrative. As we have seen in the case of Cyprus, this narrative was based on a collective Greek Cypriot identity. In the case of India, the Indian Prime Minister, Narendra Modi, developed his controversial career in his home state of Gujarat, where he managed to make sickle cell a central reference point for poor tribal families in South Gujarat (Modi, 2011), and thus position screening-for-prevention as a political act in their favour. Once he became Prime Minister of the whole of India, sickle cell prevention and high-tech cures were framed by Modi as part of the overall modernizing project of India (*Times of India*, 2014). In Brazil, the constellation of relevant factors was different again. Factors included an (alleged) uncritical acceptance by community activists of US cultural imperialism, which successfully transferred to Brazil hypodescent definitions of race, the so-called "one-drop rule", whereby having one drop of black blood makes you black (Bourdieu and Wacquant, 1999). The Brazilian context also included the post-1985 emphasis on human rights in reaction to the military dictatorship endured by the populace before that date. Moreover, in Brazil, the Lula da Silva government encouraged the linking of sickle cell rights to wider political rights of African-Brazilians in health and education. This produced a particular Brazilian context (Creary, 2018), one focused on newborn screening to save sickle cell infant lives, not prenatal screening to reduce births. As we saw in Chapter 4, the US sickle cell screening of the 1970s is regarded as a failure because it proposed segmented screening on the basis of the analytically weak concept of race, without recognizing the pre-existing widespread racism facing African-Americans and their further stigmatization by such ill-informed screening policies. And, as we have seen in Chapters 5 and 6, it has been possible subsequently to further prosecute racist social policies indirectly in Anglophone countries through the mediator of sickle cell.

Sickle cell screening: gender, ethnicity and disablement

Amartya Sen, the Indian economist-philosopher, has developed an approach to development studies that has come to be known as the capabilities approach (Sen, 1981). The devastating famines of, say, Ireland (1845–1849) Bengal (1943) or Ethiopia (1985), were not characterized by food shortages per se but by the lack of *entitlements* of local peoples to the means to obtain food. People were free to buy or obtain food but lacked the means or entitlement to do so. Crucially, though, this freedom is a liberal or nominal freedom. No-one prevented people buying food, but they lacked the positive freedom (capability) to actually buy or access food. This notion of a liberal negative freedom becomes important when trying to understand the rationale given for the prenatal screening programmes in a country like England, which followed increasingly neoliberal economic policies over the 40-year period from 1979. As the UK sociologist Beverly Skeggs (2014) notes, it is the same illusory liberal freedom as that of the worker "free" to enter a wage-labour contract. As she further notes, liberal contract laws are an enabling complement to capitalist wage-labour relations and depend upon notions of who is a "proper" (belonging to oneself or *propertied*) person, with women, racialized groups, the poor and disabled people all construed as outside such proper personhood. Thus, in neoliberal societies, such as the UK, antenatal screening raises issues of personhood with respect to gender, racism and disablement (Dyson, 2005).

Gender

To begin, let us take gender relations. The US sociologist Barbara Katz Rothman (1994) was among early critics of the expansion of genetic prenatal testing, arguing that this process was gendered in important ways. First, such screening focused on the woman who was thereby placed at the centre of a moral dilemma precisely *not* of her choosing. Rothman points out the irony that genetic screening in liberal democracies, based on notions of choice, ends with many women saying they felt they had no choice, being positioned by screening into bearing a burden of responsibility. Second, the uncertainty of a genetic carrier mother as to whether or not she might carry a foetus with a genetic condition, such as sickle cell, led Rothman to develop the concept of the "tentative pregnancy": no longer a state of enchantment, to be enjoyed precisely for the unfolding of an unknown, but to be worried and stressed over, and not emotionally invested in, just in case. Third, while genetic screening ostensibly increases nominal choice, real choices are structured by gendered power relations: a situation in which a male partner might leave, threaten to leave, or otherwise be unsupportive in the event of a disabled child being born. Finally, merely by virtue of being a programme in existence, screening communicates the message that the condition is regarded sufficiently seriously by the state to invest resources in it. Furthermore, this takes no account either of improvements in the biomedical treatment available, or any enabling policy legislation that challenges discrimination against people living with, for example, sickle cell or thalassaemia. Where treatment improves life expectancy such that key culturally valued norms (growing into adulthood, gaining educational qualifications, becoming parents and grandparents, securing employment) are increasingly met by people living with SCD or thalassaemia, at what point does the life expectancy and life quality of someone living with a genetic condition become so improved, medically and socially, that the original rationales for screening are themselves undermined?

Thus, the policy focus of prenatal screening has often been on the mother (Rapp, 2000). Given the focus of rhetoric on the ethical principle of autonomy, genetic screening, as we have seen, places mothers in the invidious position of responding to moral dilemmas not of their choosing (Rothman, 1994). Fathers' alleged lack of commitment to such testing has been regarded as a policy problem (Atkin *et al.*, 2015), since without the biological father being tested health professionals cannot know if the parents constitute a carrier couple and therefore cannot assess the likelihood of a baby having SCD. In the UK, in relation to sickle cell screening, this brings the issue of racism to the fore.

Racism

Since they are at the intersection of racist and gender discrimination, black women have been placed in an especially challenging position with regards to abortion rights (Roberts, 1997). In the USA, in a context where African-American men are disproportionately incarcerated; where children are still symbolically valued as representing the survival of the race by low-income women facing racism (Hill, 1994); where there is historical evidence of unwanted sterilization of African-American women (Davis, 1981) and in a context where there has been overrepresentation of black women in controversial long-acting forms of birth control (Roberts, 1997), black women have historically had to struggle to *have children* as well as not to have children. Freedom to choose with regard to abortion and reproductive rights, while still a value held by black women, especially younger women identifying strongly with black feminism consciousness (Simien and Clawson, 2004), is therefore not a neutral proposition to put to black women in any multi-ethnic society. Many Black British women, offered sickle cell screening, will be conscious of some of these historical legacies.

In England, if a pregnant mother is offered a blood test to see if she is a sickle cell genetic carrier, and if she is found to carry sickle cell trait, then the father is invited to be screened. If both biological parents are genetic sickle cell carriers, then the parents are offered prenatal diagnosis to see if the foetus has SCD (a 1-in-4 chance in each and every pregnancy). If the parents opt for prenatal diagnosis and the foetus has SCD, then the parents are offered the option of a medical termination of pregnancy. Although sickle cell prenatal screening extends the screening nexus to all men, White British men have no problem dissociating themselves from the issue as not relevant to them (Reed, 2011). By contrast, black fathers undergoing prenatal sickle cell screening have to struggle against stereotypes, such as being caricatured as lacking family commitment (Atkin *et al.*, 2015).

Fathers feel social pressure to be present for antenatal clinic appointments and at the birth, or at least to publicly account for the obstacles impeding this commitment. When, as part of prenatal care, they come up against sickle cell screening, they feel they have to "do the right thing" and display the "correct" disposition to sickle cell testing (Dyson *et al.*, 2016b). This disposition is to be docile. In a restricted sense, docile might consist of being obedient to health instructions handed down. In another sense, docile can be taken to mean teachable. Teachable also implies being passive or active as professional contingencies demand. Sometimes those being screened are expected to be passive (as when taking instruction from the doctor or from a midwife offering prenatal sickle cell screening) and other times to be proactive in actively seeking knowledge (for example, to question health professionals further so that the health professionals can assure themselves the client is now informed about sickle cell and thalassaemia).

However, when fathers are faced with other challenges in their lives (keeping a job, seeking asylum, getting health services to recognize their child's sickle cell illness when service providers are unfamiliar with the condition), this further complicates how they react to sickle cell testing (ibid.). When "invited" to gendered spaces such as antenatal clinics (an "offer" they find difficult to refuse if they are to counteract racist and sexist stereotypes imposed on them), they therefore have to juggle several forms of "display" to ensure their encounter with the health services runs smoothly. Sickle cell testing, prenatal diagnosis and termination of pregnancy may then be experienced as services to resist rather than a provision of service offering choice. For example, one father noted that he was actively included in discussions between health professionals and the mother. He contrasted this with his friend who, seemingly because he had not concurred with prenatal diagnosis and selective termination, was reported to have been deliberately excluded from such conversations, with health professionals refusing to speak directly with him when he answered the phone (ibid.). Another father specifically used the phrase "being good" (in the sense of being well-behaved) to describe his disposition when he acceded to prenatal diagnosis, citing the rhetoric of policy-makers identified by Hoedemaekers and ten Have (1998) that he was being socially appropriate in preventing suffering of a future child with SCD.

In England, prenatal screening for genetic conditions is often promoted to people on the basis that the services are providing "informed reproductive choice". However, some fathers get caught on a slippery slope in which, in order to be seen to be "doing the right thing", they have to struggle to resist genetic screening, prenatal diagnosis and medical termination of pregnancy that, at a complex intersection of racism, migration, citizenship, and gender relations, they may not actually welcome (Dyson *et al.*, 2016b). As Hill (1994) reminds us in other circumstances, a social context that engenders a strong pronatalist worldview will tend to subvert a framing of a child with SCD as an allegedly flawed child. This brings us to consider processes of disablement.

Disablement

Globally, up to 400,000 people are born with sickle cell disease (SCD) every year. As will be argued in Chapter 9, the lives of many infants with SCD could be saved through newborn screening. Advocating screening for sickle cell in a generic sense (not specifying whether this refers to newborn screening or to antenatal screening) has the potential to enrol sickle cell community activists to support newborn screening (to save lives) while actually buttressing antenatal screening (to make available the choice of termination of pregnancy). Furthermore, any prenatal sickle cell screening policies that present people living with SCD as a "burden", and that the way forward is the "prevention" and "control" of SCD through prenatal diagnosis are vulnerable to the criticism that they actively discriminate against the right to life for people with SCD. Thus, in disability terms too, even the most liberal versions of prenatal screening, versions based on the neoliberal concept of "informed reproductive choice", may be flawed in a number of ways.

First, health professionals involved in prenatal screening need to recognize that choice is not a gift that it is within their power to give to their client. What the life of an unborn foetus with SCD may be like lies in the future, and depends partly upon the severity of the sickle cell, but mainly on the context into which a child with SCD may be born. This context includes:

- the extent to which falciparum malaria is endemic;
- the availability of newborn screening;
- the accessibility of basic precautionary medical measures;
- the level of material deprivation into which the child is born, and the level of societal discrimination that prevails, especially the prevalence of racism and disability discrimination.

None of these factors, all of which affect what the life of a person living with SCD might be like, can be controlled by individual health professionals. In countries where people living with SCD find themselves in racialized, or otherwise politically oppressed minorities, the life chances of a person with SCD are likely to be greatly diminished, as racism itself damages health through inequalities in social standing (Wilkinson, 1996). Simply describing the way things are in terms of the variability of sickle cell over time and between different people living with SCD reproduces the fallacy that "how things are" is how things must be. This introduces an inherently conservative bias too, implying that situations cannot be changed. Relating to things as they are and not to what they potentially might be itself constitutes a form of disability discrimination against people living with SCD, since potential improvements for disabled peoples include the development and implementation of anti-discriminatory policies for supporting people with SCD in school, employment, housing, transport and insurance.

Second, in Dyson *et al.* (2016b), one father noted that a health education leaflet he had been provided with referred to the prenatal test as "for the baby's health". The father was sufficiently well informed about newborn screening to remark that the prenatal test could not be for the baby's health because, if health professionals did indeed wish to support the baby's health, they could wait until after the birth and undertake the newborn screening test (ibid.). Since the outcome for the foetus is either continuation of pregnancy (in which case there is no material difference to their health, provided the chorionic villus sampling or amniocentesis do not provoke a miscarriage), or termination of pregnancy, it is difficult to argue that the health of the foetus is enhanced by prenatal screening. Conflating, consciously or not, *the current foetus-in-the-womb* with *a potential other baby* created subsequent to a medical termination (as in the phrase *Towards a Healthy Baby*, Modell and Modell, 1992) is to mislead the argument.

Third, the notion of informed choice is closely aligned to its sister concept of making a decision. This fails in several ways to faithfully reflect what is happening. A decision implies a type of rational actor theory (taking one assumed form of competitive anti-altruistic economic behaviour in neoliberal capitalism, and imputing such behaviour not only to all actors but to actions in other spheres of life too). The concept of "informed choice" implies a rational decision-making model of behaviour that underplays the place of emotions in life. "Informed choice" also misrepresents what unfolds as if it were an event in time, whereas what happens may be better characterized as a process. Since, as discussed above, parents may feel under moral scrutiny to "do the right thing", they may feel they cannot refuse screening, prenatal diagnosis or selective termination of pregnancy outright (Dyson *et al.*, 2016b). Instead equivocation and delay may be tactics with the consequence of "running the clock out", prevaricating until the legal time limit for medical abortion is exceeded, such that these unwanted possibilities are "timed out" without the loss of moral position that would be a consequence of outright refusal.

Making sense of being a sickle or thalassaemia carrier

Being identified as a genetic carrier for sickle cell or thalassaemia has tended to be viewed by health professionals as being about making people aware of their reproductive genetic risk of having a child with a major chronic illness such as sickle cell anaemia or beta-thalassaemia. But the majority of sickle cell or thalassaemia genetic carriers will not be in a carrier couple and reproductive risk will be of less immediate relevance to them, though it may become so for their own children. We know little about how this large majority of sickle cell/ thalassaemia genetic carriers make sense of having sickle cell or thalassaemia trait outside of genetic risk. Having sickle cell or thalassaemia trait is presented by health professionals as a "diagnosis" and both sickle cell and thalassaemia traits involve actual changes in red blood cells. Together this means that expert pronouncements that they are "healthy carriers" attempts to focus all attention on genetic risk, and not on the impact of sickle cell or thalassaemia trait on the person's concept of their own body; on how they think about relationships with other family members, or on how they make sense of trait in respect of wider community folklore (Dyson *et al.*, 2016a).

As we have seen above, life-scripts of prevention and control of thalassaemia are historically linked to the Greek-Cypriot experience of the 1970s. However, in the UK, 50 years later, the views of those of Cypriot descent are more diverse. One respondent in Dyson *et al.* (2016a), pseudonym Anne, accepts thalassaemia trait as an unremarkable part of her Cypriot identity, but when her partner has an incorrect test result rectified, identifying him as a thalassaemia carrier, the threat is to her identity as a good citizen of Cypriot extraction, an identity founded upon not raising children with thalassaemia, as much as it is apprehended as a genetic reproductive risk. In the same study, Rosa and Duman make sense of thalassaemia trait by integrating it at several levels of their life through linking thalassaemia trait to food (bodily anaemia is addressed by eating food rich in iron; family relationships are strengthened through sharing food, and social relations with the Cypriot community are cemented through the family food business being used in supporting thalassaemia charities). Giannis and Alex, by contrast, mark a departure from the claims of Beck and Niewöhner (2009) for unanimity of support for the Cyprus model by Cypriots themselves, and assertively reject the interference of the state in their reproductive views (Dyson *et al.*, 2016a).

Previous research has looked at how people create narratives to help them come to terms with chronic illness (Williams, 1984) or to resist racism (Culley *et al.*, 1999). Being a sickle cell or thalassaemia carrier is largely a benign state, with health professionals mainly focusing attention onto reproductive choice. Dyson *et al.* (2016a) found that people link the new information that they are genetic carriers in order to tell stories about themselves in three ways. First, they use it to make sense of any bodily symptoms: unless they can make sense of having sickle cell or thalassaemia trait in this way, it leaves them feeling ill-at-ease. Second, they make sense of being a genetic carrier for sickle cell or thalassaemia by using it to confirm preferred family relationships and to distance themselves from unwanted family relationships. Third, they use having a trait to reaffirm, extend or deepen their communal identity. For instance, Black British Caribbean respondents struggle for recognition in opposition to the legacy of racism in the British cultural system. They name-check key historical events, such as slavery or the Tuskegee Syphilis Experiment, to link sickle cell trait to wider community struggles. This, in turn, provides them with a rationale for being ultra-vigilant in their dealings with services. They may need to fight to ensure access to desired care-oriented aspects of the provision of services by the state. At the same time, they may need to struggle against becoming entangled in the control element of state services, especially screening, prenatal diagnosis and termination of pregnancy, services that may be perceived in control terms by black women, owing to historical attempts to control black fertility. Meanwhile, British Muslim respondents struggle not to be stereotyped by wider society as having flawed family relationships in practising consanguinity. Consanguinity, a preference for cousin-marriage held by around 20 per cent of the world's population, is not a contributory cause of thalassaemia in the manner that some health professionals repeatedly continue to imply. The focus on consanguinity by health professionals is really an attempt to deflect blame (for lack of culturally competent genetic counselling services available in appropriate languages) by pathologizing people constructed as Other. In contrast, British Muslims with thalassaemia trait make reference to the trait, to consanguinity, and to raising a child with thalassaemia in a sometimes hostile environment for British Muslims, as part of an overall ethical life (ibid.). Health professionals who only focus on the reproductive risk element of having sickle cell or thalassaemia trait emphasize informed reproductive *choice*, but informed *care* would attend to the broader concerns of people who have sickle cell or thalassaemia trait.

The implications of the Dyson *et al.* (2016a) study are that we need to attend more seriously to factors other than reproductive risk in relating to people who have sickle cell or thalassaemia trait. At present, health professionals focus on reproductive risk, but do not attend to the individual health concerns of genetic carriers. This is unhelpful as public health advice to the effect that, on the whole, sickle cell or thalassaemia trait are harmless carriers, ignores substantial variations within those who have the trait (proportion of haemoglobin that is sickle haemoglobin in the case of sickle cell trait; measurable degree of anaemia in those who are genetic thalassaemia carriers). We have such individual clinical information available, but at present the details of laboratory reports are effectively discarded and those living with sickle cell or thalassaemia trait are given cursory explanations relevant to genetic risk, but left unsupported with respect to any felt symptoms.

Conclusion

This chapter has considered the issues surrounding prenatal screening for sickle cell. The experience of screening in Cyprus in the twentieth century for thalassaemia was specific to time, manner and place. Screening policies, as with medicine more broadly, tend to be formed in the image of wider societal values, material circumstances and cultural histories. Since the values of neoliberalism partly rest on placing people outside proper personhood (Skeggs, 2014), it becomes necessary to interrogate the relation of screening to gender, racism and disablement. This reveals both mothers and fathers are positioned into morally challenging situations that they then have to expend considerable emotional energy upon. Meanwhile, little attention is paid to genetic carriers outside of genetic risk, even though the trait may have significant implications for their health, their identity and their place in their community.

In particular, this chapter raises questions about the appropriateness of the policy goal of "informed reproductive choice". First, this is not within the power of individual health professionals to give to their clients. What the life of a child with SCD will be like is in the future, and radically unknowable. Second, empiricist descriptions of current life chances of a child with SCD implicitly treat class and gendered inequalities, racism and disablement as given, introducing a conservative bias into the context of decision-making. A counterfactual assessment of what life could be like, given challenges to current oppressive conditions, would require discussion and debate of many of the issues raised in this chapter. Third, choice is a key resource in imposing a neoliberal governmentality onto a population whether they like it or not. As has been argued in this chapter, imposing a negative freedom on the many, while structurally only a few enjoy the positive freedom of entitlements, is an invidious mode of social control. Finally, as the Dutch ethnographer Anne-Marie Mol (2008) argues, there is a different logic to care compared to choice. Care is a relational concept in which caring is a reciprocal activity that varies across the life-span (Chattoo and Ahmad, 2008) and the format and content of care cannot therefore be prejudged in a screening protocol. In this sense neoliberal choice closes down opportunities for relating to one another, whereas care opens up such opportunities (Dyson *et al.*, 2016a).

This chapter has focused on prenatal screening, but in Chapter 9 the focus switches to newborn screening for sickle cell disease.

9   Newborn screening

Introduction

This chapter addresses the issue of newborn (neonatal) screening for SCD. As will become apparent, newborn screening refers to more than just a laboratory test to identify if an infant has SCD, but rather to a public health programme that screens and follows up infants through diagnosis. The chapter provides a brief introduction to a key organ in SCD, the spleen, and explains the link to newborn screening. The chapter further considers the situation before newborn screening for SCD in both more affluent and less affluent parts of the world. Challenges of screening, both in terms of technical specificity and in terms of a clear therapeutic rationale, were debated, but a 1986 study demonstrated the effectiveness of prophylactic penicillin in preventing infections life-threatening to a child with SCD. Many US states adopted screening between 1986 and 1991, though progress to universal newborn screening in all states took another 20 years. In the UK, introduction of newborn screening for different conditions at different times over half a century diverged strongly from relative incidence of births. In Africa, many pilot projects for newborn screening have been undertaken, but only one has run consistently for more than a generation. The newborn screening programme in Kumasi in Ghana has had dramatic effects, and the implications of this for how SCD is then regarded are discussed. The issue of how to inform, counsel, or otherwise take account of the many sickle cell genetic carriers identified as a by-product of screening for SCD continues to be a source of debate.

The spleen and SCD

The spleen is an organ sited in the upper abdomen below the left lung. One function of the spleen is to remove old red blood cells from the circulation. In older children with SCD, repeated obstructions of the blood supply in the spleen result in tissue scarring, and the spleen progressively loses its functionality. As we saw in Chapter 3, the enslaved person had a spleen so eroded that it was not apparent at all at autopsy. In younger children, especially from around five months to two years old, there is the possibility of an acute splenic sequestration crisis. This is when blood is trapped in the spleen causing it to enlarge to the point of filling most of the abdomen (splenomegaly).

In the acute splenic sequestration crisis, a massive drop in overall amount of blood makes it impossible for the heart to pump sufficient volume around the body. This results in a form of shock, with a risk of death within hours. Prompt treatment with fluids to expand the volume available to circulate and blood transfusions can enable the blood trapped in the spleen to move again. In less severe forms of SCD, for example, HbSC disease, there may initially be fewer successive obstructions in the spleen. When older, people with HbSC disease may exhibit a persistently enlarged spleen or retain the possibility of an acute sequestration crisis, and may have an operation to remove the spleen (splenectomy). Indeed, accounts in Ghana suggest that in the absence of: (1) newborn screening providing a definitive medical diagnosis of SCD; (2) affordable and accessible health service treatment of SCD; and (3) without parental health education about spleen enlargement in SCD, people are left with other types of non-medical cosmologies with which to make sense of their world. In one example, those with enlargement of the spleen or of the liver have been referred to as exhibiting a "demonic pot in their belly" (Dennis-Antwi *et al.*, 2011: 471), a reference to a folk belief that it is a witch's cauldron that is responsible for distending the abdomen.

Meanwhile the role of the white pulp part of the spleen is to fight infection, and those without a functional spleen, such as children with SCD, are especially vulnerable to a range of bacterial infections associated with symptoms such as blood poisoning, pneumonia, and meningitis. These two spleen-related risks are the key to understanding the potential of newborn screening for SCD. In the case of acute splenic sequestration, parents can be taught by health professionals how to feel (palpate) the spleen so that they can treat spleen enlargement as a medical emergency and seek immediate help. In the case of infections, daily doses of penicillin and appropriate vaccinations can reduce chances of contracting and dying from such infections. Health provider and parent awareness that a child has SCD can help draw attention to symptoms that require prompt treatment. Thus, it is a series of precautionary and preventive measures in relation to the usual, and the sickle cell-compromised, functions of the spleen that have developed to provide a therapeutic rationale for newborn screening for SCD.

Before newborn screening

Given the statistically very large absolute numbers currently born with SCD in Sub-Saharan Africa and India compared to births in North America and Europe (Piel *et al.*, 2013a), it seems reasonable to conclude that the overwhelming majority of infants born with SCD in the twentieth century would have been born in Africa and India, in resource-poor, rural and malarial settings, with few formal health care services. Statistics from DR Congo, Rwanda and Burundi found that out of 1,879 with SCD only 15 (0.8 per cent) were over 18 years of age (Vandepitte and Stijns, 1963). And as we saw in Chapter 3, under-fives survival with SCD in rural Nigeria was estimated at 2 per cent (Fleming *et al.*, 1979). Based on early twenty-first-century estimates of 50–90 per cent under-fives mortality for infants with SCD in Africa (Grosse *et al.*, 2011), coupled with improving survival among the much smaller numbers with SCD in the Global North, perhaps the higher end of this range, 90 per cent, best reflects a guess as to the proportion of all infants with SCD born globally in the twentieth century who may have died before their fifth birthday. Most infants with SCD who died would have been indistinguishable from those dying from the leading causes of premature infant death overall, including pneumonia, infections, malnutrition and malaria. Most infants with SCD who survived beyond five years would not necessarily have a diagnosis. Without a formal diagnosis, many would have proceeded through life without specific knowledge that they had SCD, and many would have died undiagnosed (Ohene-Frempong and Nkrumah, 1994). For example, an author living with SCD, born in 1960 in Nigeria, recounts numerous SCD symptoms and illness episodes before gaining a diagnosis later in life (Tamedu, 2005). Even at the time of writing, in a malaria-endemic environment without specific interventions such as newborn screening, nearly 70 per cent of those with SCD admitted to hospital in Kenya were undiagnosed until that admission (Macharia *et al.*, 2018).

An infant with SCD will not show SCD-related symptoms immediately. This is because, at birth, infants have a high proportion of foetal haemoglobin (HbF), a type of haemoglobin that combines very readily with oxygen. HbF is the main haemoglobin produced by the developing foetus between months two and nine of pregnancy. This foetal haemoglobin is only gradually replaced by adult haemoglobin, or alternatively, of course, by sickle haemoglobin in someone with SCD, by around 3–6 months. This has two significant implications for our concern in this chapter with newborn screening. First, and provided they do not succumb to malaria, it means the symptoms associated with SCD are inhibited from developing in very young infants in the first two months of life. Second, it means that there are much lower quantities of haemoglobin S to try to detect and to diagnose the infant. Early screening for SCD at birth was undertaken using samples from the umbilical cord (van Baelen *et al.*, 1969), but using the dried blood spot technique, developed by US microbiologist Robert Guthrie for phenylketonuria (PKU), was adapted for use in SCD diagnosis by the early 1970s (Garrick *et al.*, 1973). Difficulties in definitive diagnosis through electrophoresis owing to the presence of large amounts of HbF meant that confirmation through a second test, initially using a different form of electrophoresis (and later a complementary technique to the primary test), became a standard of newborn screening for SCD.

Recognizing SCD through the onset of symptoms in the first two years of life was reportedly a feature of studies in Africa before it became a feature of studies in the USA (Haggard and Schneider, 1961: 785). In their US series of 54 infants with SCD, early presentation (before six months) was associated with respiratory infection and a disproportionately high fever, and presentation before two years was associated with enlarged spleen or liver, or with dactylitis (swelling of hands and/or feet) (ibid.). Preventive interventions appear at this stage to have been confined to the initiatives of committed physicians and community activists, and were initially aimed at older children. For example, the New York clinic of Jamaican-born physician Yvette Francis, largely serving a black population in South-East Queens, had by 1970 screened 20,000 children for SCD with the aim that preventative care, such as prescribing antibiotics, could rectify a situation whereby most contact of SCD children with health services was as an emergency rather than as ongoing comprehensive care (Francis *et al.*, 1970; *New York Times*, 2016).

Newborn screening in the USA and the UK

We saw in Chapter 8 how the issue of whether or not to target (restrict) antenatal screening for sickle cell by ethnic group, or to offer screening to all irrespective of apparent ethnicity (universal screening) was the subject of policy debate and research into the twenty-first century in multi-ethnic societies such as the USA and the UK. Similar debates accompanied developments in newborn screening for SCD in those countries.

Grosse *et al.* (2005) argue that, before eventually implementing universal newborn screening, policy-makers in the USA and the UK gave greater credence to concerns of screening specialists about the various limitations and problems of ethnically-targeted newborn screening, than to health economics analyses per se. As Grosse *et al.* (2010) have pointed out, ethics and economics are entangled since expenditure on newborn screening entails an opportunity cost in not being able to undertake expenditure on another (health) initiative. It is arguable that political decisions rather than any insurmountable technological problems, may also explain the uneven pattern of adoption of newborn sickle cell screening by the 50 US states and the District of Columbia, since adoption of universal newborn screening varied from the first state (1975 in New York State), accelerating after the publication of the trial demonstrating that penicillin could save SCD lives (Gaston *et al.*, 1986) to the final US state to adopt newborn screening (2006 in New Hampshire) taking over 30 years to become universal in all states (Benson and Therrell, 2010). This disparity suggests political and social factors were also at play.

In the UK, although newborn screening for the inherited disorder phenyl-ketonuria (PKU) using the Guthrie dried blood spot was adopted from the late 1960s, it was not until 2006 that universal newborn screening for SCD was fully implemented in England. This may be because in both the UK and the US racialized minority groups struggle to secure equitable services in a situation where prevalence is conceptualized in contingent ways, to suit particular policy or political preferences. Expected prevalence of a condition can be calculated based on using the whole population as the denominator, or in a racialized, segmented form, using, for example, a minority ethnic group as the denominator. More importantly some tests may be introduced without publicly debated requirements to meet any threshold tests at all. This flexibility in framing populations in universal or segmented ways is important: it permits policy decisions to be made contingently and arguably to the advantage of the ethnic majority. When it has suited the UK state, it has focused on racialized segments of the population.

Racialization refers to the process of taking a situation where material circumstances determine the level of illness in a population (for example, tuberculosis in a resource-poor population such as Jewish immigrants to the UK in the nineteenth century) and treating this observable health differential as if it were a consequence of systematic genetic differences between groups (and, by implication, a product of genetic inferiority). Some standard statistical tests, such as Pearson's product-moment correlation and Spearman's factor analysis were deliberately created with an anti-Semitic motivation to "prove" the genetic inferiority of the Jewish population (MacKenzie, 1979; Gould, 1996). A comparable process of racialization was a feature of UK health policy in the twentieth century too, as various diseases of poverty, such as rickets or tuberculosis, or diseases of subordinated social standing (such as hypertension and heart disease, see Wilkinson, 1996), have been wrongly ascribed to ethnic minority groups, defined in opposition to a presumed homogeneous, presumed indigenous, white-skinned population, thereby racializing the former groups (Pearson, 1986; Nazroo, 1999). Moreover, poverty itself may be racialized: post-Second World War immigration to the UK from the Caribbean, largely to take up poorly paid, dangerous, or anti-social forms of work (night work, shift work, piecework) stratified migrants into relative poverty. Subsequently explaining such poverty of that and successive generations of Black British Caribbean people by reference to ascribed ethnic characteristics of a group is an example of racialization (Miles, 1982). Racialization, and its codification through the bureaucratic use of UK Census categories, falsely constructs bounded "ethnic groups" to whom genetic differences are then assigned, when genetic variations, as Livingstone (1962) pointed out, can only accurately be described as clinal.

However, when we consider newborn screening, the policy consequences of working with racialized segments of the population has worked in an inverse way. As Figure 9.1 shows, universal screening for phenylketonuria (PKU) using dried blood spots began in the 1960s when whole-population prevalence of PKU in the UK was 100 per million births. At that time, the British Black Caribbean group was the largest fraction of Britain's black population. Later figures, derived from newborn screening matched with UK Census categories, suggest a 1 in 8 carrier rate in 2007–2009 for the Black British (Caribbean) population (Streetly *et al.*, 2010). This suggests that, at the time PKU screening was introduced, the Black British Caribbean population may have had an SCD birth prevalence rate of 3,906 per million, or nearly 40 times the level of PKU. By the time universal screening for SCD was implemented in England in 2006, the overall prevalence of SCD in the *entire* newborn population was 400 per million, four times the level of PKU. Segmenting the British Black African population in 2006, and considering an expected newborn SCD numbers just for that group, yields an excepted newborn prevalence of 5,102 per million, or 50 times the PKU rate (ibid.). And yet it took less than another decade for four further very

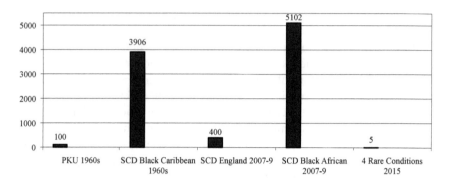

Figure 9.1 Estimates of prevalence at birth of PKU and SCD in whole and segmented populations in England, 1960s–2015.

Notes

Black British (Caribbean) expected birth prevalence 1960s was calculated on the basis of projecting back a 1 in 8 sickle cell-relevant carrier rate in Black Caribbean babies born in England in 2007–2009 (Streetly *et al.*, 2010: 628) to the 1960s, assuming no significant changes in gene frequency, random within-group unions, and no selective terminations 1 in 8: $[8 \times 8 \times 4] = 1$ in 256 expected births or 3,906 per million.

Black British (African) prevalence was calculated on the basis of 1 in 7 sickle cell-relevant carrier rate in Black African babies born in England in 2007–2009 (Streetly *et al.*, 2010: 628), assuming random within-group unions, and no selective terminations 1 in 7: $[7 \times 7 \times 4] = 1$ in 196 expected births or 5,102 per million.

rare conditions to be added to the newborn screening tests. In other words, just a few years after universal sickle cell newborn screening in England was implemented, SCD newborn prevalence in the Black British (African) population was over 1,000 times as prevalent as these rare conditions. This suggests that the uneasiness expressed by sickle cell community activists (Clare, 2007) and key sickle cell health workers (Dyson, 2005) has some basis: a sense that because SCD was (erroneously) seen as an ethnically bounded disease, as a black disease, it has had to meet incidence thresholds not demanded of other, rarer, conditions.

The Wilson-Jungner criteria on screening (Wilson and Jungner, 1968) have been regarded as both a gold standard of assessing screening, but more recently as a basis for ongoing debate and development of emerging screening criteria (Andermann *et al.*, 2008). The original criteria contain many phrases open to interpretation. The condition should be an "important health problem", but the criteria do not specify important to whom, nor a specific way of measuring importance. Brosco and Paul (2013: 987) suggest that PKU was of "marginal public health importance" but fulfilled an important emblematic role in medicine and science, garnering support of an unlikely alliance both of opponents of genetic determinism (PKU as a genetic condition can be treated by diet, an environmental intervention) and by advocates of genetic screening. As we have seen, screening for PKU (1 in 10–15,000 births) was implemented from the late 1960s onwards using dried blood spots. The importance of bacterial infections in

SCD childhood deaths was already known to clinicians (Francis *et al.*, 1970); newborn screening for SCD was technically possible not long after (Garrick *et al.*, 1973), though the key randomized controlled trial on the efficacy of penicillin in preventing SCD infant deaths (Wilson and Jungner's second criterion: "an accepted treatment for patient with recognized disease") was published somewhat later (Gaston *et al.*, 1986).

However, PKU screening became established for emblematic reasons and irrespective of prevalence (Brosco and Paul, 2013). In the UK, between 1986–2006 (the latter year marking the point when rollout of universal newborn screening for SCD was completed in England), both prevalence of SCD and costs of screening featured in key policy documents (Modell and Anionwu, 1996; Zeuner *et al.*, 1999; Davies *et al.*, 2000), barriers to becoming an "important health problem" not faced by PKU screening. Newborn screening services for SCD were not implemented until SCD was four times as prevalent as PKU *in overall population prevalence.* Ethnically bounding a disease like SCD, but then implicitly requiring that its prevalence exceeds thresholds across the unsegmented whole population, has thus proved an effective means of delegitimizing claims for SCD services over the second half of the twentieth century and into early twenty-first-century UK.

In contrast to antenatal screening, where, as we saw in Chapter 8, there may be tensions about the extent to which this may be regarded as a social good, there is a much stronger moral case for newborn SCD screening. Although no randomized controlled trials on the possible benefits of diagnosis of SCD at birth have been conducted (and now, ethically, could not be), there are reasons for believing that early diagnosis may lend itself to diverse medical and care interventions contributing beneficially to infants with SCD.

First, in comparing deaths pre- and post-1972, Powars *et al.* (1981) attributed improved outcomes to successful treatment of pneumonia septicaemia, arguing that this is easier to identify if health workers are already sensitized to look out for such a condition because one knows the infant has SCD, and the implications of a child with SCD who exhibits fever. Second, Vichinsky *et al.* (1988) noted a 1.8 per cent mortality rate for those infants with SCD diagnosed as newborns, which, combined with extensive education of parents and access to medical care, represented a reduced mortality compared to an 8 per cent mortality rate for those not diagnosed until after three months old.

In Jamaica, studies covered two separate periods of newborn screening for SCD. In the Jamaican Sickle Cell Cohort Study (1973–1981), parental health education to recognize and feel (palpate) the enlargement of the spleen and act on it as a medical emergency more than doubled numbers of episodes of acute splenic sequestration recognized, and reduced deaths as a proportion of episodes from 28 per cent to 3 per cent. A subsequent newborn screening programme (1995–2006) reduced deaths as a proportion of episodes to 0.53 per cent (King *et al.*, 2007: 121). The symptom-specific reduction in deaths suggests the possibility that parental education on spleen and spleen enlargement may represent an additional contribution of newborn screening to reducing early childhood deaths associated with SCD. The possible contribution of parental education on splenic sequestration is also suggested by the experience of the state of Minas Gerais in Brazil. There newborn screening began in 1998 and though overall SCD child mortality was about 6 per cent in an area where malaria is not endemic, one-third of the SCD deaths that did occur were attributed by post-mortem interviews with the families to splenic sequestration, with the authors consequently calling for better education (Fernandes *et al.*, 2010).

Around the turn of the century in the USA, the introduction of vaccinations (7-valent pneumococcal conjugate vaccine) for infants was associated in time with a decline in both the rate of invasive pneumococcal disease in infants with SCD (Halasa *et al.*, 2007) and with a reduction in respiratory-related deaths in infants and children with SCD (Yanni *et al.*, 2009, Lanzkron *et al.*, 2013). In summary, while it would stretch the evidence to claim definitively that various steps of newborn screening (sensitizing health professionals and carers to symptoms and treating those symptoms; penicillin, education on splenic crisis and vaccinations) each contribute to a reduction in morbidity and mortality, short of conducting a randomized controlled trial that would require the sacrificial deaths of some infants with SCD to demonstrate complete evidence, numerous studies taken together do attest to the worth of newborn screening for SCD. A summary is given in Table 9.1.

The importance of enrolment of children with SCD into comprehensive care following identification has frequently been stressed. However, what constitutes comprehensive care depends on the environmental context and may change over time. For example, in malarial contexts, it would seem plausible that malarial chemoprophylaxis, which has been shown to reduce malarial parasites in the blood of children with SCD (Eke and Anochie, 2003) should be part of comprehensive care of infants with SCD as part of newborn screening. Likewise, insecticide-treated bed nets (Figure 9.2), which aim to reduce access of biting mosquitoes to humans, have been shown to reduce childhood malaria, and infants with SCD, as has been repeatedly stressed, are very vulnerable to death from falciparum malaria. Furthermore, Killeen *et al.* (2007) report that good whole-population coverage with insecticide-treated bed nets was even more effective than targeting mothers and infants, and Hawley *et al.* (2003) suggest that there is a community effect in use of bed-nets in that those living nearby to those using bed-nets, but not using bed-nets themselves, also benefit from malarial protection. Taken together, Killeen *et al.* (2007) and Hawley *et al.* (2003) illustrate an important principle, namely, that an initiative involving all of a population may be the best way to improve the lot of a segment of that population. As we shall see in Chapter 11 on sickle cell in schools, this is a proposed principle through which a school policy on sickle cell might be effective.

What constitutes comprehensive care also alters over time. More recent additions to the list of key interventions improving morbidity include blood transfusions to prevent strokes in young children with SCD (Adams *et al.*, 1998), the use of hydroxyurea, a re-purposed cancer drug which increases levels of foetal haemoglobin and is associated with fewer sickle cell painful episodes in some

Table 9.1 Possible contributions of newborn screening to outcomes for infants with SCD

	Key issue	Reference
Cord blood screening enabled monitoring of haemoglobin level and blood transfusion	Screening enables a therapeutic intervention in principle	Van Baelen et al. (1969)
Diagnosis of infant with SCD, close medical supervision of SCD child with fever, and successful treatment of pneumococcal septicaemia decreased SCD mortality	Possible contribution of diagnosis, observation and treatment of infection with antibiotics	Powars et al. (1981)
Early diagnosis (cord blood screening) associated with increased hospital use and fewer deaths than late diagnosed group	Possible contribution of increased parental awareness	Nussbaum et al. (1984)
Penicillin prophylaxis reduces morbidity and mortality in infants with SCD	Efficacy of prophylactic penicillin in *preventing* infections in SCD infants	Gaston et al. (1986)
Lower mortality rate in those SCD infants diagnosed before 3 months old compared to those diagnosed later	Possible contribution of increased parental awareness	Vichinsky et al. (1988)
Early identification plus comprehensive care reduced case fatality rate for pneumonia septicaemia from 40% to 10% compared to early identification with no comprehensive care.	Possible contribution of increased health worker awareness	Lobel et al. (1989)
In a Jamaican cohort, parental education to detect enlarged spleen and act on it as a medical emergency was associated with reduced deaths per episode of acute splenic sequestration.	Possible contribution both of increased parental and health worker education on splenic sequestration	King et al. (2007)
The rate of invasive pneumococcal disease among children with SCD who are aged <5 years has decreased markedly since the introduction of routine administration of PCV to young children.	Possible contribution of vaccines to reduced morbidity in SCD infants	Halasa et al. (2007)
Association in time of introduction of a 7-valent pneumococcal conjugate vaccine with reduction in specific infection-related deaths in infants with SCD	Possible contribution of vaccines to reduced mortality in SCD infants (as part of overall reduction in deaths of all children)	Yanni et al. (2009)

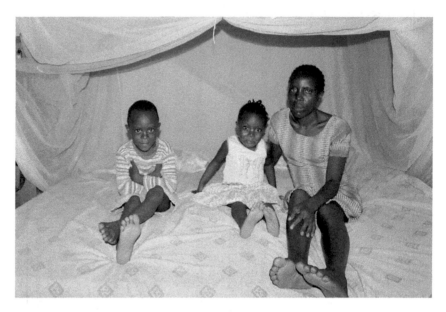

Figure 9.2 Malaria nets in use, Lagos State, Nigeria, 2017.
Source: With permission of Funso Balogun and Ayoola Olajide.

people with SCD (Charache *et al.*, 1995) and the use of Transcranial Doppler Screening in infants from around two years old, which can predict which young people have higher blood flow in the brain liable to make them at higher risk of stroke (Adams *et al.*, 1992).

Newborn screening in Africa and India

A key moment in the development of newborn screening for SCD in the Global North was the publication of a randomized controlled trial showing the efficacy of penicillin prophylaxis (*prophylaxis*: treatment given to prevent disease) in preventing deaths from infection in infants with SCD (Gaston *et al.*, 1986). For a while, there were arguments that the utility of penicillin prophylaxis should not be automatically assumed to be transferable from American and European contexts to Africa or India (Serjeant, 2005; Kizito *et al.*, 2007; Obaro, 2009). However, in a large study in Kenya, Williams *et al.* (2009) suggested that the infections most affecting African children, principally *Streptococcus pneumoniae*; non-typhi *Salmonella* species and *Haemophilus influenzae* type b, were the same range affecting infants with SCD in more affluent settings. They concluded that inclusion of appropriate vaccines within the childhood immunization schedules of African countries could greatly improve survival of children with SCD.

As we saw in Chapter 3, the 1970s Garki Malarial Study for the World Health Organization revealed that in a rural, resource-poor area of endemic malaria, in the absence of developed health care services, the numbers of infants with sickle cell disease dying before the age of five years was estimated to be as high as 98 per cent. More recent studies of under-fives mortality associated with SCD in Africa have suggested a range between 50 and 90 per cent (Grosse *et al.*, 2011). The health technology of newborn screening is of great importance in reducing rates of mortality and morbidity, whether in North America and Europe (Gaston *et al.*, 1986) or in Africa in DR Congo (Tshilolo *et al.*, 2009); Burkina Faso (Kafando *et al.*, 2009); Benin (Rahimy *et al.*, 2009); Angola (McGann *et al.*, 2015), and in India (Panigrahi *et al.*, 2011). One of these studies has also demonstrated the health economics case for the viability of newborn screening in an African nation-state (McGann *et al.*, 2015). However, comparatively little attention has been paid to the social consequences and potential of newborn screening for SCD in Africa and India.

At the time of writing, no African country has a national universal newborn screening programme for SCD. This is astounding as one early pilot screening project, using cord blood samples, was undertaken in what is now the DR Congo as far back as 1969 (Van Baelen *et al.*, 1969). At the time of writing in 2018, none of the pilot projects discussed above had been scaled up to be a comprehensive, ongoing, national programme, constituting routine service provision. To date, such initiatives have been localized to one hospital or region and/or have been time-limited research or pilot projects.

The reasons for this are numerous but plausibly include the uneven nature of capitalist development globally (Carter and Virdee, 2008), leaving many countries resource-poor; the operations of the banks of the Global North, and multilateral agencies such as the World Bank and the IMF, in keeping African countries debt-laden (George, 1988); and the corruption of some African elites in failure to build sickle cell health infrastructure as promised (Fulwilley, 2011). There are also a number of ways in which sickle cell as a health policy issue has been rendered relatively invisible.

First, there is the dominance of a mind-set that associates resource-poor settings with infectious diseases (principally diarrhoeal diseases, TB, HIV and malaria), rather than the chronic illnesses characteristic of the Global North. Since SCD is a chronic illness, albeit one also characterized by several types of acute episodes, it did not fit readily into dominant twentieth-century narratives of the health priorities in the Global South.

Second, SCD is a genetic condition. The practice of clinical genetics in affluent countries (at least until cancer genetics was realized) consisted of the identification of very rare genetic conditions. Applying a clinician-intensive model to the case of sickle cell, with carrier rates of up to 25 per cent and SCD prevalence rates at birth of up to 2 per cent in parts of West and Central Africa, means that SCD is not rare in those areas, and, considered within a clinical genetics model derived from practice in the Global North, would make a clinical genetics approach to sickle cell appear expensive in a resource-poor context.

Third, in situations where there are limited resources with which to build hospitals and train medical specialists, approaches to health care have focused on potable water and effective latrines; on primary rather than hospital care; on low cost interventions such as vaccinations, oral rehydration fluids and key generic drugs; and on training of local primary health workers stationed at decentralized health worker posts. In such situations imagining quality laboratory resources may not appear a first-line priority, even if the community-based health worker, recruited from within the local community, might represent a good model for the outreach workers needed to communicate newborn tests results to parents of newborn with SCD in Africa and India.

Fourth, early twenty-first-century conceptualizations of global disease refer to epidemiological transitions, in which the chronic diseases of the Global North (heart disease, strokes, cancers, chronic respiratory disease and mental illness) also increase in prevalence in the Global South. Research funds follow such diseases but ironically miss sickle cell, a major non-communicable disease of Africa and India, out of account. Of course, building on the insights of Martin (1999) about health priorities, heart disease, strokes, hypertension, diabetes and cancers are all of course conditions through which it is possible to repatriate the profits of pharmaceutical companies, medical technology companies and clinical research expertise to the Global North.

SCD has been by-passed as a priority because: (1) it is not an infectious disease (though infections do form a major part of its symptomatology); (2) as a genetic condition the lens through which SCD is seen has been the clinical genetics perspective; (3) the presumption was that it was too technologically expensive for settings underdeveloped by the Global North to be resource-poor; and (4) the notion of an epidemiological transition mimics the assumption of progress related to economic growth related to diseases of affluence. All of these framings have contributed to the ongoing marginalization of SCD.

This marginalization has been associated with attempts to target screening in order to reduce presumed costs of universal screening. In Mali, for example, targeted sequential screening, in which pregnant mothers are given a sickle cell solubility test and then only infants where the mother has sickle cell trait are screened for SCD at birth, has been shown to miss more than one in six infants with SCD largely because the sickle solubility test fails to identify mothers who are haemoglobin C genetic carriers who subsequently give birth to infants with haemoglobin SC disease (Diallo *et al.*, 2018).

Meanwhile, universal newborn screening is technologically possible in an African context. In epidemiological terms, newborn screening, if nested in an appropriate health care system, holds out the promise of saving millions of lives of infants with SCD in the course of the twenty-first century (Figure 9.3) (Piel *et al.*, 2013b). Newborn screening for SCD is also feasible in health economics terms (McGann *et al.*, 2015). The one programme that has been running for more than a generation is in Kumasi in Ghana, and from which it is argued we can infer important lessons for the social consequences of newborn SCD screening in Africa, is the subject of the next section.

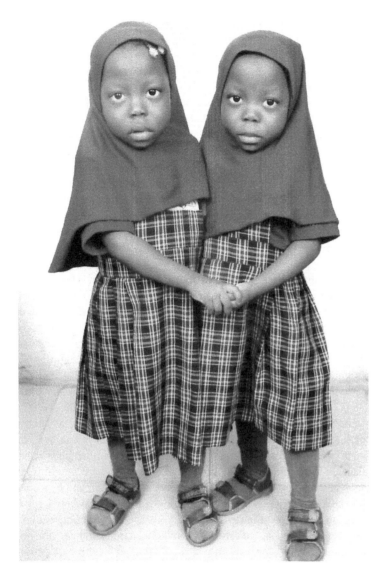

Figure 9.3 Identical twins with SCD.

Source: With permission of Funso Balogun and Ayoola Olajide.

Newborn sickle cell screening in Kumasi, Ghana

Kumasi is the second city of Ghana, situated in the Ashanti region. A pilot newborn screening programme was established by the US-Ghanaian Professor of Paediatrics, Kwaku Ohene-Frempong, with a health communication specialist Jemima Dennis-Antwi, beginning in 1995. Originally developed with a National

Institutes of Health grant, the programme has been in operation for over 20 years (1995–). A feature of the programme has been the use of outreach health workers to follow up mothers of those identified as having SCD, including in some rural areas around Kumasi. Of the 87 per cent who were followed up and enrolled in a SCD care programme, there was a 95 per cent under-fives survival rate (Dennis-Antwi *et al.*, 2008). Given that the Garki Malaria Study in Nigeria in the 1970s modelled a 98 per cent under-fives death rate for infants with SCD (Fleming *et al.*, 1979), this reversal is remarkable. Furthermore, the length of time the programme was in continuous operation has permitted cohorts of children with SCD to grow into adults with SCD. In this respect, the programme represents both a unique situation (any other newborn screening programmes just beginning will not see SCD cohorts develop for another decade) and an indication of how the global SCD experience might be transformed by newborn screening in the future (Piel *et al.*, 2014). More than a decade after the programme began, a study of fathers' reactions to having a child with SCD was conducted (Dennis-Antwi *et al.*, 2011). There are several important learning points that derive from this study.

There has arguably been a tendency to exoticize folk beliefs in Africa and to contrast this with the progress of science and technology of the Global North (Edelstein, 1986). Nzewi (2001) describes a large overlap between children with a modern SCD diagnosis and those who in African folklore are *malevolent ogbanje*: children from the spirit world placed within households to undermine families. Nzewi refers specifically to *ogbanje* in the beliefs of the Igbo in SE Nigeria, but Ebomoyi (1988: 37) suggests similar categories of spirit children are in evidence in the traditions of the Yoruba in SW Nigeria (*abikus*); the Binis of the Niger Delta (*igbakhuan*) and the Hausas of Northern Nigeria (*dan-wabi*).

In such traditions, a grossly enlarged spleen or liver may become a witch's cauldron distending the abdomen. Legs covered with ulcers that fail to heal, or scarred from such persistent ulcers become chopping boards upon which witches and wizards dispatch their spiritually-acquired meat. Treatments are sought from spiritual healers and from herbalists, and may involve scarification and exposing the child to the smoke of an open fire. A first point of the Dennis-Antwi *et al.* study is that it is too simple to point to such traditions as part of "culture". Too often situations are attributed to culture when material circumstances are not accounted for (Ahmad, 1996): poverty, a lack of schools or health care provision, a lack of entitlement to such education or health treatment provision, and a lack of public health measures such as newborn screening all frame the situation in question. The point is made that in such circumstances health professionals can augment their status by contrasting their (technical, rationalist, scientific) knowledge with such beliefs, which can thereby be characterized as backward, ignorant or based on superstition. Quite apart from the different cosmologies that the realms of science and magic signify (see Chapter 2), the contrast functions partly as a discursive device through which the person can augment their identity as a professional, to themselves, to policy-makers and to funders. In short, the contrast drawn is part of a process of identity formation as a professional. In this sense, both indigenous beliefs and scientific knowledge are equally constructed from available human and non-human resources.

It was found that, when interviewed, parents of children with SCD did indeed refer to the supernatural and to practices such as scarification, spirit children and herbalism (Dennis-Antwi *et al.*, 2011). However, and crucially, these were referred to indirectly as discourses used by others (and implicitly not believed by the parents themselves) or used in the past (and no longer regarded as typical of contemporary practice in twenty-first-century Kumasi). Likewise, local health professionals placed great store by the sometimes extreme negative first reactions of parents to the news that their child had SCD. What health workers failed to recognize was that such despair was transient and not a permanent feature of parental reactions. Indeed, the claim that fathers regularly abandoned their SCD children was, on closer inspection, found to be generally untrue once the commitment of fathers who had to work at a distance in other regions or abroad, and a minority who had separated from the mother but continued with financial support for the family were accounted for. In contrast, both mothers and fathers of children with SCD developed child-rearing practices contrary to discourses of despair (ibid.). Thus, they acted contrary to expectations that children with SCD would "die today, die tomorrow" and purchased medicines for their care and sent their SCD children to school, in opposition to claims that such an education would be wasted. They learned how to be the carers of a child with SCD through praxis, and shared this praxis with other parents. An important concluding suggestion of the study was that part of funding for newborn screening should be allocated to help establish and run support groups for parents and their children with SCD (ibid.).

Thus, the study found that parents of children with SCD refer to supernatural discourses of despair around SCD, but do not necessarily subscribe to them themselves. This is not to say that indigenous knowledge was simply false and scientific belief true. Both indigenous knowledge and science assemble long chains of relations, comprising humans, non-humans and ideas, and building towards an accountable knowledge (see Latour, 2013), though indigenous knowledges precede science in working with the intimate connections of humans, ancestors and non-humans to climate and place (Todd, 2016). Rather than an absolute gap between indigenous knowledge and science, the similarity in structure makes a shift in allegiance from one to another possible. Thus, expressions of distress at the birth of a child with SCD are transient and complemented by modes of resilience, including the praxis of caring for a child with SCD and sharing that praxis with others. Part of what makes the change in outlook possible is the provision of newborn screening. The material difference that this makes is that it can create a whole cohort of young people with SCD, perhaps 1–2 per cent of each age cohort overall, who stand as an immediate embodiment, contradicting discourses that associated SCD with early death and lack of potential. As such, the Ghanaian example stands as a marker of potential futures for those living with SCD: what might be possible should newborn screening for sickle cell become established and widespread in Africa and India. The next section takes up the issue of sickle cell in India.

Sickle cell disease in India

In 2011, CNN-News18, an Indian English-language news television channel based in Noida, Uttar Pradesh, published a short news article online entitled "Six Die of Cholera in Kerala". The article reported questions raised by local politicians, and, as might be expected with regard to a water-borne disease such as cholera, reported on issues of access to water and sanitation. However, a further element of the report drew my attention. The article read, without any apparent criticism: "Health authorities say the tribals are affected with sickle cell anaemia and are prone to fall sick" (CNN-News18, 2011).

This example seemed to me to encapsulate all that is wrong when marginalized groups have a genetic condition strongly associated with them. The authorities fail to put in place a water and sewerage infrastructure that would prevent water-borne illness. They then deflect blame by drawing on the stereotype that deaths from cholera occur, not because all may be at risk of cholera, and especially those with compromised water and sanitation environments, but because of high rates of sickle cell anaemia. Even in groups with the highest prevalence of the sickle cell gene, the proportion affected by SCD would rarely surpass 2 per cent, and so cannot be a plausible explanation, as this does not account for the health of the other 98 per cent of the population who do not have SCD. Raising the topic of sickle cell (implicitly relying on a confusion between those who are carriers and those who have SCD, making such infants more susceptible to infectious diseases) is a classic misuse of sickle cell to draw attention away from the broader responsibilities of health authorities. It also draws on a reductionist conception of genetics. As Rose and Rose (1986) pointed out, being genetic logically equates neither with inalterability nor with social justice. Many health conditions, including genetic ones, can in principle be ameliorated by changes to the environment.

The association of sickle cell with African origins has meant a relative neglect of India as a site of SCD (Chattoo, 2018). Overall, India has the third highest number of global births of sickle cell anaemia in the world after Nigeria and DR Congo, with the states of Karnataka, Tamil Nadu and Maharashtra most affected (Piel *et al.*, 2013a).

It is noteworthy that the numbers cited in Piel *et al.* (ibid.) refer only to sickle cell anaemia (HbSS) and do not include other forms of sickle cell disease (sickle beta-thalassaemia; haemoglobin SD-Punjab Disease; haemoglobin SE disease), many of which will be relevant to India, and estimated numbers would need to be increased by around 20 per cent to account for these other forms of SCD. When these numbers are added, estimated numbers of those born annually with SCD in India surpasses 40,000 (ibid.).

Just as, globally, sickle cell has been associated exclusively with African origins, so in India a parallel problem of over-associating sickle cell with tribal groups has been in evidence. However, it is clear that SCD affects *all* communities in India (Jain *et al.*, 2012; Tewari and Rees, 2013) and is not confined to scheduled castes and scheduled tribes, though it does indeed have a high prevalence in some, but not all, of those groups (Ghosh *et al.*, 2015). In any case, as we saw in Chapter 7, although newborn screening programmes might commence in selected groups, there are many ethical and social problems with targeted screening (Dyson, 2005) and, in the USA and the UK, universal newborn screening, rather than ethnically-targeted newborn screening was found to be more appropriate (Grosse *et al.*, 2005).

There are many health issues facing scheduled castes and scheduled tribes that are likely to be determined by levels of poverty, the extent of social inequalities, and to a lack of access to basic health-protecting infrastructure and health services. A general principle of community development is that people are very adept at identifying both their overall priorities (not necessarily health, compared to family, housing and work opportunities) and their health-specific priorities. In the absence of newborn screening, infant deaths owing to SCD (respiratory tract infections, diarrhoeal diseases and malaria) will likely go unattributed to SCD in the absence of a diagnosis, as was previously the case in Africa (Ohene-Frempong and Nkrumah, 1994).

Notwithstanding the fact that all communities in India may be affected by SCD, the reported rates of SCD in some scheduled castes and scheduled tribes are high – for example around 1 in 50 and 1 in 86 births respectively in central India (Jain *et al.*, 2012), comparable to other high SCD prevalence areas of the world, such as Nigeria or Ghana. Moreover, newborn sickle cell screening has been shown to be feasible in the Indian context (Jain *et al.*, 2012; Panigrahi *et al.*, 2011). A research team has found universal newborn screening for SCD to be cost-effective in health economics terms in Angola (McGann *et al.*, 2015), a country with a per capita GDP broadly similar to that of India.

However, much of the research and policy focus in India has been on prenatal screening (Chattoo, 2018), rather than newborn screening, with the assumption that this can "prevent" the "burden" of SCD on populations (Patra *et al.*, 2011). A recent study of neonatal SCD screening in India (Upadhye *et al.*, 2016) continues to refer to the "health burden", while failing to foreground the fact that the newborn screening programme reported had itself resulted in only 8 per cent deaths after a three to four year follow-up. As discussed above, under-fives SCD mortality in resource-poor areas ranges from 50–90 per cent, so a mortality rate of only 8 per cent at around four years represents a powerful and positive public health intervention. Neither is this explainable solely by reference to the purportedly less severe Indian sickle cell haplotype, since the same authors continue to note severe (but treatable) symptoms in Indian infants with SCD.

If the views of scheduled tribal and caste groups are to be given central place in health development, as basic community development principles suggest they should be, then we can only adequately judge the attitude of scheduled tribal and caste groups, or indeed the views of any community affected to SCD, once we have given them the opportunity to see what the lives of those living with SCD are like years after the implementation of universal newborn sickle cell screening, where such screening has made possible the safe survival of the overwhelming majority of young people living with SCD into adulthood. Again, what is possible exceeds the empirical. What is possible depends upon the historically configured arrangements of humans and non-humans, technologies and policies, science and politics. Indeed, one might surmise that, once newborn screening is in place, attention is more likely to turn to how best to support young people living with sickle cell disease to attend and to achieve in school (Dyson *et al.*, 2010a, 2010b) and in moving to employment, parenthood and other valued social statuses.

What about sickle cell trait newborns?

Unless specific technological adjustments are made to hide the results, newborn screening for SCD also identifies infants with sickle cell trait, genetic sickle cell carriers of sickle cell. From the outset there were concerns expressed over technical aspects of the electrophoresis in use, including that the test might identify infants with Sickle Cell-Hereditary Persistence of Foetal Haemoglobin (HbS-HPFH), a very mild form of SCD (Rees *et al.*, 2010), and raise parental anxieties unnecessarily (Rubin and Rowley, 1979). At the same time articles considered that such results created another opportunity for education around genetic risk for current parents and the child in the future. A key ethics issue here though is that the children themselves have not given consent for the test, the result of which may be recorded in medical records without their knowledge.

A further concern is whether to communicate carrier test results to parents and, if so, what information should be given and how. The province of Ontario in Canada, which has an SCD birth prevalence of around 1 in 2,500 and a carrier prevalence of 1 in 60 births, informs the parents that a test result is available upon request but does not automatically convey the result to them (Miller *et al.*, 2010). In England, the test results are given to the parents, but practice varies whether this is through a face-to-face meeting, a telephone conversation, written information or a combination of these, and whether the information comes from a generic heath worker or a specialist sickle cell/genetic professional (Kai *et al.*, 2009). Information on sickle cell trait is apprehended not by individuals in isolation but within the context of broader family influences (Ulph *et al.*, 2011) and parents express the view they need greater support in communicating sickle cell test results to wider family and eventually to their child (Ulph *et al.*, 2015). Genetic information such as sickle cell trait status, when linked to parental trait status, potentially raises the issue of unexpected paternity, and in England the policy is for local areas to have a policy, though without specific guidance on what such a policy should entail. In Kenya, a thoughtful response to such potential dilemmas was to start with community-derived ethics in which the local populace was consulted in discussion groups about how to proceed with respect to information about sickle cell genetic carriers (Marsh *et al.*, 2013), leading to a strengthening of community views not to undertake paternity tests at all, in contrast to alternative courses of action, such as to undertake such tests, with or without disclosure of results to fathers.

There are specific controversies with respect to whether or not sickle cell trait has significant clinical consequences. Studies have found that some sickle cell community advocates articulated dissenting views and insisted that sickle cell trait has real symptoms (Clare, 2007; Miller *et al.*, 2010; Dyson *et al.*, 2016a). Many different versions of the significance of sickle cell trait are in circulation within the community, and different screening programmes highlight different cautions with respect to sickle cell trait, creating challenges for communicating with parents of carriers (Miller *et al.*, 2010).

In England, the policy with regard to carrier infants is that the GP (general practitioner, or primary care doctor) and the health visitor should be informed within six weeks. The information is provided to the GP, but analysis of GP records shows that conclusive information is missing in a significant proportion of primary care records (Little *et al.*, 2017). Often primary care documentation records the fact of newborn screening, and may specify a non-carrier result, though sometimes non-carrier status has to be inferred from lack of a recorded positive test result. Such record-keeping variations make a substantive difference in trying to assess if sickle cell trait is associated with conditions such as venous thromboembolism, a condition where blood clots form in a vein (Little *et al.*, 2017). To date, we know something of the preferences of the parents with respect to information about their carrier infant (Kai *et al.*, 2009; Ulph *et al.*, 2011; Ulph *et al.*, 2015), but some questions raised decades ago, such as by what specific pathway an infant with sickle cell trait might be offered genetic counselling in the future, and the uncertainties and complexities of any clinical implications of sickle cell trait (Laird *et al.*, 1996), have still not been addressed.

We know that, historically, sickle cell trait has been used to effect discrimination (Duster, 2003) but that most public health advice reports sickle cell trait as benign, largely in an attempt to damp down such discrimination (Hampton *et al.*, 1974; Carter and Dyson, 2015). However, there are lay reports of symptomatic sickle cell trait in North America (Miller *et al.*, 2010), the UK (Dyson *et al.*, 2016a) and in developing countries (Fulwilley, 2011); medical literature on (very rare) carrier genotype with disease phenotype (Rees *et al.*, 2010); and clinical literature making links between sickle cell trait and complications including venous thromboembolism (Little *et al.*, 2017), chronic kidney disease (Naik *et al.*, 2017) and (the very rare) renal medullary cancer (Alvarez *et al.*, 2015). There are also rare complications reported under certain environmental conditions, such as splenic infarction with SCT at altitude (Nair *et al.*, 2017); required caution in administering anaesthetics (Laird *et al.*, 1996) and arguments and counter-arguments about the possible relevance of sickle cell trait during intense exertion (Le Gallais *et al.*, 2007), the latter issue discussed at length in Chapter 5. We also know what parents think about how and when information about sickle cell carrier infants should be conveyed (Kai *et al.*, 2009). Information is currently lacking about what young people, who, according to policy standards, should have been tested in infancy, and who may have sickle cell trait, feel about having been tested using a process that revealed their carrier status and the communication of that carrier status to parents. Furthermore, since the status of sickle cell trait as benign but constituting a reproductive risk is complex, we do not know to what extent young people wish to engage with these complexities and what difference this might make to their views on carrier identification.

Conclusion

In conclusion, newborn screening programmes for sickle cell disease, when embedded in robust health care systems, seem to be extremely powerful programmes, capable of greatly reducing early deaths and illness associated with SCD, whether in North America and Europe, or in Africa, India and Brazil. To anticipate a theme of subsequent chapters, what health care around newborn screening requires us to do for infants with SCD, whether this be in terms of provision of malaria nets and malarial prophylaxis, in relation to provision of comprehensive health care free at the point of use, or with respect to vaccinations, is to implement a public health measure that reduces SCD mortality and morbidity but which often does so through measures that are of benefit to the whole infant population or simply to the whole population overall. The potential of newborn screening for SCD, operating within a well-functioning health care system, to save millions of SCD lives seems to me to be very real. It also stands in stark contrast to the over-inflated claims of those advocating that sickle cell screening (undefined, but meaning pre-conceptual or prenatal screening) can "eradicate", "fight" or "stamp out" sickle cell. Furthermore, when cohorts of young people with SCD are enabled to survive, then not only do negative discourses decline – discourses that sickle cell entails a certain and early death, that a child with SCD is not worth investing in, that they cannot find employment and become parents themselves – but the very existence of adults with SCD stands as a challenge to such negativity. We can then turn our attention to how to challenge discrimination against people with SCD (the focus of Chapter 10) and to how to support young people with SCD in their schooling and education (the subject of Chapter 11) and in their adult lives.

Meanwhile, the continued indeterminacy of sickle cell trait frustrates professionals who cannot tolerate ambiguities, and who yearn to give a simple public health message that sickle cell trait is harmless. It may be that we need to develop new categories which recognize that the ambiguity of sickle cell trait may denote an accurate reality (see Morton, 2017). Moreover, while calling for sickle cell trait research sounds tempting to try to resolve such ambiguities, it risks taking away from research monies from the eminently more serious SCD. Sickle cell trait seems to represent a classic case whereby working with a permeable knowledge boundary between professionals and interested community members is appropriate. In this way, claims for real effects of sickle cell trait can be taken seriously by professionals; warnings that misattribution to sickle cell trait risks masking other underlying causes of symptoms may be taken seriously by community members, and both professionals and sickle cell genetic carriers can become attuned to the types of misuse of sickle cell trait covered in Chapters 6 and 7.

10 SCD and the social model of disability

Introduction

In previous chapters we have established that sickle cell disease (SCD) represents a major global public health challenge, with estimates of up to half a million born annually by 2050. While some World Health Organization policy documents stress the "burden" of SCD and means to enact policies of "prevention" and "control", an alternative perspective is provided by the social model of disability. Although traditionally this model eschews identification with illness, in fact there is much to commend its adoption with respect to SCD. In this chapter, I look at the main features of the social model of disability and discuss the limitations of such a model. The limitations partly explain why racialized groups in general, and those living with SCD in particular, may have problems recognizing their own challenges within this model. We can explore this further through an examination of the theory of stigma, and through a case study of living with SCD and depression in Nigeria, a study which attempts to apply the social model of disability to SCD.

The social model of disability

In the UK, the phrase *social model of disability* has been associated with the disabled sociologists and with the journal *Disability and Society*. At its most basic, the model has five key components. First, in traditional ways of thinking, the issue, or more pejoratively "the problem", is seen as being located within the person concerned. This is an essentialist view in which disabled peoples are conceived in isolation from their environment and reduced to being labelled in terms of a condition, which is thought to define them in their entirety. For example, people living with SCD are sometimes labelled "sicklers" as if this reduction of their whole person to one emblematic symptom encapsulates all that they are. Second, in this traditional view, the disabled person is conceived as tragic, passive, and to be pitied for their situation, often positioned as a "sufferer" who is in need of charity to help them. Third, disabled peoples are frequently excluded in society – excluded from schools, from using public transport, from obtaining paid employment, and *in extremis* excluded from society itself by being sequestered in institutions, or from life itself by being subject to prenatal diagnosis and selective termination. They may also be excluded from the processes of research (Oliver, 1992). Fourth, professionals who work with disabled peoples may be regarded as beyond criticism or even as having saint-like qualities by virtue of working with marginalized peoples. My own earliest academic article contributed to the emerging critique of such assumptions (Dyson, 1986). Finally, the traditional view takes for granted what is normative in any given society: who is allowed to do what; what people should look like, or how people should behave.

The social model consists of a political strategy to improve disabled people's lives by inverting these principles. First, the problem is not inside the person but in the physical and collective environment. Thus the problem is not that the wheelchair user cannot climb stairs but that adaptations have not been provided or that laws have not been passed to ensure accessible buildings. In this instance a person is dis-abled by their environment (*dis*-abled: verb transitive, something done to the person, not a description of their state of being). The social model is a relational model and seeks changes to the environment that can be *en*-abling. Furthermore, the disabling barriers and enabling environments may be attitudinal as well as physical. Second, the social model emphasizes the agency of the disabled person: what they have achieved, what they can do and what they could potentially do were environments altered to be enabling. Third, the social model stresses inclusion of disabled peoples: in decisions about their lives, in designs of services for them, and in research into disabled people's lives. This concept of inclusion is captured in the phrase "nothing about us without us". This leads into the fourth challenge made by the social model: the very services and professionals, ostensibly developed for disabled peoples, may in fact be contributing to their oppression, and one way of avoiding such oppression is for disabled peoples to themselves take the lead in defining their own challenges and designing the appropriate responses to those challenges. Fifth, the logic of the social model suggests that what is normative in any given society may need to be challenged. This involves understanding and working with the concept of stigma, a concept around which the latter part of this chapter is based. The five points cited above, taken together, produce an orientation in which a disabled identity is transformed into a positive selfhood whose characteristics of motor, sensory or mental differences are embraced as affirmative of their value.

Challenges to the social model of disability

Even the original advocates of the social model of disability stress that it is a political campaigning strategy and not a comprehensive sociological theory (Oliver, 2013). We therefore need to consider the limitations of the social model of disability, but also to consider its enduring strengths in the face of such criticisms.

The first criticism is that it sets up an unsustainable distinction between the social and the natural, a feature of modernist thinking criticized by French philosopher Bruno Latour in his work, *We Have Never Been Modern* (Latour, 1993). Much everyday interaction termed "social interaction" actually entails mediation through animals and/or objects. Indeed, technologies and helper animals, in being the non-human mediators of human experience, could be the basis of enabling environments for disabled peoples. In this sense it might better be described as a collective model of disability.

The next criticism is that the social model of disability deals poorly with the body-in-pain (Hughes and Paterson, 1997). Part of the very reason for the social model is to stress that social discrimination can be the cause of pain: a key feature of the case study on SCD in Nigeria in the latter part of this chapter. However, this does not address pain that arises irrespective of human collective activities. SCD is a good example: no matter how much we improve collective circumstances or create precautionary environments that reduce triggers to sickle cell painful crises, people with SCD still experience severe pain of several types.

The social model also opposes the notion that disabled peoples represent a care burden on their families. If families are primary care-givers for some disabled peoples, then, in the absence of other mediating factors, they may exert a great deal of control over disabled peoples' lives. Sometimes this control may be experienced as oppressive and, within the social model, disabled peoples would wish to reserve the right to see the family as a potential source of such oppression. However, in multi-ethnic societies like the USA and the UK, most people living with SCD are black, and facing racism is a key experience in their lives. As such, the family may be a key resource in offering advice, life-skills, and protection against racism. Thus black disabled peoples, including those living with SCD, may not be in the same position as white disabled peoples to offer trenchant criticism of their own families.

Part of the social model is to confront normative notions of the human body. Thus, those born around 1960, as a result of the thalidomide drug scandal, were born with shortened limbs, termed, in disabling language, "birth defects". However, the assumption that this represents an incapacity is disabling, for people may write with a pen (using the clamp of the outside chin lowered against the shoulder to grip the instrument), paint (with the brush held in the mouth), or to pick up objects from the floor (taking off footwear to grasp and retrieve items between clenched toes). A disability rights view is that people are not reducible to an assumed standard anatomy and function of a "normal" body. But part of a racist ideational system is that it reduces black people to *only* their bodies (Shilling, 1993) and denies them any interiority, and sense that they have psychological depth (Skeggs, 2014) caricaturing black people as intuitive and spontaneous rather than deep-thinking. When, with SCD, a black body is scarred, in pain and invaded by medical technologies, then the UK installation artist Donald Rodney (1961–1998), himself living with SCD, provided one response. If a racist society reduces him to his black body, and that body is in pain, its surface scarred through operations and subjected to myriad medical technologies, then Rodney marshalled his own body, his own scars, his own body tissue and fluids, and medical technologies such as his own X-rays, all brought together in his art in a challenge to British society, a society conceived of as diseased because of its racism (Hylton, 2003).

A further key value enshrined in the social model is independence: independence from the control by others of their lives, autonomous and self-directing in one's own life, and free from reliance on those who might stigmatize them. Ironically, this emphasis dovetails too readily into the aggressive self-reliance and blame-attributing culture of Anglophone neoliberalism, leaving behind a trail of devastated lives of those who, despite (often weak, spurious and unenforced) claims of adjustments, are disabled by their bodies as much as society. However, in people who are under pressure, perhaps from a combination of poverty and resisting racism, the value is more likely to be found is *inter-dependence* rather than independence. Over the life-course people may be care-givers at one point of their lives and care-receivers at another. They may value such inter-dependence as it plays out over time (Chattoo and Ahmad, 2008). In resource-poor communities, all will eventually face periods where they depend absolutely on others, and those facing racism will depend on others for advice, practical strategies of resistance, emotional succour and even physical protection. The disability movement's emphasis on independence as a self-evident value is thus arguably one reason why it has struggled to reach out to racialized minority communities, and why people living with SCD may not readily subscribe to a disabled identity.

Some of the above criticisms of the social model, coupled with the nature of the SCD experience itself, help explain why people living with SCD do not make SCD a central part of their identity (Atkin and Ahmad, 2001; Dyson *et al.*, 2010b). Living with SCD, a highly variable condition, involves being periodically assailed by waves of extreme pain, undermining one's sense of autonomy. In such circumstances bracketing SCD in one's everyday life (until forced to confront it during a sickle cell painful episode) is a key tactic, in opposition to foregrounding SCD as a central part of one's identity.

Notwithstanding the very real drawbacks to the social model as a comprehensive theory, there remains much in the social model as a campaigning strategy that could be of use to people with SCD, not least in avoiding sentimentalizing SCD in order to raise charitable funds. For example, Tapper (1999) notes that in the US context of racism, it was not possible for the African-American SCD community to take advantage of the strategy of the television charity telethons which raise large sums of money for a particular cause. This is because telethons achieve their effect at the expense of requiring those living with the target condition to cast themselves in the role of tragic, passive supplicants, the better to evoke sympathy and elicit charitable funds.

Much of the remainder of the chapter centres on working through the implications of the social model of disability with respect to two particular contexts. The chapter draws further on the example from Ghana introduced in Chapter 9, but also introduces a new case study: those living with SCD and depression in Nigeria. Nigeria has the world's largest SCD population, and Nigerian SCD births are likely to increase from 100,000 per year to 150,000 annually by 2050.

Meanwhile depression was projected by the WHO to become the second leading contributor to global health challenges by 2020. One factor that has not been the focus of attention thus far has been the extent to which SCD is frequently experienced in combination with other long-term conditions (termed co-morbidities in medical terminology). In the absence of transcranial Doppler (TCD) scanning and blood transfusion, people with SCD may undergo strokes. The long-term effect of repeated damage caused following acute painful episodes may lead to long-term organ damage and, just to take one example, damage to the pancreas may lead to diabetes. People with SCD also have very high rates of asthma. Another well-documented correlate of ongoing pain is depression, and it is thus not surprising that people living with SCD may exhibit high levels of depression for this reason alone. However, some previous medical and psychological research on SCD and depression is unhelpful, limited to merely describing correlations of SCD symptoms, or service utilization, with depression. Moreover, it is potentially harmful to the extent it links alleged psychological maladjustment to SCD with depression.

Stigma

In this section I consider the sociological concept of stigma in relation to sickle cell disease. Like many sociological concepts, it has passed into everyday usage but, as Carter (2000) has pointed out, the use of concepts within a social scientific community requires greater precision, not least because the concepts stand in a logical relationship with other social scientific concepts. The section begins with a brief exposition of the original meaning of the term stigma when used sociologically and, in particular, its development by the US sociologist whose work brought the term to wider attention, Erving Goffman. It then draws attention to limitations in the manner in which stigma has come to be used in popular language and, by contrast, what a usage of "stigma" might look like if it is to remain congruent with the original meaning. This original meaning of the term stigma is then used to examine the possibilities for challenging stigma with specific reference to the experiences of those living with SCD.

In order to illustrate the points made, reference is made to two empirical studies. One is a study of fathers' reactions to the birth of a child with sickle cell disease (SCD) in Kumasi in the Ashanti Region of Ghana, and involved focus groups with health workers and mothers as well as in-depth interviews with fathers of children with SCD. As we saw in Chapter 9, the point of this study was to show that, contrary to naïve conceptions of culture (see Ahmad, 1996), the supposed African "culture" that allegedly stigmatizes SCD breaks down when a combination of factors emerges, such as the regular survival of whole cohorts of newborns with SCD. The second study is of adults living with both depression and SCD in Lagos State in South-West Nigeria (Ola *et al.*, 2016). This entailed administration of a validated depression scale identifying those from a sickle cell clinic who exhibited moderate depression, followed by in-depth interviews and focus groups with those living with SCD and depression.

The point of this study was to demonstrate the plausibility of the proposition that there are social pathways to depression and that, in the case of SCD, these pathways relate to the manner in which stigma is enacted, and may be countered using the same insights.

The trouble with the everyday usage of the sociological term stigma is not only is it inaccurate but it has deleterious consequences for how we think about SCD and the practical steps that may be taken to ameliorate the life of someone living with SCD. I would argue that, in popular usage, stigma has come to mean little more than the person is being discriminated against. Thus the following quotation of an adult living with SCD in Nigeria might mistakenly be referred to in order to buttress the proposition that the condition of SCD causes the person to be stigmatized (in this case, clearly, severely stigmatized):

> People say negative things to you and you are not happy to move with them. You pretend to live; you are a living dead; you can't live like others because of the restrictions: 'Don't do this, don't do that'. It is a terrible disease; you are not happy to tell people you have SS. It is killing; you lie to people because of sickle cell. They call you all sorts of names your parents did not give you: "ogbanje", "sunwonan" "wasting money", "it would have been better to have her pregnancy terminated". I always feel bad. "You are lazy, you are pretending", I get embarrassed, I become lonely and ashamed, I get depressed and cry.
>
> (Cited in Ola *et al.*, 2016: 30–31)

This linking of sickle cell as a medical condition, which ostensibly directly leads to stigma, can be found in sickle cell health care workers, as illustrated by the quotation from this health worker in Ghana: "In the Ghanaian society any ailment which is associated with high level of morbidity, mortality and chronicity is *automatically* stigmatised" (Ghanaian health worker, cited in Dennis-Antwi *et al.*, 2011: 474; author's emphasis).

However, this assumption that sickle cell mechanistically results in stigma may also be found in the wider health literature. For example it is claimed that "Young adults with sickle cell disease (SCD) are at risk for health-related stigmatization due to the many challenges of the disease" (Jenerette and Brewer, 2010: 1050); or that "The physical manifestations of SCD, such as smaller stature, late maturation, or disfigurements secondary to the disease can lead to feelings of stigma" (Moskowitz *et al.*, 2007: 64); or even that the (alleged) stigma of sickle cell attracts a "courtesy stigma" (to use a phrase in stigma theory developed by Goffman himself) for sickle cell trait: "SCT children also showed affection of all domains as compared to normal children, which was perhaps due to the stigma of the disease" (Patel and Pathan, 2005: 567). Moreover, parents of children with SCD may themselves take up such flawed conceptions of stigma. One mother is cited as saying "my family's got [SCD], so we shouldn't let many people know because it will stigmatize us" (Burnes *et al.*, 2008: 215). In all of these examples, professional, academic or lay, the concept of stigma is used inappropriately. We need to return to the original sociological text to understand why this is the case.

According to Goffman (1968), stigma represents a special discrepancy between *actual* identities (what people can do) and *imputed* or *virtual* identities (projections by another person, consisting of what limitations others presume they have). I propose a generous reading of Goffman, one that does not conflate imputed and virtual identities. If the actual is taken in the same sense as Bhaskar's (2008 [1975]) realm of actualized experience, then the stigmatizer imputes empiricist limitations onto the person. Meanwhile, that person's virtual identity, what they could do were they placed in an enabling assemblage (DeLanda, 2016), may require as yet non-actualized but real enabling mechanisms (Bhaskar, 2008 [1975]) to be brought into play. This may entail thinking counterfactually: thinking counter to the empirical facts and imagining what could be brought into actuality by altering the prevailing conditions or circumstances.

For Goffman, the distinction between actual and virtual is important because stigma is primarily about *relationships* and not about traits/characteristics/attributes somehow located deep at the core of people, constituting their essence. These relationships are social relationships to the norms and expectations of a society. It follows therefore that the operation of stigma will vary over time and place. Compare the work of Hill (1994), who examined the situation of mothers of people with SCD in the early 1990s in low-income families in the USA. A number of contextual factors operated so as to minimize the chances that SCD was stigmatized. Children with SCD, who were eligible for medical insurance and hence treatment, did not require the family to spend a month's income at a time on every illness episode. Before cuts in social security (the more apposite term for what are now mislabelled "welfare" payments), having a child would have constituted one sustainable source of income for a poor family. Access to US public schools would not have depended on the family's ability to pay school fees. Furthermore, the history of chattel slavery in the USA, which meant forcible separation of married couples, the rape of enslaved women and the appropriation of children as slaves meant the destruction of stable black families, but consequently then led to a lasting hyper-valuation of children as representing symbolic survival. Thus, the SCD mothers in Hill's study did not hear the implications of those counselling them against having further children; they did not accept that children with SCD were somehow "imperfect", because, like all children, young people with SCD represented the continued survival of African-Americans in adversity.

We can contrast this to a situation in many West and Central African countries, where health services are organized on a fee-for-service basis, meaning that families of a chronically ill child are faced with repeated payments for health care (Figure 10.1). This material situation may help explain the enduring power of the idea of the "malevolent *ogbanje*" (Nzewi, 2001), the notion that an ill child has been placed into the family in order to undermine its financial well-being (Dennis-Antwi *et al.*, 2011). In the absence of newborn screening for SCD, and in the presence of falciparum malaria, under-fives SCD mortality in Africa may be high, and the notion that it is therefore not worth a family investing in the

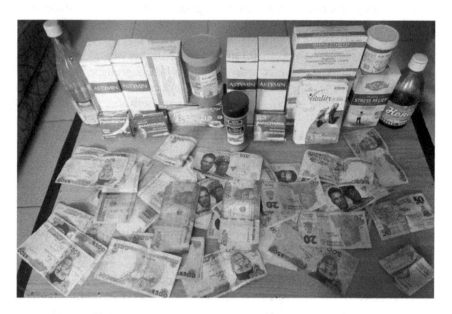

Figure 10.1 A month's family income for SCD medicines.
Source: With permission of Funso Balogun and Ayoola Olajide.

future of an SCD child, and certainly not worth the costs of sending them to school, may flourish. The pronatalist views of many African cultures, in which having a child to continue the family lineage is extremely important, does not override these other material factors until West Africans find themselves in a different social context such as the UK. In England, there is universal newborn screening for sickle cell, health care for children with SCD free at the point of care, and state-funded schools that do not charge school fees, and, coupled with the desire to have children to secure one's place in a country to which one has migrated, the family pressures to continue the family lineage reassert themselves. In such different circumstances the issues may be more about resisting unwanted offers of prenatal diagnosis of SCD and termination of pregnancy (Dyson *et al.*, 2016b).

From these examples we can conclude that stigma is not directly related either to the condition of SCD, or directly to its symptoms. Instead stigma is generated in the relationship that other people presume that people with SCD hold with respect to fulfilling the norms and expectations of a particular society. As we shall see, part of this also involves the relationship of someone living with SCD to the historically and culturally specific concept that people have about what constitutes "imperfections" in that society. Having outlined the importance of the original sociological usage of the term stigma, we now turn to consider how this sociological conception opens up ways in which discrimination against those living with SCD may be challenged.

Challenging stigma, part 1

The first possible way to challenge stigma would be to simply demonstrate that, contrary to the assumptions of those effecting the stigmatization, people living with SCD empirically meet norms and expectations of their society, contradicting the assumptions of others that they do not. Such norms might include an expectation that a child will live into adulthood, attend school regularly, be able to have children themselves, take up employment, and so on. In Africa, children with SCD may be stigmatized because it is assumed they may not live into adulthood, but in England where there is neonatal screening, treatment and social security (in the UK, state-funded payments paid directly to the mother to cover some costs of raising a child), the majority do live into adulthood. Telfer *et al.* (2007) cite a 99 per cent survival rate of young people with SCD to age 16 in their cohort in East London. Although focused on reasons for school absence, Dyson *et al.* (2010a) demonstrate that young people with SCD attend school on over 90 per cent of possible school days. People with SCD can clearly become mothers, and Chakravarty *et al.* (2008), for example, note over 4,000 births to women with SCD in the USA between 2002 and 2004. Examples of the employment of people with SCD were included in Chapter 9.

In short, there is often empirical evidence that contradicts the assumptions of those undertaking the stigmatizing. It is possible to demonstrate that people living with SCD *can* do and achieve things despite prejudiced assumption on the part of others that people with SCD cannot. One enduring assumption is that people with SCD do not grow old. But Ballas *et al.* (2016) have formally noted the presence of several octogenarians in the community of people living with SCD, and the world's oldest living person with SCD is currently 93 (Figure 10.2). This leads us to the second consideration of how stigma may be challenged.

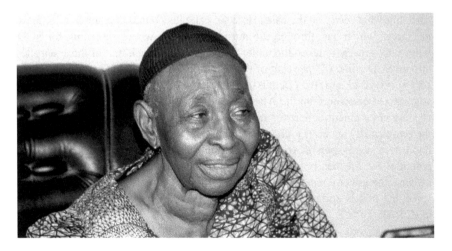

Figure 10.2 Alhaja Onikoyi-Laguda turns 93.
Source: With permission of Funso Balogun and Ayoola Olajide.

Challenging stigma, part 2

There is a second way in which stigma may be contested. This is to draw on the implications of the social model of disability (Oliver, 1998). As we have seen, the social model of disability involves relocating the issue from something intrinsic to the person concerned, to look instead at the impact of the collective environment. This is the sense in which it is the rest of us who *dis-able* the wheelchair user by not engaging in inclusive forms of building design in the first place. Although young people living with SCD do not make their SCD a central part of their identity (Dyson *et al.*, 2010b), "the disadvantages associated with haemoglobinopathies are often socially imposed as young people find themselves excluded, because of the inflexible attitudes of the wider society" (Atkin and Ahmad, 2001: 624). Thus it is not only the physical and collective environments that dis-able people with SCD but the attitudes of others in that they fail to create situations that *en-able* people living with SCD. Thus, from the perspective of the social model of disability, people with SCD could in principle meet societal norms and expectations, were reasonable adjustments made to way that we organize our society.

The relatively recent improvements in life expectancies of people with SCD in the Global North remind us that such increased survival is partly a product of a particular level of income and health services availability and that such survival would not characterize the population living with SCD in Sub-Saharan Africa, where currently only a minority with SCD are estimated to live into adulthood (Grosse *et al.*, 2011). The point, however, is to question not what is currently the case, but what could be the case, were adjustments, perhaps substantial adjustments, made to the way society is organized. If it is indeed the case, as Grosse *et al.* (2011) note, that there is a mortality rate of 50–90 per cent of under-fives with SCD in Africa, then the question to pose is not what *is* the case, but what *could be* the case. Here we can cite again the example of Kumasi in Ghana, which has, through the introduction of newborn screening for SCD, reportedly greatly reduced the under-fives death rate, such that of those enrolled into an SCD clinic (87 per cent of those identified by neonatal screening), 95 per cent survived to age five (Dennis-Antwi *et al.*, 2011). If children with SCD are stigmatized elsewhere on the African continent, it is partly because the national or state government concerned has failed to implement newborn screening, and the (empirically accurate) judgements that others make about the survival likelihood of a young person with SCD are not necessary judgements because the potential for life has not been actualized, and it has not been actualized only because the government has failed to provide for newborn screening, a newborn screening that is eminently affordable even in the African context (McGann *et al.*, 2015).

Likewise, one could consider the issue of mothers with SCD becoming pregnant and having children of their own. Smith *et al.* (1996) noted that, prior to their study, advice was frequently geared to persuade SCD mothers not to have children because of the dangers to their health and those of the unborn child.

However, such evidence was based on naïve forms of empiricism, for some studies compared the births to mothers with SCD to all births to women in the USA, thereby comparing a group largely experiencing the negative effects of poverty, racism, and lack of access to good quality health services, with more affluent white mothers. However, even the comparator of SCD mothers and all other African-American mothers represents a conceptually inadequate comparison. This is because, as Smith *et al.* (ibid.) argue, if care staff are neither knowledgeable nor trained with specific respect to take care of an SCD pregnancy, then greater mortality and morbidity will be in evidence than if SCD-knowledgeable and SCD-trained staff care appropriately for the woman. Again, simply to describe a correlation between SCD pregnancies and birth outcomes is itself discriminatory to the extent that it represents a "current-state-of-affairs" as a scientific truth, in contrast to an approach that recognizes the potential of changes in the collective environment (in this case, changes in health staff knowledge and training). Of course, this evidence also implies that were we to create a society in which African-American women were not living in poverty, were not subject to racism, and were all able to access full medical insurance, then birth outcomes would be better both for African-American women in general and for women living with SCD as a (largely overlapping) sub-set of all African-American women. A similar argument may be made with regard to schooling and SCD. As we will see, young people with SCD do miss schooling in the UK (Dyson *et al.*, 2010a) but it is not necessary to conclude that this is "because of" their SCD. This is taken up further in Chapter 11.

In a similar vein, one could examine the employment and work situations of adults living with SCD. But the capacity to undertake paid work depends on schools having robust, enabling policies that ensure school inclusions so as to make the best of a person's abilities, and careers advice that does not recommend completely unsuitable employment roles for someone with SCD. For example, one young person with SCD, not achieving strongly at school, was a talented artist, but was given the careers advice to become a bricklayer. As a physically demanding job this would be unsuitable for someone tired through chronic anaemia. As an outdoors occupation this would be potentially dangerous to be exposed to winds cooling the sweat of physical work (see Dyson *et al.*, 2011). Inclusion in the workplace is also dependent on a whole set of anti-discrimination laws that require employers to make reasonable adjustments to enable those with SCD to obtain and keep a job, and which prevent employers using illness episodes to effect dismissals (De *et al.*, 2016). To take an African example, the road traffic in the Lagos metropolis is notoriously crowded. The minibuses which many use to get around do not stop to take on board passengers, for fear they would not get moving again amidst the chaotic traffic. Prospective passengers must jump on to the minibus as it is moving. However, this leaves the person with SCD who has painful recurrent leg ulcers unable to use the urban transport system as it is currently configured. In order to make transport accessible to people with SCD with leg ulcers (or indeed with severe strokes, or with necrosis of the hips), reasonable adjustments to the transport environment would be required. This might mean lanes of traffic reserved for buses at the expense of cars; a law requiring buses to halt to take on passengers; a policy to make buses accessible for wheelchairs; and the attitudes of bus drivers reconfigured so as to regard their job as a duty to pick up passengers with SCD rather than an inconvenience. All of this in turn would require political will to pass the necessary laws, and for the attempts to enact and enforce those laws not to be countered by vested interests opposed to the ideas, for example, the owners of bus companies, or other motorists.

All of this brings us in turn to the recognition that stigma (and indeed bus design) are ultimately a political issue, it is about power. However, it is rare that an individual can successfully challenge long-term structured interests by themselves, and successful challenge requires the strength of a group. A first stage in this may be to ensure that sickle cell organizations are themselves constituted in such a way that people living with SCD feel that their interests are being faithfully represented:

> I support L because if we go as a group and we are the ones who bear this pain, people will listen to us and they will be glad to help. We need to work as a group. Even people at the sickle cell centre will be willing to work with us since we would be reckoned with as a group. As single persons we may not be able to do this alone.
>
> (Unpublished data from Ola *et al.*, 2016)

In this quotation, the person with SCD in Nigeria expresses a view suggesting that the sickle cell NGO concerned does not adequately represent the local people with SCD because none of the employees of the NGO are themselves people living with SCD:

> People should try and encourage people with sickle cell. They should not be saying that "these people, their life is too short, we cannot accommodate them, we won't give them job, and things like that." Some relations are even afraid to marry people with sickle cell. They believe that they would die during childbirth or they will die not long after childbirth. These are attitudes of people generally against people with sickle cell. So when you live in these kinds of attitudes, you will become afraid, you will not be confident. You will start to worry a lot. You will not want to mix with people. We need a lot of encouragement. People with sickle cell can live long, they can become good manager at work, they can contribute well to the society but they need the encouragement and support of people in the society.
>
> (Cited in ibid.: 32)

However, just as Brown and Harris (1978) suggest that social isolation of young mothers in urban settings may lead to depression, there are potentially social causes of depression in those with SCD in a country, such as Nigeria. Testimonies of those living with SCD and depression refer to extensive discrimination by others. Being widely and extensively stigmatized was interpreted by people living with SCD themselves as contributing to their depression. They also recount situations where this negativity is suspended by virtue of their various achievements, interactions and accomplishments (pride in work or educational achievements, or pride in giving birth and raising a child when no-one thought they could). But stigma is a relationship to societal norms not a consequence of SCD, and, upon coming together in groups, people with SCD recognize that what they would like changed are social arrangements, the very way society is organized. Broad social relations are thus argued to contribute to depression in people living with SCD. There is thus a need for *social strategies* (laws and policies relating to schools, transport and employment) to challenge attitudes and collective environments resulting in stigma and depression in persons living with SCD in Nigeria.

Challenging stigma, part 3

The third level at which stigma may be challenged is the most difficult of the three. This is because the challenge consists of asserting that the very norms and expectations of a given society are themselves flawed, oppressive, discriminatory, inappropriate or even morally wrong. Nollan (2016: 128) reports that as SCD became more known in Memphis, some black leaders had concerns "that there was a certain stigma attached to sickle cell disease and that ... delving into it was a plot to make the race look bad". This may explain why challenging stigma is such a challenge in the case of SCD. For, in the case of SCD, this requires a challenge to the power of disability discrimination in effecting stigma, in addition to a challenge to the power of racist discrimination.

One norm or expectation that characterizes certainly much of European and North American societies, but possibly the majority of societies in the world, is that the human body is a site through which broader moral and social concerns are enacted (Turner, 2008). One obvious example of this is the tendency to assign moral worth or moral disapprobation to the very physical features of the body, to the extent that people are expected to have the perfect body. For example, Dyson and Boswell (2009) cite the case of a prison doctor disbelieving that a female inmate had SCD since she did not exhibit the skinny frame anticipated by the doctor as a typical somatic feature of sickle cell. Furthermore, in Ghana, "In Twi language, children with SCD are described as *woayo ndwedwendwedwe*, meaning stunted in growth and likened to sugarcane in its knotted or segmented form" (Dennis-Antwi *et al.*, 2011: 467) and this is a source of both identifying those living with SCD, and the basis for stigmatizing them: they (allegedly) fail to live up to the ideal body. The 6'10" Nigerian actor with SCD, Bolaji Badejo, introduced in Chapter 4, was reportedly chosen for the seminal role of *Alien*, precisely because the director of the film thought that, once in costume, no-one would readily believe the body-shape (tall, spindly and insect-like) could be that of a human (Figure 10.3). In both instances people impute negative assumptions about the person. Based on their alleged deviation from

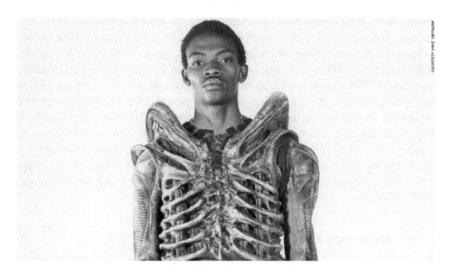

Figure 10.3 Bolaji Badejo: the 6'10" Nigerian actor who played *Alien*.
Source: Reproduced with permission of Mike Sibthorp.

what is considered an ideal body-shape, people living with SCD may be discrimi-nated against by others or may be publicly shamed. Here is a case upon which many might agree: the ideals of our society are themselves flawed, and this results in much human misery as people resort to extremes to try to approximate the so-called perfect body (Orbach, 2009). In such circumstances, one response may be to resist the very norms and expectation of society in order to try to reduce the levels of ano-rexia, bulimia, and lowered self-esteem that come with such societal norms.

One might find some level of agreement on the undesirability of what has been called "body fascism" (Pronger, 2002). However, if we consider a more controver-sial example, we can see more readily how stigma is intimately bound up with power and politics. A central norm and expectation of European and North Amer-ican societies is that adults should be independent and, either implicitly or expli-citly, should achieve this independence through paid work or employment.

Much contemporary neoliberal social policy has been centred on the implic-itly moral good of someone who works and the implicit moral blame attached to people who do not. This has led to applying "remedial" strategies to disabled peoples/those with chronic illnesses to help them achieve this socially desirable state, while stigmatizing those who fail to achieve, or aspire to, the subject of "productive" employee (Roulstone and Barnes, 2005). Unfortunately for those living with SCD, those very characteristics, such as assertiveness, likely to be of use in effectively mastering their SCD, have been shown to be inversely related to the prospect of achieving paid employment in the USA (Bediako, 2010).

Other authors are examining critically the norm that work is morally "good". For example, the idea that people can take control of their own career in a neoliberal capitalist economy has been called into question (Atkinson, 2010). Others have noted the undesirable, ecology-destroying and health-damaging nature of much contemporary employment (Graeber, 2013), leading to rejections of work as a social good (Frayne, 2015). Still others have pointed out that much work is devalued because it is the (usually female) labour of those engaged in caring work for future, current and ex-workforce members (Skeggs, 2014). Hence, in line with our broader argument, the stigma that an adult living with SCD cannot be regarded as a full and proper member of society because their illness means they cannot obtain or keep work can be challenged in three ways. First, this assumption can be challenged by documenting those living with SCD who are undertaking work or paid employment (Figures 10.4 and 10.5).

Second, it can be countered by pointing to the way in which employment, environment or employer practices could be adjusted to facilitate greater inclusion of people living with SCD into the workforce. But, third, one could begin to

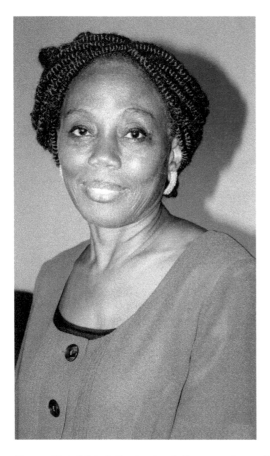

Figure 10.4 Adebola Benjamin, civil servant, Lagos State, Nigeria.
Source: With permission of Funso Balogun and Ayoola Olajide.

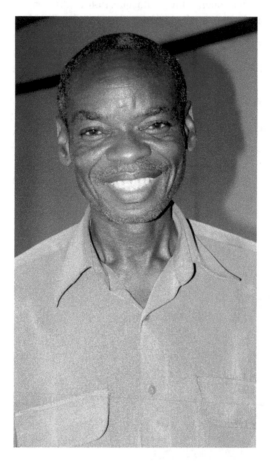

Figure 10.5 Ayoola Olajide, journalist, Lagos State, Nigeria.
Source: With permission of Funso Balogun and Ayoola Olajide.

question the appropriateness of making independence defined by work a central value of society in the first instance. Of course, this would require us to recognize that those enacting stigma are often the powerful, that is, the stigmatizers are in positions in which they can subordinate, regulate or exclude people with SCD on the basis of this power (Link and Phelan, 2014).

Conclusion

The social model of disability has certain drawbacks of particular relevance to SCD. In particular, the social model accounts inadequately for the bodily experience of pain, a key issue in SCD. Moreover, SCD sits at the intersection of racism and disability discrimination. In particular, the social model emphasis on independence is at odds with resource-poor communities experiencing racism, for whom the family may be a buffer against racism, and for whom inter-dependence may be more highly valued than independence. However, this has meant that the very real benefits of the social model as a campaign strategy have been denied to the SCD community. A challenge to discrimination is possible, one in which, for example, depression is not seen merely as somehow a natural co-morbidity of SCD, but one whose genesis is located in the discriminatory atti-tudes of others in society, and one which could therefore be challenged by people living with SCD working together in groups.

Likewise, some medical and psychological literature is mistaken in treating the origins of stigma as deriving from SCD itself. Rather, we must consider that the origins of stigma are in the societal roles and expectations that are assumed by the community to be inevitably broken when someone has SCD. Notwith-standing the complexity of SCD in that sometimes it operates as an acute illness, sometimes as a chronic illness and sometimes more akin to a disability, and that people living with SCD tend not to make SCD a central part of their identity (Atkin and Ahmad, 2001), the social model of disability offers some important insights in understanding and challenging stigma. The social model of disability addresses itself to the imputations that others make about people based solely on the fact that they have SCD. The social model can help by demonstrating that: (1) these assumptions by the community are wrong (both in the sense of factu-ally in error and wrong in a moral sense); (2) that these assumptions by the com-munity could be shown to be wrong if we made reasonable adjustments in society; and (3) that norms/expectations vary within and between societies and over time, and it is perfectly possible to argue that at least some of the norms and expectations of our own societies are flawed, oppressive or immoral.

However, any of the three aforementioned types of challenges to stigma involve addressing oneself to power. This means that change may not be forth-coming unless people living with SCD work as groups towards that change. Individualistic strategies may further isolate already vulnerable people and may themselves become damaging. In Chapter 11, we look in detail at one case of how one social policy, specifically, a policy for schools, could underpin a better life for those living with SCD in the UK and globally.

11 Sickle cell and social policy

The case of SCD and schools

Introduction

In this chapter I focus on one particular aspect of the lives of young people with SCD: their experiences at school. This is principally because this is the example I have to hand. Where sickle cell is marginalized as a research priority, and where sociology is under serial attack as a legitimate discipline (Dyson and Atkin, 2012), the opportunity to pursue funded research on sickle cell and social policy issues, such as education, employment, housing, insurance, transport, or family care has been limited. In meeting conditions of employment in a neoliberal university, securing research grants is a priority, and funding for screening and genetic carriers has been more readily accessible than funding for research with people living with SCD.

Research on sickle cell in school is a good place to start to redress this imbalance of research priorities, because, as we saw in Chapter 4, SCD was considered a disease of childhood until the mid-twentieth century in the Global North, and to this day remains associated with early childhood death in the Global South. In resource-poor settings with high SCD infant mortality, it may be that some young people with SCD are denied access to education at all. Where, following newborn screening, the majority of children with SCD can be nurtured through to age five, the issue of education for those living with SCD comes into view, though as will become apparent, those students with SCD do not necessarily feature prominently in the concerns of the education authorities. The chapter challenges the clinical and psychological framing of much research on school-aged young people and SCD, and outlines a particular context for thinking critically about silent strokes and SCD. The chapter then considers a body of empirical research in England, published between 2010 and 2014, comprising a national study of the experiences of young students living with SCD. This in turn led to the production of a guide to school policy on sickle cell and to attempts to develop equivalent resources in other countries. Throughout the chapter the focus is on how the social model of disability can usefully be applied to the issue of sickle cell in schools.

Challenging the framing of sickle cell in schools research

The majority of research on sickle cell and schools within the Global North has adopted the very disabling framework that was criticized, using the social model of disability, in Chapter 10. Abuateya *et al.* (2008) provide an overview of such criticisms of previous research on sickle cell and school-aged people living with SCD. Within much previous work, SCD is treated as a taken-for-granted condition, only the amelioration of which can improve the SCD experience at school. Both medical and psychological literature are implicated in this critique. Their focus is on the internal characteristics of the young person with SCD: either on their physical symptoms or on their psychological adjustments to those physical symptoms. In both instances, this ignores the basic possibilities of the social model: that negative experiences may be as much a product of collective arrangements as of SCD, and that while improved SCD treatments might indeed aid school attendance, school inclusiveness depends on the school environment and the school ethos, not on the individual characteristics of the young person with SCD. Moreover, while to focus primarily on the internal characteristics of young people with SCD is itself disabling, the psychological concept of maladjustment is especially pernicious, effectively blaming the person living with SCD for their experiences. Abuateya *et al.* (2008) note that much extant research also ignores the manner in which schools in the USA or the UK are situated within a broader experience of racism in wider society, an experience that does not require racism to be activated in situational interaction within the classroom to have an impact on the lives of young people with SCD at school in England (see Dyson *et al.*, 2014).

Meanwhile, studies on sickle cell in schools in the Global South have, to date, failed to foreground the experiences of young people living with SCD in their school lives. Rather such studies have tended to concentrate on knowledge of non-SCD students of their genotype (Owolabi *et al.*, 2011); on factual information about SCD, on attitudes of non-SCD pupils to those living with SCD, and on the degree to which non-SCD students hold stigmatizing attitudes towards those living with SCD (Bazuaye and Olayemi, 2009; Ola *et al.*, 2013; Olakunle *et al.*, 2013), or else studies focus on knowledge of genotype in relation to the issue of prenatal screening and prevention (Ebomoyi, 1988; Abiola *et al.*, 2013; Serjeant *et al.*, 2017).

The attention in the Global South, as in the Global North, has generally not been on support for the young person living with SCD. Evidence from the US suggests that an intensive intervention with schools can produce improvements in teacher and fellow pupil attitudes (Koontz *et al.*, 2004), but even such promising results demonstrate only short-term effects, and have yet to be built up to a comprehensive programme across schools nationally.

Silent strokes and SCD

The problem of focusing on an assumed "condition", rather than on circumstances which are dynamic, alterable and to be questioned, is encapsulated in the extensive research on silent strokes: a body of work which predominates in research linking schooling and sickle cell. As we saw in Chapter 1, haemoglobin is the protein responsible for carrying oxygen in red blood cells. In someone with SCD, the body compensates for lower haemoglobin levels by increasing blood flow to the brain. This in turn increases the risk for people with SCD of developing overt strokes, but also what are termed silent cerebral infarcts or silent strokes.

As the term silent stroke implies, the young person with SCD may show no overt symptoms, and silent strokes can only be properly be detected using a magnetic resonance imaging (MRI) scanner. Clearly silent strokes are important, though subtle, symptoms associated with SCD. These successive, smaller injuries to the brain potentially affect academic performance and ability to perform tasks. One-third of a large multicentre sample of children with SCD had undergone silent strokes, the proportion increasing with age (DeBaun *et al.*, 2012).

Transcranial Doppler (TCD) scanning to measure the rate of blood flow, in order to identify those children at higher risk of overt stroke, and place such children on long-term exchange blood transfusion regimes, has been a major contributor to reducing overt strokes in young people living with SCD (Adams *et al.*, 1998). In young people with SCD with normal TCD measurements and previous silent stroke, red blood cell transfusions may improve quality of life, but are reported to make little or no appreciable difference to IQ (Estcourt *et al.*, 2017).

Let us, however, consider a meta-analysis of 17 studies comparing SCD children with and without silent strokes (Kawadler *et al.*, 2016). In this meta-analysis, SCD children with silent strokes had a mean percentage points decline attributed to silent strokes of 6 IQ points compared to SCD children without silent strokes. The same study also noted that young people with SCD who did not exhibit silent strokes, as measured on an MRI scan, themselves showed a reduction of 7 IQ points compared to controls without SCD. The latter data leads the authors to conclude that factors other than silent strokes must play a significant factor in cognition in those living with SCD, including socio-economic factors.

However, there exists data on the experience of black pupils in England that provides a dramatic contrast to such clinical studies. The evidence concerns the falls in school performance of black pupils compared to local authority averages in ten areas of England (Gillborn, 2008). Across these ten education authorities, the decline in black pupil performance between age 11 and age 16 ranges from a fall of 8 to a fall of 29 points (mean =19.5 points) compared to the national average scores (ibid.: 101). Indeed, in one local education authority where scores were also available at school entry aged 5, black pupils commenced school 20 percentage points *ahead* compared to their white socio-economic peers, were 2 per cent behind by age 11, and 21 per cent points behind by age 16 (ibid.: 100). Thus, reasons to do neither with initial school entry ability of black pupils, nor with overall socio-economic status of a local authority area, account for a fall of 41 per cent points, over six times the average impact clinical authors attribute to silent strokes in young pupils with SCD.

This leads me to suggest that there are three important criteria by which to judge studies on silent strokes. One is the extent to which the study acknowledges the overall small contribution attributable to silent strokes to any decline in school performance compared to social factors. The second is to note that silent strokes have greater impact on school achievement rather than on ability per se. Hence it is plausible that performance is affected by school absences, and the social model of disability suggests that the inclusiveness of the school environment can reduce absences (Koontz *et al.*, 2004). The third is to assess whether the silent stroke study is linked to any practical educational intervention to help the young person with SCD make up any ground lost. The original purpose of IQ tests was not to label children and segregate them into separate schools or classes, but to identify and intervene with practical help. Subsequent misuse of IQ tests to discriminate in US immigration policy and their perversion into an alleged global, inherited, fixed characteristic (see Gould, 1996) have obscured this original purpose of IQ tests. Where the clinical study of silent strokes in pupils with SCD is not linked to practical intervention with that same SCD group studied, this creates a danger of inertia: what is to prevent teachers attributing poor subsequent performance to silent strokes in a form of self-fulfilling prophecy? Silent strokes may indeed be associated with a small but significant cognitive decline. But there is nothing to say that any such decline is necessary and could not and should not be remedied by an educational intervention. In short, the value of such clinical research lies ultimately in whether it is linked to educational programmes that prevent or reverse any cognitive decline identified.

Sickle cell in schools in early twenty-first-century England

Between 2006 and 2011, I led a team of researchers examining the experiences at school of young people living with SCD in England. Previous research (Black and Laws, 1986) had identified the salient issues: knowledge of which children had SCD was a prerequisite to providing adequate reasonable adjustments, but early registers confused SCD and sickle cell trait, and operated without the knowledge of parents. This failed the parents on two grounds. First, it failed them on the ethical grounds of lack of consent. Second, it failed them on anti-racist grounds in not recognizing the additional legitimate suspicion that secret registers would arouse in the black community (see Chapter 7). The Black and Laws (1986) study did not attract the attention it deserved, and other early works on sickle cell in schools were critical commentaries not based on original research (Dyson, 1992). A particular concern that motivated the study was that the social model of disability had hitherto had little impact on how people thought about SCD as an issue (Atkin and Ahmad, 2000b) and that the way forward would involve reconciling the real clinical consequences of SCD with not only the social model of disability, but with an understanding of how racism interposed itself in the lives of young people with SCD (Dyson *et al.*, 2007a).

The hints of how a social model of disability might find traction when applied to the situation of SCD in schools were already visible in outline in the existing literature (Dyson *et al.*, 2007a). When teachers were unaware the young person had SCD, they stereotyped them as different, invoking inappropriate labels such as HIV or problem drug use (Noll *et al.*, 1992; Noll *et al.*, 1996). Lack of support from teachers was cited as a reason that young people with SCD had difficulties in completing school (Thomas and Taylor, 2002). Absences from school in young students living with SCD were associated with educational attainment at school, but crucially not with performance of tests of academic skills per se, suggesting school absences undermine achievement but not academic potential. Even early advocates of strong heritability of IQ accepted environmentally achieved improvement in IQ tests of 20 points to be compatible with their model of heritability (Eysenck v Kamin, 1981), and any evidence of IQ decline would in any case have to be of comparable magnitude to be remarkable, since anything less is within the powers of motivated and adequately resourced educators to put right.

Since the thrust of the argument to follow is that some solutions to the challenge of sickle cell in schools involve collectivist actions, it seems worthwhile considering a particular decline in such collectivism in the context of the education system in England. In the twentieth century, local education authorities, overseen by democratically elected local councillors, had numerous benefits. Organization of education provision through local education authorities enabled economies of scale in purchasing; facilitated medical assessments of pupils; provided a nurturing staff development process for teachers, and made possible innovations in the curriculum, for example, around multiculturalism (Lowe, 2002).

Local education authorities could have had particular relevance for students with SCD, where there may be few or isolated individuals with SCD within one school, but considerable numbers at the level of the whole local school population. This appears to have been the benefit that enabled the former Inner London Education Authority (ILEA) to produce a written school policy circular for sickle cell in 1989, just one year before the abolition of ILEA in 1990 (Dyson *et al.*, 2008). The development of school policies, innovation in the curriculum, and specialist advice are all potential functions of a local education authority of potential relevance to young pupils with SCD. Individual schools may not have the expertise, resources or political will to effect change. In Chapter 7, it was noted that collecting data in (ethnic) categories that are conceptually weak and/ or failing to collect relevant data at all, render sickle cell invisible for the purposes of screening services (Dyson *et al.*, 2007b). Likewise, failure to collect appropriate data about young people with SCD in schools results in an institutionalized arrogance in which some local authorities in England felt able to assert that they had no students with SCD in their schools, even when they were in an area designated high SCD prevalence by the equivalent local health services (Dyson *et al.*, 2008). Conversely one local authority, although ranked only 122nd out of 150 local authorities in England for the proportion of black pupils in the district area (a proxy for SCD numbers necessary before the advent of a National Haemoglobinopathy Register in the UK) could identify five young people with SCD in their schools. Numerous areas in the top 100 for proportion of black pupils did not know if they had any such students; did not know the numbers of such students they had under their jurisdiction, or, *in extremis*, denied they had any pupils with SCD (ibid.).

Other responses of local authorities to what action they were taking on SCD support was met with reference to generic documents on supporting pupils with medical needs in schools. While representing a successful minimalist defensive strategy to deflect blame (the debased currency of organizational culture that is engendered within neoliberalism), such generic guidance failed students with SCD in several respects. First, it did nothing to help teachers appreciate the multi-system nature of SCD, which may generate numerous and superficially disparate symptoms, symptoms thereby liable to be disbelieved. Second, it failed to frame SCD as a preventable illness, and to change the school environment to reflect the need to avoid extremes of temperature; enable intake of fluids; facilitate frequent toilet breaks; avoid emotional upset, stress or bullying; avoid strenuous exercise; avoid cold, wet and windy conditions, and provide time out spaces when young people were in pain. Third, in contrast to conditions such as diabetes, epilepsy and asthma, it did nothing to address a situation where teachers and other pupils alike lacked even rudimentary knowledge about what sickle cell was. Fourth, in an issue later confirmed by our own empirical data (Dyson *et al.*, 2010a), it did not address the episodic nature of much of school absence associated with SCD. Fifth, the generic policy guidance did not engage with the benefits of the social model of disability: that improvements were best sought in challenging disabling attitudes and environments and instantiating positive framing of the potential of young people with SCD, coupled with enabling environments. Finally, although the one factor teachers might venture as knowledge about SCD was its association with black people, the extant policy guidance recognized neither the gendered not the racialized nature of disabling experiences. Being called lazy when tired from ongoing premature destruction of red blood cells occurs in a context where laziness is a long-standing racist stereotype applied to black people; being a boy with priapism (a painful persistent erection of the penis, unrelated to sexual feelings, but with a potential outcome of impotence if left untreated) carries greater significance in the context of racist ideas of black men's sexuality and sexual anatomy; a reluctance to engage in extreme exercise is framed differently where racist expectations of academic underachievement for black boys are coupled with a heightened expectation of success on the sports field (Dyson *et al.*, 2008). Moreover, as our later empirical study was to show, the issues that *were* addressed by generic guidance available to schools (emergencies and pharmaceutical drugs) were handled extremely badly by schools in the case of SCD. Young people with SCD were often subjects of demeaning situations of being put on public display while awaiting an ambulance (Dyson *et al.*, 2011). Denying a young person their insulin injection or their asthma inhaler would rightly be regarded as an abrogation of a school's duty of care to the young person. But three-quarters of schools in England were apparently content with a situation in which a young person with SCD was denied access to painkillers for middle or moderate acute painful episodes or for the ongoing residual pain between acute episodes (Dyson *et al.*, 2010a).

Since the study of local authorities in England in 2008, powers have been further devolved to individual schools, or to unelected chains of academy schools, and the lack of a local authority able to act for the collective good of young people with SCD, without undermining the profession of teaching, has further eroded the possibilities to improve the situation for young people with SCD at school. That situation is challenging indeed for young people living with SCD.

In a survey of 569 young people living with SCD in England, young people with SCD reported missing considerable time from school. On average, they missed 16 days a year owing to SCD-related illness alone, a level that exceeds the 15 days beyond which schools have a statutory duty to make alternative arrangements. However, the episodic nature of the school absences, typically in short periods of 2 or 3 days, meant that a narrow interpretation of the guidance (not taking action, for example, unless the absences comprised more than 15 days "in a row") was being used. This led to young people with SCD being unsupported. The majority of students with SCD reported that they were not helped to catch up their missed schooling (ibid.).

Neither were schools very good at instituting precautionary measures that might prevent young people with SCD becoming ill while at school. Half the children reported not being allowed to use the toilet when needed and not being allowed water in class; a third reported being made to take unsuitable exercise or being labelled lazy when tired from the severe anaemia associated with their SCD (ibid.) (Figure 11.1). Schools were therefore failing to take simple measures that would enable young people with SCD to remain well at school.

Neither did schools institute sufficient precautions to minimize the environmental triggers that might precipitate a sickle cell painful episode. Some 54 per cent of young people with SCD cited the school temperature (too hot or too cold) as a trigger to a sickle cell crisis, and 43 per cent mentioned unsuitable exercise

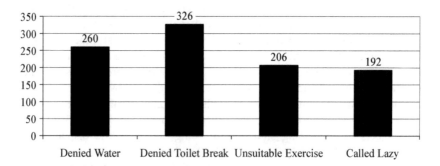

Figure 11.1 Reported experiences of young people with SCD at school.
Source: drawn from data in Dyson *et al.* (2010a).

as an antecedent to a painful episode. Being emotionally upset was also noted as a precursor of an illness episode: 30 per cent had been upset by a teacher, 25 per cent by another pupil (ibid.). One key factor around which bullying by other students was centred was being taunted for having yellow eyes. Jaundice develops if there is excess bilirubin in the body. Bilirubin is a yellow pigment that is formed by the breakdown of dead red blood cells in the liver and SCD is one of the causes of jaundice. Another issue was being bullied for "being skinny". People with SCD have higher metabolisms than others and burn more calories. This might usually become more noticeable in less affluent countries (see Chapter 10). However, with the imposition of austerity politics in the UK after 2010, and the accompanying growth in families needing food banks to survive, this may be an increasing feature of the SCD experience. A further focus of bullying was around being a "slowcoach", a reference to those whose physical exertions were undermined by their severe anaemia.

A common response to such lack of support to young people with SCD is to call for greater teacher awareness. This focus on awareness assumes that if only teachers knew about SCD, then appropriate support would automatically follow. The evidence suggests otherwise. Whether or not teachers reportedly knew that the student had SCD made no significant difference to reported negative experiences at school. Indeed, for some sub-sets of teachers, notably PE teachers, knowledge a child had SCD made it *even more likely* they would push them to undertake unsuitable exercise, call them lazy, deny them water or prevent toilet breaks (Dyson *et al.*, 2010b). This does indicate that there is the world of difference between hearing a term "sickle cell" and a deep appreciation of what that term means with regards to specific symptoms, especially when the person with SCD may look well to an outside observer.

A second dimension to the rationalist line of argument is to suppose that if only young people with SCD were to own their condition, tell others that they had SCD and what it entails, that this would result in improved school relations. Most young people with SCD favoured disclosure to teachers, because they hoped teachers would know what actions to take if they became ill and would make allowances for school absences. Some young people with SCD disagreed, citing instances of attracting unwarranted attention or of experiencing disabling attitudes (ibid.). Attitudes to disclosing to peers were ambivalent between acknowledging the reality of their sickle cell, and not wanting it to be a central part of their identity (Dyson *et al.*, 2011). Overall, about a third of students with SCD favoured disclosing their SCD to others at school, about a third were vehemently against this, and the final third were ambivalent and could see merit in both courses of action (Dyson *et al.*, 2010b). Since a major strategy of young people with SCD is not to make SCD a central part of their identity, and only reluctantly to acknowledge its reality when confronted with pain, (Atkin and Ahmad, 2001), this is at odds with the embracing of a disabled identity as a positive strategy, as would be suggested by the social model of disability.

A further factor to consider is the position of the teachers. As will have become apparent throughout this book, SCD is a complex issue. It can be thought of within numerous frames of reference: an acute illness (the painful episodes); a chronic illness (the ongoing anaemia and chronic pain); a public health issue to which preventive (avoiding triggers to pain) and precautionary measures (drinking water) may be applied; and as an illness that may be experienced as a co-morbidity. However, and crucially, it may also be conceived within a framework of disablement, in which (notwithstanding that the sickle cell body may sometimes itself be disabling) challenging the physical and collective environment could greatly improve the lives of those with SCD. The range of medical symptoms associated with SCD is daunting to keep abreast of, even for a physician. Teachers, though, are trained to be educators not medical practitioners. Furthermore, they have students with other chronic illnesses such as diabetes, epilepsy and asthma. They have children with myriad learning needs such as dyslexia, autism and learning disabled young people. They have to respond to pressures of working with children whose first language is not that of the school system. They have pressures with respect to government inspectors of schools, targets for their classes in examinations which feed into highly publicized league tables of achievement, and increasingly extensive interim monitoring targets and audits related to these broader targets. They also face potentially libellous remarks on social media from their pupils to which they have no redress, and sometimes violence from pupils. One union, representing teaching assistants, records 30 per cent of school support staff being injured through violence at school, with 57 per cent of that violence reportedly coming from pupils (*Guardian*, 3 June 2017). They also endure a unique pressure from politicians and wider society: anything that goes wrong with the current generation of pupils is the fault of schools and teachers: from teenage pregnancies, use of illegal drugs, to knife crime – the blame for all of life it seems can be laid at the door of teachers. In short, teachers are anguished. Despite this, many teachers in England support the increasing numbers of children in poverty in tangible ways, buying them food, clothes, bedding and even paying for family funerals (*Guardian*, 1 May 2018).

A lack of control over the terms and conditions of their own work is in evidence in the UK education system, where an imposed national curriculum, standardized testing and league tables of schools deny teachers opportunities to exercise professional judgement (see Ball, 2003). The work of the US sociologist Julius Roth (1966) is instructive here. Roth argues that where workers do not have control over the flow and pace of their work, nor any say in setting the ultimate goals of their work, nor any control over the way in which they organize their work processes, and where targets are then externally imposed on workers, we should expect the following developments *as normal behaviour* (see Dyson and Dyson, 2014). In the UK education context described, such factors include attempts to disengage from the original purposes of work in favour of strategies to short-cuts, circumventing the true purpose of the work (education in this case) in favour of a strategy to meet the imposed targets. One could become very judgemental of the school that, faced with a young person with SCD struggling psychologically to the extent he had attempted suicide, and being bullied by four other students, was not supported. Instead the school permitted those doing the bullying to continue to attend school, but offered the student with SCD six weeks of "study leave" around exam time. This had the effect of removing the student with SCD (who was achieving very weakly at school) from the school roll at the very time that standard educational tests were being administered, thereby slightly improving the position of the school in competitive league tables and school rankings (Dyson *et al.*, 2012). Or, bearing in mind the work of Roth (1966), one could conclude that such behaviour is actually normal behaviour when workers, in this case, teachers, are placed in oppressive conditions of work. This defensiveness is also behind the reported reaction of teachers to attempts by parents, usually mothers, to engage them on the specific needs of their child with SCD. The response of teachers tended to be twofold: don't make claims for your child as special among other children, and don't make claims for your child over and above the needs of all the other children I have responsibility for at school. This leaves parents (mothers) with an uphill, emotionally draining battle to engage teachers on the needs of young people with SCD in school (Dyson *et al.*, 2011; Dyson *et al.*, 2014).

Overall, young people with SCD were found to be regularly positioned awkwardly between the demands of their doctors, who advised on how they could remain well through self-care and taking appropriate precautions, and the practices of the school with its emphases on routines and consistent attendance. Even where good practice was in evidence in schools, the school concerned tended to address just one aspect of sickle cell in isolation and this was not consolidated into comprehensive school policies (Dyson *et al.*, 2011).

Therefore, what is required, it seems, is for an approach that recognizes that not all young people wish to disclose their SCD publicly and one that does not require teachers, who in England are anguished as a result of unbearable pressures on them and their occupational roles, to know extensive details about a highly complex condition. A change in wider school environments is required so that young people with SCD are supported irrespective of whether or not they want to speak out about their sickle cell, and whether or not teachers can bring to mind details about SCD as a medical condition (Dyson *et al.*, 2010b).

A guide to school policy on sickle cell

With the passing of the *Brown v Board of Education* judgment in the USA in 1954, bussing of children to desegregated schools meant that children with SCD might more readily be encountered by white teachers. In 1972, Lemuel Diggs was involved with the Memphis Sickle Cell Council's attempts to ensure young people living with SCD were supported at school so that teachers did not mistake anaemia for laziness and understood that strenuous exercise might precipitate a crisis (Nollan, 2016: 142). For more than half a century such a rationalist and individualistic approach to the issue has been both the dominant policy response, but a response that has shown few positive effects.

A feature of accounts of young people living with SCD at school is the breakdown of any reasonable adjustments when these are focused on individual behaviours. Sometimes this is because information degrades. The school may have been told that a young person with SCD needs to be well-hydrated and requires additional toilet breaks, but this information may not be passed on from the head teacher to the classroom teacher, nor when the young person moves class or moves school, nor when a substitute teacher is taking the class. A school may have agreed that a young person with SCD may keep their gloves/hat/scarf/coat on in class in order to keep warm, but this does not prevent many reported tensions as another teacher, or a teaching assistant or a school administrator, unaware of this informal arrangement, insists the person with SCD is breaking school uniform policy. Furthermore, such inter-personal tensions, *and* the repetition of them, *and* the anticipation of such incidents, *and* the emotional energy in challenging such recurrences, may each contribute the stress experienced by a young person with SCD, stress that, in itself, may precipitate a crisis. Being emotionally upset by a teacher was cited as a trigger for a sickle cell painful episode by one-third of young people with SCD (Dyson *et al.*, 2010a).

In response to the evidence from the sickle cell in schools' research programme, a *Guide to School Policy and Sickle Cell* was produced, and released as an open education resource in 2011, being updated in 2016 (Dyson, 2016). The guide was aimed not at classroom teachers and teaching assistants but at those with the power to influence school policy: school governors, head teachers, teachers with lead responsibility for children with medical conditions, heads of school nursing services and local Boards of Education or their equivalents. The guide provided examples of good practice that involved initiatives operating in the background, based on changes to the whole school or to a complete process within the school, rather than focusing on individual knowledge and behaviour of teachers. For example, one school developed an early evening catch-up session with a teacher present. Young people with SCD had told us that worksheets sent home were of limited value since they could not connect the worksheet to other learning, nor could they ask for the advice that might enable them to proceed through the worksheet if they became stuck. The twilight catch-up session, available for all young people who had missed school for any reason, enabled the person with SCD to make up educational ground, but without drawing attention to them as different from their peers.

An all-boys school with shorts as part of the school uniform was disciplining a young boy with SCD who tried to wear long trousers to cover the tights (pantyhose) he was also wearing to give him an extra layer of insulation from the cold. Eventually the school governors changed the school uniform for the whole school, enabling the young boy with SCD to wear long trousers indistinguishable from his peers. One school used a computerized timetabling system to ensure the class with the SCD pupil was never timetabled into their portacabin classrooms which were too hot in summer and too cold in winter. Another school negotiated with the local swimming pool to raise the temperature of the air and water when the class with a young person with SCD attended. Though positive initiatives in the spirit of the social model of disability – fostering inclusion through making reasonable adjustments to the environment – each individual school had only undertaken one such initiative. Hence it was an aspiration of the guide to persuade schools to adopt a suite of such initiatives and not just one.

In the sickle cell and schools research programme, a survey of 200 schools where there was a young student with SCD also found only 43 per cent had an individual education, health and care plan in accordance with government policy. The *Guide to School Policy and Sickle Cell* therefore also included a model individual care plan with suggestions as to who might be involved in drawing up such a plan and with generic guidance (such as not to use ice for sports injuries) on SCD. The plan also had space for individual-specific symptoms and complications to take account of the variability of symptoms between different young people with SCD.

The guide was developed as an open education resource (using a form of Creative Commons Copyright, CC-BY-SA), with the specific intention that others not only could use the guide freely but also that it could be adapted to suit specific needs. In the event, the guide was adapted with Nigerian educators, doctors and nurse counsellors and translated into Yoruba, Hausa and Igbo. It was also adapted to the situation in the state of Minas Gerais in Brazil and translated into Portuguese. An adaptation was undertaken to make the guide relevant to the context in Freetown, Sierra Leone, inspiring a sickle cell school song in Krio in the process (Macauley, 2018). More tangentially it stimulated the US Centers for Disease Control and Prevention to develop their guide (CDC, 2014) and acted as a catalyst to the Toronto District School Board to implement a policy for children with all medical conditions.

Conclusion

We saw in Chapter 10 that the key to understanding SCD lies in thinking counterfactually. A similar argument may be made with regard to schooling and SCD. As we have seen, young people with SCD do miss schooling in the UK (Dyson *et al.*, 2010a) but it is not helpful to conclude that this is "because of" their SCD. Schools have many ways in which they could (and arguably should) be inclusive environments not just for young people with SCD but for other disabled young people living with a chronic illness. As we have seen, environmental and social triggers to episodes of illness include being denied water or toilet breaks; being compelled to undertake unsuitable exercise; being upset by a teacher or pupil; being forced to be outside in inclement weather; bullying that is not challenged by the school; refusal to take responsibility for administration of mild painkilling drugs; and exclusion from school if administered mild painkilling drugs. Individual teachers already have too many complex educational and institutional issues to address to be able to be knowledgeable about each and every illness, disability or special learning needs of all their pupils. Moreover, some young people do not wish to disclose their SCD to others. For these reasons an approach that simply aims to raise awareness of sickle cell among teachers is insufficient to make a difference in reducing discriminatory behaviours and actions against young people with SCD at school (Dyson *et al.*, 2010b).

Instead a policy is required that supports young people with SCD in school by making adjustments at the whole school level without drawing attention to young people with SCD as somehow different from their peers (Dyson, 2016), a policy that does not place the onus on teachers to remember details about SCD and its myriad symptoms, a policy that, in line with the social model of disability, adjusts the collective environment of the school. A school environment and culture can be devised that *en-ables* young people with SCD to attend school regularly, to achieve academically and to be socially included, thereby enabling them to flourish.

Conclusion

In this book I have attempted to show that there is much to think about with respect to SCD beyond important work in basic and clinical science. In the early chapters of the book, I tried to stress that sickle cell is first and foremost a genetic adaptation to malarial pressures and not an essential correlate of black skin. It is a complex as well as variable condition, and Chapter 1 discussed how the simplifications devised for community education do sickle cell a disservice in two crucial respects. First, the shape of the red blood cell that has given sickle cell its very name (in the Global North) has meant that not only were SCD and sickle cell trait inadequately distinguished (since both were associated with sickling in the sickle solubility test) but also that other key mechanisms, for example, the ongoing premature destruction of red blood cells then associated with anaemia, and with increased blood flow to the brain, with implications for strokes, are not considered. Second, the focus on sickled cells blocking narrow blood vessels ignores a host of interactive, generative and cumulative physiological processes, as much, if not more important than the mechanics of blocking. But the emblematic role of the sickle shape and the blocking mechanisms in community education permits the types of discourse that conflate SCD and sickle cell trait to flourish in popular media, journalism and everyday understanding of sickle cell. This has deleterious consequences. A more nuanced understanding would not permit the assertion of a relationship of sickle cell trait to sudden deaths, whether in state custody, military training or professional sports training, to pass unremarked.

A concern with complexity led us to the themes of Chapter 2, and a consideration of the ways in which SCD is influenced not only by a gene on chromosome 11, but what comprises a whole genome and how genomic expression is related to the whole organism of a human being. The human organism is itself nested in several environments, for instance, genomic environments in which the capacities of one gene to spread in a geographical region partly depend upon the epigenetic effects of other genes present in that region. The interaction of genes associated with sickle cell and with thalassaemia represents one such process of mutual influence. The human being is also in physical relationships in which weather patterns and levels of pollution help determine the SCD experience. Finally, what the life of someone with SCD may be like depends on the collective relations in which they find themselves. Whether they can study, travel or work depends as much upon the inclusiveness of the school environment, the accessibility of public transport systems and the flexibilities shown by employers, as it does on SCD itself.

In Chapter 3, it was noted that the human body is an historical record of the evolution of non-humans. The protozoan *Plasmodium falciparum*, the *Anopheles gambiae* mosquito, the Green Sahara of 7,300 years ago, the forest canopies of West/Central Africa and the cultivation of yams are just some of the non-humans implicated in the development of the gene associated with sickle haemoglobin. This "long history" of sickle cell also draws our attention to the changing nature of humans and their environments. Changes sometimes happen without what Harman (2018) characterizes as human correlationism, as malarial pressures wrought changes in the size and genetic structure of human populations. Whether we consider the human genome, the physical geography of the Sahara, or the level of social development in the Jigawa district, we cannot look at the present and read off that the human body, the topography of a region or the character of human societies remain the same. This is important. Appeals to natural states of being, primordial attachments of peoples to lands, and the notions of Man and of Nature as equally unchanging are, in my view, the staple of regressive politics.

One day a new tale of sickle cell will be written from the critical perspectives of those living with SCD. Furthermore, given the global distribution of SCD, this will likely foreground perspectives from the Global South. The purpose of Chapter 4, a "short history" of sickle cell, was to try to be reflective about the manner in which black people have been stratified into lower socio-economic positions in North America and Europe, and have been racialized on the basis of the resulting poverty. A combination of the fact that the USA was a dominant twentieth-century global force in medical treatment and research, coupled with the enduring poverty and racialization of many of those living with SCD in the USA, has bequeathed a particular set of concerns and framings of our understanding of SCD. These understandings do not define the global experience of SCD and they will not define the future of sickle cell. They remain important, however, in understanding how we have arrived where we are.

These framings have shown up not only in our understanding of SCD, but in the manner in which sickle cell trait has come to be the focus of controversies. In Chapter 5, it was argued that the combination of the simplifications of sickle cell had to do with the shape of the red blood cells and their role in mechanically blocking the narrow blood vessels, coupled with the racialized lens through which African-Americans, the largest group affected by SCD in the USA, are seen, has deleterious consequences. These consequences are that the role of sickle cell trait in sudden death is amplified in ways consonant with the prosecution of racist social policies. In professional sports, the financial interests in expropriating student athlete unpaid labour and the autonomy of sports coaches to compel student athletes to undertake dangerous activities are not subject to critical scrutiny. Instead, sickle cell trait is marshalled as an alternative explanation. There is compelling evidence that, with the appropriate suite of precautionary measures in place, notably attention to Wet Globe Bulb Temperature, that student athletes or military recruits in training need not develop exercise-related illness. It is by minimizing the pool of students/recruits who develop exercise-related illness in the first place that is the key to reducing sudden deaths in sports or military training. Focusing on sickle cell trait enables autonomous sports coaches the freedom to require student athletes to undergo dangerous training regimes without precautions, thereby putting their lives, but not sport business profits, at risk. Meanwhile, with climate change, we will all need to become cognizant of wet globe bulb temperatures.

If the evidence for a compelling link between sickle cell trait and sudden death was weak in the case of sports, it was weaker still with respect to sudden death in contact with officers of the state. Chapter 6 reviewed cases of sudden death in police and prison custody that were attributed to sickle cell trait. The focus in state talk on the trait, rather than on use of chokeholds, positional asphyxia, extreme prolonged restraint associated with muscle breakdown, conductive electrical devices, pepper sprays, or other forms of assault on the person, was regarded as disingenuous. Furthermore, a response to the enduring nature of these displacement tactics by officers of the state, away from their actions to the genetic constitution of their victims, had been attributed to "institutional racism". As this chapter made clear, this is a flawed concept, which conflates intended behaviours at the level of situated activity and discriminatory outcomes at the level of contextual resources. While racism, as a set of ideational elements present in the cultural system of a society that may be taken up and employed by particular individual actors, may become widespread and unchallenged in organizations (i.e. racism has become institutionalized in an organization), this is a different concept from institutional racism. This concept, now widespread in UK social policy discussions, conflates agency and structure into a confused mix. With the concept of institutional racism, organizational leaders can project racism as intractable and beyond their control and individual members of the organization can deflect blame to an amorphous entity that is the organization itself. Analytically, the concept is weak. Politically, the concept permits racism to continue unchecked, with ongoing disastrous consequences for those living with sickle cell trait.

In Chapter 7, I reflected on the putative link between race, ethnicity and decisions about resource allocation to sickle cell, especially with regard to prenatal screening and sickle cell. The chapter began by criticizing the framing of sickle cell in Europe as to do with migration and migrants, noting that commentaries had alleged the "new" arrival of the haemoglobinopathies every decade for the past 60 years. The historical circumstances of the emergence of sickle cell in the USA in the twentieth century, and the contemporary tendency of the Anglophone academy to racialize the world, ran into difficulties when it became apparent that attempts to target sickle cell screening were problematic because they mixed external constructs, such as sickle cell genetic carriers, with internal constructs, namely, the folk classifications of race. Ethnicity categorization could never wholly capture the proportion of a population who carried genes associated with sickle cell or thalassaemia (Dyson, 1998). It was possible to conduct empirical research that estimated the proportion of genetic carriers missed in a selective screening programme based on an ethnicity-type question (Dyson *et al.*, 2006). Unfortunately, the use of ethnic categories cemented flawed conceptions of distinct biological races in the minds of professionals and clients alike, with some professionals even subverting the purpose of the research based on their own folk knowledge of who "really" needed to be screened for sickle cell (Dyson *et al.*, 2007c). Newborn universal screening in England revealed that, in terms of original definitions of populations at higher risk of carrying genes encoding variant haemoglobins, the white British population was equally a high risk group.

The cognate chronic illness of beta-thalassaemia major was considered in Chapter 8. Here it was noted that the historically-specific circumstances of post-war Cyprus, then still a British colony, led to the population acceding to a model of carrier identification, and later to prenatal diagnosis and selective termination of foetuses affected by beta-thalassaemia major, as part of a thalassaemia "prevention and control programme". The chapter noted how this was consonant with the time, place, material circumstances, the level of medical treatment, and the culture of Cyprus. However, it was strongly argued that those same combinations of factors were largely different in Sub-Saharan Africa, and that SCD differed in important ways from beta-thalassaemia, not least in the possible survival of some people with SCD in the absence of biomedical treatments, and the potential of newborn screening for SCD to enable lives to be saved. Even more importantly, the issue of prenatal diagnosis and selective termination raised issues of gender, racism and disablement. The focus of prenatal screening placed the mother in an invidious and paradoxical position: forced to live her life through the narrowness of neoliberal choices. This entails having a choice over having a disabled child, but being denied choice over partner constancy, family poverty and social treatment of the child with SCD. In North America and Europe, the birth of a child with SCD is in the context of societal racism and family experiences may be beset by struggles over resisting adversarial immigration and nationality laws; securing precarious employment, and countering racist assumptions through the emotional work of displays and performances necessary to survive in a racist society (Dyson *et al.*, 2016b). The selective termination of disabled children promoted as one of the neoliberal choices of antenatal screening presupposes what should not be claimed in advance: what the life of a young person living with SCD might be like. The chapter concluded by considering genetic sickle cell or thalassaemia carriers, whose reports of symptoms associated with the trait status are not taken seriously outside of genetic reproductive risk. *Informed reproductive care*, which, being relational, cannot be pre-judged by protocols, is asserted as a more appropriate goal of antenatal screening than the discredited neoliberal notion of choice.

Chapter 9 began with a brief exposition of the role of the spleen and an explanation of why the functions of the spleen are central to the purpose of newborn screening for SCD. Newborn screening is not merely the technology to diagnose a newborn with sickle cell disease, but the bringing together of health measures to ensure their subsequent well-being. Both in the USA and in the UK the formal implementation of universal screening for SCD for all newborn children lagged significantly behind the availability of the appropriate technology to do so. In malarial areas of the world, without extensive formal health services, estimated under-fives mortality for children with SCD is extremely high: perhaps as low as 2 per cent survival in the worst case scenario. Various frameworks that have emphasized sickle cell in relation to clinical genetics, or as requiring expensive technologies, in opposition to vaccinations for infectious diseases, have combined to prevent the strong development of sickle cell services in Africa, at least until the third decade of the twenty-first century. One particular initiative stands out. Newborn sickle cell screening in Kumasi, Ghana, conducted from 1995 onwards, began to produce cohorts of young people living with SCD. These young people literally embodied other ways of being with sickle cell that did not necessarily entail early deaths, attributions to the supernatural world or extensive discrimination against the person with SCD. A more optimistic future for infants with SCD in Africa, and in India is possible if newborn screening, embedded in robust health care provision, is adopted by whole states or whole nation states. Meanwhile, more thought is required in assessing how to relate to those identified as sickle cell genetic carriers by such newborn screening programmes.

Although many living with SCD have rejected the label disabled, for the understandable reason that black people already have a daunting array of negative labels attached to them, this has isolated people with SCD from the possible political benefits of applying a campaigning social model of disability to SCD. This was the subject of Chapter 10. The chapter outlined the basic features of the social model of disability, before considering some of its drawbacks: chiefly that its emphasis on independence is in tension with the need for interdependence in resource-poor communities fighting racism. Moreover, extreme versions of the social model, which locate all pain in social relationships, ignore the acute and chronic pain of SCD located at the heart of the body. The chapter examined the sociological concept of stigma in relation to a study of living with depression in Nigeria. This revealed that depression is not merely a by-product of SCD symptoms, but can be located in the oppressive and discriminatory social relations in which people living with SCD find themselves in Nigeria. By bringing a proper understanding of stigma to bear, namely, that stigma involves relationships to the norms and expectations of a particular society, challenges to discrimination can be more effectively conceived. First, it is possible to demonstrate that people with SCD can achieve in education, employment and longevity, contrary to disabling assumptions. Second, they could so achieve, were reasonable adjustments to be made to societal arrangements. And third, it is possible to conceive of the norms of any society as subject to challenge for their role in subordinating certain peoples: the expectations of a normalized body image, or of an independent utterly self-reliant worker, are equally challengeable as values that dis-able people.

Chapter 11 illustrated one application of the social model of disability, with particular reference to the experiences of young people with SCD at school. In some countries the struggle may be for the entitlement of someone with SCD to attend school at all in the face of discriminatory assumptions that an investment in education for someone with SCD represents a resource wasted. In England, the quality of school experience for someone with SCD is at stake. The chapter outlined the issue of silent strokes in SCD, but noted that these contribute only marginally to educational disadvantage compared to a combination of racism and poverty. The decline of local government agencies, such as local education authorities, had removed sources of innovation regarding school inclusiveness, downgraded curriculum innovation of relevance to racialized minority pupils, and produced an impetus to exclusion of black and/or disabled pupils, those with SCD included. Existing government guidance on supporting pupils with medical conditions was overly narrow, missing the preventive and precautionary measures required for SCD. Pupils with SCD missed schooling, with inadequate support to catch up, and were made ill unnecessarily by teachers and other pupils alike. Rationalist assumptions that raising teacher awareness would be sufficient were shown to be flawed, and what was required were changes to the school environment that enabled support for the students with SCD, without requiring extensive knowledge from hard-pressed teachers, and without drawing attention to the young person with SCD as different from their peers. Not all young people with SCD were willing to adopt a "poster-child" attitude in becoming assertive, outward-going spokespeople for their condition, even those who might have the energy to do so. A *Guide to School Policy on Sickle Cell* was presented as an alternative way forward. The production of this guide in the form of an open education resource was an attempt to make such a resource available globally.

The book began by noting that popular communications about sickle cell institutionalized misunderstandings about key physiological mechanisms, and suggested that permeable boundaries between the activities of researchers and community activists would produce better science. Sickle cell exerts its effects through assemblages of greater or lesser scale, from genes, through genomes and organisms, to environments. A history of sickle cell that moves beyond any one society, and moreover beyond humans themselves, reveals that the human body changes in conjunction with its non-human symbionts; the landscape changes with and without humans; and that neither a fixed body nor a fixed location characterizes human, nor indeed non-human, experience. The aggressive assertions of blood-and-soil that seek to negate human and non-human history are what underpin the misuses of sickle cell trait to draw attention away from the expropriation of unpaid student athlete labour and from the causes of sudden deaths in contact with state officials. More prosaically, sickle cell screening services have also developed, or been slow to develop, in the context of racism. Racism depends on an aggressive empiricism that claims to be able to point to an essence in the here and now. The singular essence of each person living with SCD lies in the future, and counterfactual reflecis required on what assemblages need to be brought into being to enable people with SCD to flourish. This means thinking counterfactually, beyond the empirical facts. Sickle cell could thus be a key resource in thinking non-anthropocentrically, in resisting racism, and in developing new ways of living.

Epilogue

The story of sickle cell can alert us to a number of key insights: about the role of non-human actors (protozoans, insects, ecologies) in shaping the human body in history (Dyson, 2018); the limitations of race-thinking (Dyson, 2005), and the benefits of such intellectual tools as generative notions of causality and counter-factual thinking. But, to conclude, I wish to highlight just two challenges. These challenges are real and will impact on us whether we acknowledge them or not, and irrespective of the silence of our politicians. These are, respectively, human-induced climate change and mass human migration. Strictly speaking, of course, climate change is rich, white, Global North, male-induced climate change (Seab-rook, 2016), and so, on nearly every dimension, principally *not* the culpability of the majority living globally with SCD. And yet it is on the Global South, includ-ing those living with SCD, upon whom the earliest impacts are falling. This, together with the vast global inequalities in wealth exacerbated by neoliberal globalization policies; the dislocation of wars, and indeed climate change itself (Missirian and Schlenker, 2017), will compel millions to move from their homes in the twenty-first century.

It is with respect to these two era-defining changes – migration and climate change – that sickle cell provides helpful insights. Recall that sickle cell gene is the product of changing ecologies, arising either in the period of the Green Sahara, which, as the name suggests, was fertile before its subsequent extensive desertification, or with the removal of the forest canopy in favour of slash-and-burn agriculture in West Africa. Recall too that the ostensibly natural savannah grasslands of Northern Nigeria at the time of the WHO malaria study in the 1970s would once have been the site of a pre-colonial, flourishing, Hausa civili-zation. Ecology and topography often outlast a single human generation, and so may wrongly be conceived of as natural and fixed, but nonetheless are subject to change, with or without human mediation. Neither is the human body fixed (Robb and Harris, 2013). It changes over time in interaction with the environ-ment, and sickle cell, as one genetic response to malarial pressures, is one such rebound creation of environmental flux.

The climate, the ecology, the human red blood cell, the mosquito, and the protozoan parasite do not stay the same, but alter in ongoing and complex ways. Their respective influence may or may not be reciprocal, and the impact may or may not be symmetrical, that is, of comparable significance for both parties. But what this does establish is that neither blood nor soil is primordial. Continued belief in *primordialism*, that is, an appeal to the fixed nature of both human bloodlines and geographical borders, of blood and soil, a set notion of which humans belong to which habitat, would be to remain, as Latour (2016) puts it, trapped in two bubbles of unrealism:

> [N]o one has explained clearly enough that globalization is over, and that we urgently need to re-establish ourselves on an Earth that has nothing to do with the protective borders of nation-states any more than the infinite horizon of globalization. The conflict between the utopia of the past and the utopia of the future must not occupy us any longer. What matters now is finding a way to bring together two kinds of migrants: those forced by the ecological mutation to find a new world by crossing borders and those forced to do the same without even having moved, and whom borders can no longer protect.

Where parts of the world become less habitable for humans, owing to desertification, extreme wet globe bulb temperatures or failing agriculture, the numbers migrating with the sickle cell gene (Piel *et al.*, 2014) will be small compared to the many thousands with genes associated with sickle cell likely to migrate in the twenty-first century. But note also that, on this real twenty-first-century Earth, those who don't move will be subject to equally powerful changes. Any map of the sea will eventually, but literally, *over-lap* the cities of London, New York, New Orleans, Miami and Rio de Janeiro. Areas of the Global North that were not malarial may become so, as changes in temperature and rainfall in currently temperate parts of the world may nurture mosquitoes and malaria in the future. Territories will not only disappear but, faced with mass migration, either human characters in territories will change and diversify, as many more people learn to share the living space of the Global North, or the character of the humans in those territories will be revealed and immigration internment, squalid refugee camps, neglectful deaths and murderous deportations will prevail. Early signs of the fate of refugees with SCD are not encouraging (Dyson, 2009).

What comes next is, of course, radically indeterminate and unknowable. But the realities of climate change and mass migration, changes that highlight the changing nature of human bodies and of the Earth itself, suggest that sickle cell as an issue will at last become less subaltern and more real in the future.

References

Abiola AO, Ojika BO, Mannir B, *et al.* (2013) Effect of health education on the knowledge and attitude to sickle cell disorder and screening practices among school of nursing students in Sokoto, Nigeria. *Nigerian Quarterly Journal of Hospital Medicine* 23(1): 65–68.

ABNA News (2012) Tragic photos of Bahraini youth. Available at: http://en.abna24.com/service/bahrain/archive/2012/01/28/293135/story.html (accessed 7 November 2018).

Abuateya H, Atkin K, Culley LA, Dyson SE and Dyson SM (2008) Young people with sickle cell disorder and education: A knowledge review. *Diversity in Health and Social Care* 5(2): 123–135.

ACLU (American Civil Liberties Union) (2008) Letter to Winn Parish District Attorney. Winfield, LA, July 16.

Adamkiewicz TV and Piel FB (2014) Divergence from Hardy Weinberg Equilibrium in newborn screening cohorts for sickle hemoglobin. *Blood* 124(21): 1389.

Adams RJ, McKie VC, Hsu L, Files B, Vichinsky E, *et al.* (1998) Prevention of a first stroke by transfusions in children with sickle cell anemia and abnormal results on transcranial Doppler ultrasonography. *New England Journal of Medicine* 339(1): 5–11.

Adams RJ, Mckie V, Nichols F, Carl E, Zhang DL, *et al.* (1992) The use of transcranial ultrasonography to predict stroke in sickle cell disease. *New England Journal of Medicine* 326(9): 605–610.

Ahmad WIU (1996) The trouble with culture. In: D Kelleher and S Hillier (eds) *Researching Cultural Differences in Health.* London: Routledge, 190–219.

Ahmad WIU and Atkin K (1996) Ethnicity and caring for a disabled child: the case of sickle cell or thalassaemia. *British Journal of Social Work* 26(6): 755–775.

Ahmed SG, Kagu MB, Abjah UA, and Bukar AA (2012) Seasonal variations in frequencies of acute vaso-occlusive morbidities among sickle cell anaemia patients in Northern Nigeria. *Journal of Blood Disorders and Transfusion* 3:120. doi: 10.4172/2155-9864.1000120.

Aisiku IP, Smith WR, McLish DK, Levenson JL, Penberthy LT, *et al.* (2008) Comparisons of high versus low emergency department utilizers in sickle cell disease. *Annals of Emergency Medicine* 53(5): 587–593.

Alexander, JC (2010) The celebrity-icon. *Cultural Sociology* 4(3): 323–336.

Al Juburi G, Laverty AA, Green SA, Phekoo KJ, Bell D, *et al.* (2013) Socio-economic deprivation and risk of emergency readmission and inpatient mortality in people with sickle cell disease in England: observational study. *Journal of Public Health* 35(4): 510–517.

Allison AC (1954) Protection afforded by sickle cell trait against subtertian malarial infection. *British Medical Journal* 1: 290–294.

Allison AC (1964) Polymorphism and natural selection in human populations. *Cold Spring Harbor Symposia on Quantitative Biology* 29: 137–149.

Alonso-González P (2016) Between certainty and trust: boundary-work and the construction of archaeological epistemic authority. *Cultural Sociology* 10(4): 483–501.

Alvarez O, Rodriguez MM, Jordan L and Sarnaik S (2015) Renal medullary carcinoma and sickle cell trait: a systematic review. *Pediatric Blood and Cancer* 62(10): 1694–1699.

American Anthropological Association (1998) Statement on 'Race'. Available at: www.aaanet.org/stmts/racepp.htm.

American Society of Hematology (2012) Statement on Screening for Sickle Cell Trait and Athletic Participation. Available at: www.hematology.org/Advocacy/Statements/2650.aspx.

Amos RJ (2015) A rendezvous with sickle cell and slavery in New Orleans. Available at: https://sicklesense.wordpress.com/2015/05/08/a-rendezvous-with-sickle-cell-and-slavery-in-new-orleans/ (accessed 7 November 2018).

Andermann A, Blancquaert I, Beauchamp S and Déry V (2008) Revisiting Wilson and Jungner in the genomic age: a review of screening criteria over the past 40 years. *Bulletin of the World Health Organization* 86(4): 241–320.

Andersch MA, Wilson DA and Menten ML (1944) Sedimentation constants and electrophoretic mobilities of adult and fetal carbonylhemoglobin. *Journal of Biological Chemistry* 153(1): 301–305.

Anderson P (2008) The division of Cyprus. *London Review of Books* 30: 1–34.

Anderson SA (2012) The junction boys' syndrome. *The Journal of Strength and Conditioning Research* 26(5): 1179–1180.

Angastiniotis M, Corrons J-LV, Soteriades ES and Eleftheriou A (2013) The impact of migrations on the health services for rare diseases in Europe: the example of haemoglobin disorders. *The Scientific World Journal* (2013) Article ID 727905 http://dx.doi.org/10.1155/2013/727905.

Angastiniotis M, Kyriakidou S, and Hadjiminas M (1986) How thalassaemia was controlled in Cyprus. *World Health Forum* 7: 291–297.

Angastiniotis M and Modell, B (1998) Global epidemiology of hemoglobin disorders. *Annals of the New York Academy of Sciences* 850(1): 251–269.

Anionwu EN (1993) Sickle cell and thalassaemia: community experiences and official response. In: WIU Ahmad (ed.) *'Race' and Health in Contemporary Britain*. Buckingham: Open University Press, 76–95.

Anionwu EN (1996) Ethnic origin of sickle and thalassaemia counsellors: does it matter? In: D Kelleher and S Hillier (eds) *Researching Cultural Differences in Health*. London: Routledge, 160–189.

Anionwu EN (2016) *Mixed Blessings from a Cambridge Union*. London: ELIZAN Publishing.

Anionwu EN and Atkin K (2001) *The Politics of Sickle Cell and Thalassaemia*. Buckingham: Open University Press.

APHL/CDC (Association of Public Health Laboratories and Centers for Disease Control and Prevention) (2015) *Hemoglobinopathies: Current Practice for Screening, Confirmation and Follow-Up*. Silver Spring, MD: APHL. Available at: www.cdc.gov/ncbddd/sicklecell/documents/nbs_hemoglobinopathy-testing_122015.pdf.

Archer MS (1995) *Realist Social Theory: The Morphogenetic Approach*. Cambridge: Cambridge University Press.

Arnaiz-Villena A, Elaiwa N, Silvera C, Rostom A, Moscoso J, *et al*. (2001) The origin of Palestinians and their genetic relatedness with other Mediterranean populations. *Human Immunology* 62(9): 889–900.

Aspinall PJ (2013) When is the use of race/ethnicity appropriate in risk assessment tools for pre-conceptual or antenatal genetic screening and how should it be used? *Sociology* 47(5): 957–975.

Aspinall PJ, Dyson SM and Anionwu EN (2003) The feasibility of using ethnicity as a primary tool for antenatal selective screening for sickle cell disorders: pointers from the research evidence. *Social Science and Medicine* 56(2): 285–297.

Atkin K and Ahmad WIU (1998) Genetic screening and haemoglobinopathies: ethics, politics and practice. *Social Science and Medicine* 46(3): 445–458.

Atkin K and Ahmad WIU (2000a) Pumping iron: compliance with chelation therapy among young people who have thalassaemia major. *Sociology of Health and Illness*, 22(4): 500–524.

Atkin K and Ahmad WIU (2000b) Living with sickle cell disorder: how young people negotiate their care and treatment. In: Ahmad, WIU (ed.) *Ethnicity, Disability and Chronic Illness.* Buckingham: Open University Press, 45–66.

Atkin K and Ahmad WIU (2001) Living a 'normal' life: young people coping with thalassaemia major or sickle cell disorder. *Social Science and Medicine* 53(5): 615–626.

Atkin K, Ahmad WIU and Anionwu EN (1998a) Screening and counselling for sickle cell disorders and thalassaemia: the experience of parents and health professionals. *Social Science and Medicine* 47(11): 1639–1651.

Atkin K, Ahmad WIU and Anionwu EN (1998b) Service support to families caring for a child with a sickle cell disorder or thalassaemia: the experience of health professionals, service managers and health commissioners. *Health* 2(3): 305–327.

Atkin K, Berghs M and Dyson SM (2015) "Who's the guy in the room?" Involving fathers in antenatal care screening for sickle cell disorders. *Social Science and Medicine* 128(2015): 212–219.

Atkinson W (2010) The myth of the reflexive worker: class and work histories in neo-liberal times. *Work, Employment and Society* 24(3): 413–429.

Bahrain Center for Human Rights (2013) Sickle Cell Disease and the Government Crackdown in Bahrain. Available at: www.bahrainrights.org/sites/default/files/field/image/Sickle%20Cell.pdf (accessed 7 November 2018).

Ball SJ (2003) The teacher's soul and the terrors of performativity. *Journal of Education Policy* 18(2): 215–228.

Ballas SK (2009) The cost of health care for patients with sickle cell disease. *American Journal of Haematology* 84(6): 320–322.

Ballas SK, Bauserman RL, McCarthy WF, Waclawiw MA and the Investigators of the Multicenter Study of Hydroxyurea (2010) The impact of hydroxyurea on career and employment of patients with sickle cell anemia. *Journal of the National Medical Association* 102(11): 993–999.

Ballas SK, Gupta K and Adams-Graves P (2012) Sickle cell pain: a critical reappraisal. *Blood* 120(18): 3647–3656.

Ballas SK, Pulte ED, Lobo C and Riddick-Burden G (2016) Case series of octogenarians with sickle cell disease. *Blood* 128(19): 2367–2369.

Bar-Or O and Rowland TW (2004) *Pediatric Exercise Medicine: From Physiologic Principles to Health Care Application.* Leeds: Human Kinetics Europe.

Bauman Z (1992) Survival as a social construct. *Theory, Culture & Society* 9(1): 1–36.

Bautista A (2010) College football's serial murderer: sickle cell trait. *Marquette Sports Law Review*, 21(1). Available at: https://scholarship.law.marquette.edu/sportslaw/vol.21/iss1/14.

Bazuaye GN and Olayemi, EE (2009) Knowledge and attitude of senior secondary school students in Benin City Nigeria to sickle cell disease. *World Journal of Medical Sciences* 4: 46–49.

BBC (2013a) Bahrain police jailed over death of activist in custody, 13 March 2013. Available at: www.bbc.co.uk/news/world-middle-east-21769901.

BBC (2013b) Sarah Mulenga died after trainee paramedics' 'failings', 14 May 2013. Available at: www.bbc.co.uk/news/uk-england-london-2251947.

Beaudevin C (2013) Old diseases and contemporary crisis: inherited blood disorders in the Sultanate of Oman. *Anthropology and Medicine* 20(2): 175–189.

Beck S (2016) The loving care of postcolonial subjects: doctors, medicine and epidemiological interventions in Cyprus. *The Cyprus Review* 28(1): 101–120.

Beck S and Niewöhner J (2009) Localising genetic testing and screening in Cyprus and Germany. In: P Atkinson, P Glasner and M Lock (eds) *Handbook of Genetics and Society*. London: Routledge, 76–93.

Bediako SM (2010) Predictors of employment status among African Americans with sickle cell disease. *Journal of Health Care for the Poor and Underserved* 21(4): 1124–1137.

Bediako SM, Lavender AR and Yasin Z (2007) Racial centrality and health care use among African American adults with sickle cell disease. *Journal of Black Psychology* 33(4): 422–438.

Bediako SM and Moffitt KR (2011) Race and social attitudes about sickle cell disease. *Ethnicity and Health* 16(4–5): 423–429.

Bello NA, Hyacinth HI, Roetker NS, Seals SR, Naik RP, *et al.* (2017) Sickle cell trait is not associated with an increased risk of heart failure or abnormalities of cardiac structure and function. *Blood* 129(6): 799–801.

Benjamin R (2011) Organized ambivalence: when sickle cell disease and stem cell research converge. *Ethnicity and Health* 16(4–5): 447–463.

Benson JM and Therrell Jr BL (2010) History and current status of newborn screening for hemoglobinopathies. *Seminars in Perinatology* 34(2): 134–144.

Bergin C (2016) *African American Anti-Colonial Thought, 1917–1937*. Edinburgh: Edinburgh University Press.

Bhaskar R (2008 [1975]) *A Realist Theory of Science*. London: Verso Books.

Bhopal R and Donaldson L (1988) Health education for ethnic minorities: current provision and future directions. *Health Education Journal* 47(4): 137–140.

Birmingham Mail (2014) Tyseley schoolboy died after blood transfusion delays, 30 September 2014. Available at: www.birminghammail.co.uk/news/midlands-news/tyseley-schoolboy-died-after-blood-7852830.

Birmingham Mail (2017) Toddler died after GP made 'gross failure' by failing to carry out vaccinations, 20 April 2017. Available at: www.birminghammail.co.uk/news/midlands-news/toddler-died-after-gp-made-12918260.

Black J and Laws S (1986) *Living with Sickle Cell Disease*. London: East London Sickle Cell Society.

Bloomfield GS, Lagat DK, Akwanalo OC, Carter EJ, Lugogo N, *et al.* (2012) Waiting to inhale: an exploratory review of conditions that may predispose to pulmonary hypertension and right heart failure in persons exposed to household air pollution in low- and middle-income countries. *Global Heart* 7(3): 249–259.

Bonham VL, Dover, GJ and Brody LC (2010) Screening student athletes for sickle cell trait: a social and clinical experiment. *New England Journal of Medicine* 363(11): 997–999.

Bourdieu P and Wacquant L (1999) On the cunning of imperialist reasoning. *Theory Culture & Society* 16(1): 41–58.

Bourne J (2001) The life and times of institutional racism. *Race and Class* 43(7): 7–22.

Bowman JE (1977) Genetic screening programmes and public policy. *Phylon* 38: 117–142.

Bradby H (2012) Race, ethnicity and health: the costs and benefits of conceptualizing racism and ethnicity. *Social Science and Medicine* 75: 955–958.

Braun L and Hammonds E (2008) Race, populations and genomics: Africa as laboratory. *Social Science and Medicine* 67(10): 1580–1588.

Braverman H (1974) *Labour and Monopoly Capitalism: The Degradation of Work in the Twentieth Century.* New York: The Monthly Review Press.

Bristow LR (1974) The myth of sickle cell trait. *Western Journal of Medicine* 121: 77–82.

Brosco JP and Paul D (2013) The political history of PKU: reflections on 50 years of newborn screening. *American Academy of Pediatrics* 132(6): 987–989.

Brousseau DC, Panepinto JA, Nimmer M and Hoffman RG (2009) The number of people with sickle cell disease in the United States: national and state estimates. *American Journal of Haematology* 85(1): 77–78.

Brown C (1984) *Black and White Britain: The Third PSI Survey.* London: Heinemann.

Brown GW and Harris T (1978) *Social Origins of Depression.* London: Tavistock.

Buckle AER, Hanning L and Holman CA (1964) Routine haemoglobin electrophoresis in at-risk gravid women. *BJOG: An International Journal of Obstetrics & Gynaecology* 71(6): 923–926.

Burnes DP, Antle BJ, Williams CC and Cook L (2008) Mothers raising children with sickle cell disease at the intersection of race, gender, and illness stigma. *Health and Social Work* 33(3): 211–220.

Burrows EG and Wallace M (1999) *Gotham: A History of New York City to 1898.* New York: Oxford University Press.

Carmichael S and Hamilton C (1968) *Black Power: The Politics of Liberation.* Harmondsworth: Penguin.

Carrington B (2011) 'What I said was racist – but I'm not a racist': anti-racism and the white sports/media complex. In: J Long and K Spracklen (eds) *Sport and Challenges to Racism.* Basingstoke: Palgrave Macmillan, 83–99.

Carter B (2000) *Racism and Realism.* London: Routledge.

Carter B (2007) Genes, genomes and genealogies: the return of scientific racism? *Ethnic and Racial Studies* 30(4): 546–556.

Carter B and Dyson SM (2011) Territory, ancestry and descent: the politics of sickle cell disease. *Sociology* 45(6): 963–976.

Carter, B and Dyson SM (2015) Actor Network Theory, agency and racism: the case of sickle cell trait and US athletics. *Social Theory and Health* 13(1): 62–77.

Carter B and Fenton S (2010) Not thinking ethnicity: a critique of the ethnicity paradigm in an over-ethnicized sociology. *Journal for the Theory of Social Behaviour* 40(1): 1–18.

Carter B and Virdee S (2008) Racism and the sociological imagination. *British Journal of Sociology* 54(9): 661–679.

Carter R and Mendis KN (2002) Evolutionary and historical aspects of the burden of malaria. *Clinical Microbiology Reviews* 15(4): 564–594.

Cartwright SA (1851) Diseases and peculiarities of the Negro race: Africans in America. *De Bow's Review Southern and Western States* XI. Available at: www.pbs.org/wgbh/aia/part4/4h3106t.html.

Cavalli-Sforza LL, Menozzi P and Piazza A (1996) *The History and Geography of Human Genes*. Abridged edn. Princeton, NJ: Princeton University Press.

CDC (Centers for Disease Control and Prevention) (2014) *Tips for Supporting Students with SCD*. Available at: www.cdc.gov/ncbddd/sicklecell/documents/tipsheet_supporting_students_with_scd.pdf.

CDC (Centers for Disease Control and Prevention) (2018) *Sickle Cell Trait and Damage to the Spleen*. CS265405F. Available at: www.cdc.gov/ncbddd/sicklecell/documents/FS_SplenicInfarcts_LAY.pdf.

Chakravarty EF, Khanna D and Chung L (2008) Pregnancy outcomes in systemic sclerosis, primary pulmonary hypertension, and sickle cell disease. *Obstetrics and Gynecology* 111(4): 927–934.

Charache S, Terrin ML, Moore RD, Dover GJ, *et al.* and Investigators of the Multicenter Study of Hydroxyurea in Sickle Cell Anemia (1995) Effect of hydroxyurea on the frequency of painful crises in sickle cell anemia. *New England Journal of Medicine* 332(20): 1317–1322.

Chattoo S (2018) Inherited blood disorders, genetic risk and global public health: framing 'birth defects' as preventable in India. *Anthropology and Medicine* 25(1): 30–49.

Chattoo S and Ahmad WIU (2008) The moral economy of selfhood and caring: negotiating boundaries of personal care as embodied moral practice. *Sociology of Health and Illness* 30(4): 550–564.

Chen J, Hobbs WE, Le J, Lenting PJ, De Groot PG, *et al.* (2011) The rate of hemolysis in sickle cell disease correlates with the quantity of active von Willebrand factor in the plasma. *Blood* 117(13): 3680–3683.

Christgau R (2004) In search of Jim Crow. *The Believer* 2(1): February 2004. Available: https://believermag.com/in-search-of-jim-crow/ (accessed 7 November 2018).

Christianson A, Streetly A and Darr A (2004) Lessons from thalassaemia screening in Iran: screening programmes must consider societal values. *British Medical Journal* 329(7475): 1115.

Chugg AM (2012) *The Quest for the Tomb of Alexander the Great,* 2nd edn. London: AMC Publications.

Ciribassi RM and Patil C (2016) "We don't wear it on our sleeve": sickle cell disease and the (in)visible body in parts. *Social Science and Medicine* 148(2016): 131–138.

Clare N (2007) *An OSCAR for My Troubles*. London: Neville Clare.

Clendennen GW and Lwanda J (2003) David Livingstone and Southern Africa's first recorded cases of sickle cell anaemia? *Journal of Royal College of Physicians Edinburgh* 33(S12): 21–28.

Clotfelter CT (2011) *Big-Time Sports in American Universities*. Cambridge: Cambridge University Press.

CNN-IBN News-18 (2011) Six die of cholera in Kerala, 29 June 2011. Available at: www.news18.com/news/india/six-die-of-cholera-in-kerala-380212.html (accessed 7 November 2018).

Coburn D (2004) Beyond the income inequality hypothesis: class, neo-liberalism, and health inequalities. *Social Science and Medicine* 58(1): 41–56.

Cohen RT, Strunk RC, Field JJ, Rosen CL, Kirkham FJ, *et al.* (2013) Environmental tobacco smoke and airway obstruction in children with sickle cell anemia. *CHEST Journal* 144(4): 1323–1329.

Coleman B, Ellis-Caird H, McGowan J and Benjamin MJ (2016) How sickle cell disease patients experience, understand and explain their pain: an Interpretative Phenomenological Analysis study. *British Journal of Health Psychology* 21(1): 190–203.

Coleman D and Salt J (1996) The ethnic group question in the 1991 Census: a new landmark in British social statistics. In: D Coleman and J Salt (eds) *Ethnicity in the 1991 Census, Volume 1* London: HMSO, 1–32.

Conley CL (1980) Sickle cell anemia: the first molecular disease. In: MM Wintrobe (ed.) *Blood Pure and Eloquent: A Story of Discovery of People and Ideas.* New York: McGraw-Hill, 318–371.

Cook JE and Meyer J (1915) Severe anemia with remarkable elongated and sickle-shaped red blood cells and chronic leg ulcer. *Archives of Internal Medicine* 16(4): 644–651.

Craig G (2007) 'Cunning, unprincipled, loathsome': the racist tail wags the welfare dog. *Journal of Social Policy* 36(4): 605–623.

Creary MS (2018) Biocultural citizenship and embodying exceptionalism: biopolitics for sickle cell disease in Brazil. *Social Science and Medicine* 199: 123–131.

Cronin de Chavez A (2018) The triple-hit effect of disability and energy poverty: a qualitative case study of painful sickle cell disease and cold homes. In: N Simcock, H Thomson, S Petrova and S Bouzarovski (eds) *Energy Poverty and Vulnerability: A Global Perspective.* London Routledge, 169–187.

Culley L, Dyson SM, Ham-Ying S and Young W (1999) Racisms, resistances and healing narratives: Caribbean nurses in the UK. In: S Roseneil and J Seymour (eds) *Practising Identities: Power and Resistance.* Basingstoke: Macmillan, 155–179.

Currat M, Trabuchet G, Rees D, Perrin P, Harding RM, *et al.* (2002) Molecular analysis of the β-globin gene cluster in the Niokholo Mandenka population reveals a recent origin of the β S Senegal mutation. *The American Journal of Human Genetics* 70(1): 207–223.

Davidson B (1996) *The African Slave Trade.* Oxford: James Currey.

Davies SC, Cronin E, Gill M, Greengross P, Hickman M, and Normand C (2000) Screening for sickle cell disease and thalassaemia: a systematic review with supplementary research. *Health Technology Assessment* 4(3): 1–87.

Davis A (1981) *Women, Race and Class.* New York: Random House.

Davis M and Troupe Q (1989) *Miles: The Autobiography.* New York: Simon & Schuster.

De D, Dyson SM and Atkin K (2016) Valuing people with sickle cell disease. *Occupational Health and Wellbeing* 68(9): 27–30.

Deane CR, Goss D, Bartram J, Pohl KRE, Height SE, *et al.* (2010) Extracranial internal carotid arterial disease in children with sickle cell anemia. *Haematologica* 95(8): 1287–1292.

DeBaun MR, Armstrong FD, McKinstry RC, Ware RE, Vichinsky E, *et al.* (2012) Silent cerebral infarcts: a review on a prevalent and progressive cause of neurologic injury in sickle cell anemia. *Blood* 119(20): 4587–4596.

DeLanda M (2016) *Assemblage Theory.* Edinburgh: Edinburgh University Press.

DeLanda M and Harman G (2017) *The Rise of Realism.* Cambridge: Polity Press.

Denham AR, Adongo PB, Freydberg N and Hodgson A (2010) Chasing spirits: clarifying the spirit child phenomenon and infanticide in Northern Ghana. *Social Science and Medicine* 71(3): 608–615.

Dennis-Antwi JA, Culley L, Hiles D and Dyson SM (2011) "I can die today, I can die tomorrow": lay perceptions of sickle cell disease in Kumasi, Ghana at a point of transition. *Ethnicity and Health* 16(4–5): 465–481.

Dennis-Antwi JA, Dyson SM and Ohene-Frempong K (2008) Healthcare provision for sickle cell disease in Ghana: challenges for the African context. *Diversity in Health and Social Care* 5(4): 241–254.

Diallo, DA, Guindo, A, Touré, BA, Sarro, YS, Sima, M, *et al.* (2018) Dépistage néonatal ciblé de la drépanocytose: limites du test de falciformation (test d'Emmel) dans le bilan prénatal en zone ouest africaine. *Revue d'Épidémiologie et de Santé Publique* 66(3) 181–185.

Diggs LW and Ching RE (1934) Pathology of sickle cell anemia. *Southern Medical Journal* 27(10): 839–845.

Dingwall R (2001) Contemporary legends, rumours and collective behaviour: some neglected resources for medical sociology? *Sociology of Health and Illness* 23(2): 180–202.

Draper E (1991) *Risky Business: Genetic Testing and Exclusionary Practices in the Hazardous Workplace.* Cambridge: Cambridge University Press.

Driss A, Asare KO, Hibbert JM, Gee BE, Adadmkiewicz TV, *et al.* (2009) Sickle cell disease in the post-genomic era: a monogenic disease with a polygenic phenotype. *Genomics Insights* 2: 23–48.

Duchovni-Silva I and Ramalho AS (2003) Maternal effect: an additional mechanism maintaining balanced polymorphisms of haemoglobinopathies? *Annals of Human Genetics* 67(6): 538–542.

Dunning E (1999) *Sports Matters: Sociological Studies of Sport, Violence and Civilization.* London: Routledge.

Duster T (2003) *Backdoor to Eugenics,* 2nd edn. New York: Routledge.

Duster T (2009) Ancestry testing and DNA: uses, limits – and caveat emptor. *Genewatch* 22(3–4): 16–17.

Duster T (2015) A post-genomic surprise: the molecular reinscription of race in science, law and medicine. *The British Journal of Sociology* 66(1): 1–27.

Dyson SE, Atkin K, Culley LA, Demaine J and Dyson SM (2012) School ethos and variation in health experience of young people with sickle cell disorder at school. *Diversity and Equality in Health and Care* 9(1): 33–44.

Dyson SM (1986) Professionals, mentally handicapped children and confidential files. *Disability, Handicap and Society* 1(1): 73–87.

Dyson SM (1992) Blood relations: educational implications of sickle cell anaemia and thalassaemia. In: T Booth, W Swann, M Masterton and P Potts (eds) *Curricula for Diversity in Education (Learning for All 1).* London: Routledge, 277–283.

Dyson SM (1994) *Beta-Thalassaemia: Current Carrier and Community Awareness in Manchester.* No. 2 in the DMU Haemoglobinopathy Series. Leicester: De Montfort University.

Dyson SM (1997) Knowledge of sickle cell in a screened population. *Health and Social Care in the Community* 5(2): 84–93.

Dyson SM (1998) 'Race', ethnicity and haemoglobin disorders. *Social Science and Medicine* 47(1): 121–131.

Dyson SM (1999) Genetic screening and ethnic minorities. *Critical Social Policy* 19(2): 195–215.

Dyson SM (2005) *Ethnicity and Screening for Sickle Cell and Thalassaemia.* Oxford: Elsevier/Churchill Livingstone.

Dyson SM (2007) Genetic traits as pollution: 'White English' carriers of sickle cell or thalassaemia. In: M Kirkham (ed.) *Exploring the Dirty Side of Women's Health.* London: Routledge, 270–283.

Dyson SM (2009) Sickle cell: a signifier for the New Europe. In: C Howson and M Sallah (eds) *Europe's Established and Emerging Immigrant Communities: Assimilation, Multiculturalism or Integration?* Stoke: Trentham Books, 31–45.

Dyson, SM (2016) *Sickle Cell: A Guide to School Policy.* Open education resource [CC-BY-SA 4.0], 2nd edn. Available at: www.sicklecellanaemia.org/open-education-resources/guide-for-schools-with-children-with-sickle-cell-and-thalassaemia.

Dyson SM (2018) Assessing Latour: the case of the sickle cell body in history. *European Journal of Social Theory.* https://doi.org/10.1177/1368431018754730.

Dyson SM, Abuateya, H, Atkin K, Culley LA, Dyson SE, *et al.* (2008) Local authorities and the education of young people with sickle cell disorders (SCD) in England. *International Studies in Sociology of Education* 18(1): 47–60.

Dyson SM, Abuateya H, Atkin K, Culley LA, Dyson, SE, *et al.* (2010a) Reported school experiences of young people living with sickle cell disorder in England. *British Educational Research Journal* 36(1): 125–142.

Dyson SM, Ahmad WIU and Atkin K (2016a) Narrative as re-fusion: making sense and value from sickle cell and thalassaemia trait. *Health: An Interdisciplinary Journal for the Social Study of Health, Illness and Medicine* 20(6): 616–634.

Dyson SM and Atkin K (2011) Sickle cell and thalassaemia: global public health issues come of age. *Ethnicity and Health* 16(4–5): 299–311.

Dyson SM and Atkin K (2012) Sickle cell and thalassaemia: why social science is critical to improving care and service support. In: SM Dyson and K Atkin (eds) *Genetics and Global Public Health: Sickle Cell and Thalassaemia.* London: Routledge, 192–203.

Dyson SM, Atkin K, Culley LA and Dyson SE (2007a) The educational experiences of young people with sickle cell disorder: a commentary on existing literature. *Disability and Society* 22(6): 581–594.

Dyson SM, Atkin K, Culley LA and Dyson SE (2014) Critical realism, agency and sickle cell: case studies of young people with sickle cell disorder at school. *Ethnic and Racial Studies* 37(13): 2379–2398.

Dyson SM, Atkin K, Culley LA, Dyson SE and Evans H (2011) Sickle cell, habitual dispositions and fragile dispositions: young people with sickle cell at school. *Sociology of Health and Illness* 33(3): 465–483.

Dyson SM, Atkin K, Culley LA, Dyson SE, Evans H, *et al.* (2010b) Disclosure and sickle cell disorder: a mixed methods study of the young person with sickle cell at school *Social Science and Medicine* 70(12): 2036–2044.

Dyson SM, Berghs M and Atkin K (2016b) "Talk to me. There's two of us": fathers and sickle cell screening. *Sociology* 50(1): 178–194.

Dyson SM and Boswell GR (2006) Sickle cell anaemia and deaths in custody in the UK and USA. *The Howard Journal of Criminal Justice* 45(1): 14–28.

Dyson, SM and Boswell, GR (2009) *Sickle Cell and Deaths in Custody.* London: Whiting and Birch.

Dyson, SM and Brown, B (2006) *Social Theory and Applied Health Research.* Buckingham: Open University Press.

Dyson SM, Chambers K, Gawler S, Hubbard S, Jivanji V, *et al.* (2007b) Lessons for intermediate and low prevalence areas in England from the ethnicity questions and antenatal screening for sickle cell/thalassaemia [EQUANS] study. *Diversity in Health and Social Care* 4(2): 123–135.

Dyson SM, Cochran F, Culley LA, Dyson SE, Kennefick A, *et al.* (2007c) Observation and interview findings from the ethnicity questions and antenatal screening for sickle cell/thalassaemia [EQUANS] study. *Critical Public Health* 17(1): 31–43.

Dyson SM, Culley LA, Gill C, Hubbard S, Kennefick A, *et al.* (2006) Ethnicity questions and antenatal screening for sickle cell/thalassaemia [EQUANS] in England: a randomized controlled trial of two questionnaires. *Ethnicity and Health* 11(2): 169–189.

Dyson SM, Davis V and Rahman R (1994) Thalassaemia major: counselling and community education. *Health Visitor* 67(1): 25–26.

Dyson, SM and Dyson SE (2014) The politics of health services research: health professionals as hired hands in a commissioned research project in England. *Sociological Research Online* 19(3):14.

Dyson SM, Fielder A and Kirkham M (1996) Midwives' and senior students' knowledge levels of the haemoglobinopathies. *Midwifery* 12(1): 23–30.

Eaton WA and Bunn HF (2017) Treating sickle cell disease by targeting HbS polymerization. *Blood* 129(20): 2719–2726.

Eaton WA and Hofrichter J (1994) Sickle haemoglobin polymerization. In: SH Embury, RP Hebble, N Mohandas, and MH Steinberg (eds) *Sickle Cell Disease: Basic Principles and Practice.* New York: Raven Press, 53–87.

Ebomoyi E (1988) Knowledge and attitude towards genetic screening for sickle cell disease. *Hygie: International Journal of Health Education* VII (1): 33–38.

Edelstein SJ (1986) *The Sickled Cell: From Myths to Molecules.* Cambridge, MA: Harvard University Press.

Eichner ER (1993) Sickle cell trait, heroic exercise, and fatal collapse. *Physician and Sports Medicine* 21(7): 51–64.

Eichner ER (2010) Sickle cell trait in sports. *Current Sports Medicine Reports* 9(6): 347–351.

Eke FU and Anochie I (2003) Effects of pyrimethamine versus proguanil in malarial chemoprophylaxis in children with sickle cell disease: a randomized, placebo-controlled, open-label study. *Current Therapeutic Research* 64(8): 616–625.

Elam M (1999) Living dangerously with Bruno Latour in a hybrid world. *Theory, Culture & Society* 16(4): 1–24.

Elander J, Beach MC and Haywood Jr, C (2011) Respect, trust, and the management of sickle cell disease pain in hospital: comparative analysis of concern-raising behaviors, preliminary model, and agenda for international collaborative research to inform practice. *Ethnicity and Health* 16(4–5): 405–421.

El-Beshlawy A and Youssry I (2009) Prevention of hemoglobinopathies in Egypt. *Hemoglobin* 33(Suppl. 1): 14–20.

Elder-Vass D (2015) Disassembling actor-network theory. *Philosophy of the Social Sciences* 45(1): 100–121.

El-Hazmi MA, Al-Hazmi AM and Warsy AS (2011) Sickle cell disease in Middle East Arab countries. *The Indian Journal of Medical Research* 134(5): 597–610.

Embury SH, Hebbel RP, Steinberg MH and Mohandas N (1994) Pathogenesis of vaso-occlusion. In: SH Embury, RP Hebble, N Mohandas and MH Steinberg (eds) *Sickle Cell Disease: Basic Principles and Clinical Practice* New York: Raven Press, 311–326.

Emmel VE (1917) A study of the erythrocytes in a case of severe anemia with elongated and sickle-shaped red blood corpuscles. *Archives of Internal Medicine* 20(4): 586–598.

Estate of Richardson v. Bowling Green State University, 2010-Ohio-3475. Available at: https://law.justia.com/cases/ohio/court-of-claims/2010/2005-10179-0.html (accessed 6 November 2018).

Estcourt LJ, Fortin PM, Hopewell S, Trivella M, Doree C, *et al.* (2017) Interventions for preventing silent cerebral infarcts in people with sickle cell disease. *Cochrane Database of Systematic Reviews* 5 10.1002/14651858.CD012389.pub2.

Evans-Pritchard E (1976 [1937]) *Witchcraft, Oracles, and Magic among the Azande.* Oxford: Oxford University Press.

Evening Standard (2010) Sick boy, three, dies waiting for an appointment, 15 November 2010. Available at: www.standard.co.uk/news/sick-boy-three-dies-waiting-for-an-appointment-6536099.html.

Eysenck HJ versus Kamin L (1981) *Intelligence: The Battle for the Mind.* Basingstoke: Macmillan.

Feldman SD and Tauber AE (1997) Sickle cell anemia: re-examining the first 'molecular disease'. *Bulletin of the History of Medicine* 71(4): 623–650.

Fernandes APPC, Januário JN, Cangussu CB, de Macedo DL, and Viana MB (2010) Mortality of children with sickle cell disease: a population study. *Jornal de Pediatria* 86(4): 279–284.

Ferrari R, Parker LS, Grubs RE and Krishnamurti L (2015) Sickle cell trait screening of collegiate athletes: ethical reasons for program reform. *Journal of Genetic Counseling* 24(6): 873–877.

Ferster K and Eichner ER (2012) Exertional sickling deaths in army recruits with sickle cell trait. *Military Medicine* 177(1): 56–59.

Final Call (2010) Jurors find ex-officer not guilty in Taser case. Available at: www.final-call.com/artman/publish/National_News_2/article_7413.shtml.

Fleming AF, Storey J, Molineaux L, Iroko EA and Attai EDE (1979) Abnormal haemoglobins in the Sudan savanna of Nigeria, I: prevalence of haemoglobins and relationship between sickle cell trait, malaria, and survival. *Annals of Tropical Medicine and Parasitology* 73(2): 161–172.

Foucault M (1979) *The Birth of the Clinic: An Archaeology of Medical Perception.* London: Tavistock.

Francis YF, Wethers DL and Fenwick LA (1970) The foundation for research and education in sickle cell disease: a prospectus. *Journal of the National Medical Association* 62(3): 200–203.

Frank AG (1966) The development of underdevelopment. *Monthly Review* 18(4): 17–31.

Frayne D (2015) *The Refusal of Work.* London: Zed Books.

Friend PD (1994) *So That His Death Will Not Have Been in Vain. Sickle Cell Trait: A Serious Factor to be Observed by the Military.* Holly Hill, SC: R&M Publishing.

Fry P (2011) Remembering or forgetting Mendel: sickle cell anemia and racial politics in Brazil. In: S Gibbon, RV Santos and M Sans (eds) *Racial Identities, Genetic Ancestry and Health in South America.* New York: Palgrave Macmillan, 155–174.

Fryer P (1984) *Staying Power.* London: Pluto Press.

Fujimura JH, Bolnick DA, Rajagopalan R, Kaufman JS, Lewontin RC, *et al.* (2014) Clines without classes: how to make sense of human variation. *Sociological Theory* 32(3): 208–227.

Fulwilley D (2011) *The Enculturated Gene: Sickle Cell Health Politics and Biological Difference in West Africa.* Princeton, NJ: Princeton University Press.

Gabriel A and Przybylski J (2010) Sickle-cell anemia: a look at global haplotype distribution. *Nature, Education* 3(3): 2.

Garrick MD, Dembure P and Guthrie R (1973) Sickle-cell anemia and other hemoglobinopathies: procedures and strategy for screening employing spots of blood on filter paper as specimens. *New England Journal of Medicine* 288(24): 1265–1268.

Gaston MH, Verter JI, Woods G, Pegelow C, Kelleher J, *et al.* (1986) Prophylaxis with oral penicillin in children with sickle cell anemia: a randomized trial *New England Journal of Medicine* 314(25): 1593–1599.

George S (1988) *A Fate Worse Than Debt.* Harmondsworth: Penguin.

Ghosh K, Colah RB and Mukherjee MB (2015) Haemoglobinopathies in tribal populations of India. *Indian Journal of Medical Research* 141(5): 505–508.

Gilbert GN and Mulkay M (1984) *Opening Pandora's Box: A. Sociological Analysis of Scientists' Discourse.* Cambridge: Cambridge University Press.

Gill PS and Modell B (1998) Thalassaemia in Britain: a tale of two communities: births are rising among British Asians but falling in Cypriots. *British Medical Journal* 317(7161): 761–762.

Gillborn D (2008) *Racism and Education: Coincidence or Conspiracy?* London: Routledge.

Gillham NH (2011) *Genes, Chromosomes, and Disease: From Simple Traits, to Complex Traits, to Personalized Medicine.* Upper Saddle River, NJ: Pearson Education.

Goffman, E (1968) *Stigma: Notes on the Management of Spoiled Identity.* Harmondsworth: Penguin.

Gonçalves MS, Bomfim GC, Maciel E, Cerqueira I, Lyra I, *et al.* (2003) ßS-Haplotypes in sickle cell anemia patients from Salvador, Bahia, Northeastern Brazil. *Brazilian Journal of Medical and Biological Research* 36(10): 1283–1288.

Gould SJ (1996) *The Mismeasure of Man.* Rev. ed. London: Penguin.

Graeber D (2013) On the phenomenon of bullshit jobs. *Strike!* 17 August. Available at: http://strikemag.org/bullshit-jobs/.

Grant AM, Parker CS, Jordan LB, Hulihan MM, Creary MS, *et al.* (2011) Public health implications of sickle cell trait: a report of the CDC meeting. *American Journal of Preventive Medicine* 41(6): S435–S439.

Griffiths AJF, Gelbart WM, Lewontin R and Miller JH (2002) *Modern Genetic Analysis: Integrating Genes and Genomes.* New York: WH Freeman and Company.

Grosse SD, Atrash HK, Odame I, Amendah D, Piel FB, *et al.* (2012) The Jamaican historical experience of the impact of educational interventions on sickle cell disease child mortality. *American Journal of Preventive Medicine* 42(6): e101–e103.

Grosse SD, Odame I, Atrash H, Amendah DD, Piel FB, *et al.* (2011) Sickle cell disease in Africa: a neglected cause of childhood mortality. *American Journal of Preventive Medicine* 41(6) S4: 398–405.

Grosse SD, Olney RS and Baily MA (2005) The cost effectiveness of universal versus selective newborn screening for sickle cell disease in the US and the UK: a critique. *Applied Health Economics and Health Policy* 4(4): 239–247.

Grosse SD, Rogowski WH, Ross LF, Cornel MC, Dondorp WJ and Khoury MJ (2010) Population screening for genetic disorders in the 21st century: evidence, economics, and ethics. *Public Health Genomics* 13(2): 106–115.

Guardian (2017) Most school support staff have been assaulted by pupils, 3 June 2017. Available at: www.theguardian.com/education/2017/jun/03/most-school-support-staff-assaulted-by-pupils-union-survey.

Guardian (2018) Food, clothes, a mattress and three funerals. What teachers buy for children, 1 May 2018. Available at: www.theguardian.com/education/2018/may/01/teachers-buy-children-food-clothes-mattress-funerals-child-poverty.

Gulliver G (1840) Observations on the blood-corpuscles of certain species of the genus Cervus. *Abstracts of the Papers Printed in the Philosophical Transactions of the Royal Society of London* 4: 199–200, 6 February 1840.

Gurnah A (1984) The politics of racism awareness training. *Critical Social Policy* 4(11): 6–20.

Haggard ME and Schneider RG (1961) Sickle cell anemia in the first 2 years of life. *The Journal of Pediatrics* 58(6): 785–790.

Halasa NB, Shankar SM, Talbot TR, Arbogast PG, Mitchel EF, *et al.* (2007) Incidence of invasive pneumococcal disease among individuals with sickle cell disease before and after the introduction of the pneumococcal conjugate vaccine. *Clinical Infectious Diseases* 44(11): 1428–1433.

Hall S (1997) *Race: The Floating Signifier.* Northampton, MA: Media Education Foundation. Available at: www.mediaed.org/assets/products/407/transcript_407.pdf.

Hall S (2003) Preface. In: R Hylton (ed.) *Donald Rodney: Doublethink.* London: Autograph, 6–7.

Hampton ML, Anderson J, Lavizzo BS and Bergman AB (1974) Sickle cell nondisease: a potentially serious public health problem. *American Journal of Diseases of Children* 128(1): 58–61.

Harman G (2018) *Object-Oriented Ontology: A New Theory of Everything.* London: Penguin/Random House.

Harmon KG, Asif IM, Klossner D and Drezner JA (2011) Incidence of sudden cardiac death in National Collegiate Athletic Association athletes. *Circulation* 123(15): 1594–1600.

Harris MS and Eckman JR (1989) Approaches to screening: Georgia's experience with newborn screening. *Pediatrics* 83(5): 858–860.

Hawley WA, Phillips-Howard PA, ter Kuile FO, Terlouw DJ, Vulule JM, *et al.* (2003) Community-wide effects of permethrin-treated bed nets on child mortality and malaria morbidity in western Kenya. *The American Journal of Tropical Medicine and Hygiene* 68(S4): 121–127.

Haywood C, Diener-West M, Strouse J, Carroll CP, Bediako S, *et al.* and IMPORT Investigators (2014) Perceived discrimination in health care is associated with a greater burden of pain in sickle cell disease. *Journal of Pain and Symptom Management* 48(5): 934–943.

Hedrick PW (2011) Population genetics of malaria resistance in humans. *Heredity* 107(4): 283–304.

Herivel T and Wright P (2003) (eds) *Prison Nation: The Warehousing of America's Poor.* New York: Routledge.

Herrick JB (1910) Peculiar elongated and sickle cell red blood corpuscles in a case of severe anemia. *Archives of Internal Medicine* 6: 517–521.

Hickman M, Modell B, Greengross P, Chapman C, Layton M, *et al.* (1998). Mapping the prevalence of sickle cell and beta thalassaemia in England: estimating and validating ethnic-specific rates. *British Journal of Haematology* 104(4): 860–867.

Higginbotham Jr AL (1978) *In the Matter of Color, Race and the American Legal Process: The Colonial Period.* New York: Oxford University.

Hill SA (1994) *Managing Sickle Cell Disease in Low Income Families.* Philadelphia, PA: Temple University Press.

Hill SA and Zimmerman MK (1995) Valiant girls and vulnerable boys: the impact of gender and race on mothers' caregiving for chronically ill children. *Journal of Marriage and the Family* 57(1): 43–53.

Hinton CF, Grant AM and Grosse SD (2011) Ethical implications and practical considerations of ethnically-targeted screening for genetic disorders: the case of haemoglobinopathy screening. *Ethnicity and Health* 16(4–5): 377–388.

Hochschild AR (1983) *The Managed Heart: Commercialization of Human Feeling.* Berkeley, CA: University of California Press.

Hochschild AR and Machung A (1989) *The Second Shift: Working Parents and the Revolution at Home.* New York: Viking.

Hodenpyl E (1898) A case of apparent absence of the spleen with general compensatory lymphatic hyperplasia. *Medical Record* 54: 695–698.

Hoedemaekers R and ten Have H (1998) Geneticization: the Cyprus paradigm. *The Journal of Medicine and Philosophy* 23(3): 274–287.

Hogg C and Modell B (1998) *Sickle Cell and Thalassaemia: Achieving Health Gain.* London: Health Education Authority.

Hollinger DA (2003) Amalgamation and hypodescent: the question of ethnoracial mixture in the history of the United States. *The American Historical Review* 108(5): 1363–1390.

Howarth C (2002) "So you're from Brixton?": the struggle for recognition and esteem in a stigmatized community. *Ethnicities* 2(2): 237–260.

Horton JAB (2011 [1868]) *West African Countries and Peoples, British and Native.* Cambridge: Cambridge University Press.

Horton JAB (1874) *The Disease of Tropical Climes and Their Treatment.* London: J and A Churchill.

Huck JG (1923) Sickle cell anaemia. *Bulletin of the Johns Hopkins Hospital* 34(392): 335–344.

Huffington Post (2015) Final moments of army Sgt. James Brown's life captured in graphic jail video, 18 May 2015. Available at: www.huffingtonpost.co.uk/entry/soldier-james-brown-dies-jail-video_n_7309716?guccounter=1.

Hughes B and Paterson K (1997) The social model of disability and the disappearing body: towards a sociology of impairment. *Disability and Society* 12(3): 325–340.

Hughes EC (1962) Good people and dirty work. *Social Problems* 10(1): 3–11.

Human Rights Watch (2011) Suspicious deaths in custody. Available at: www.hrw.org/en/news/2011/04/13/bahrain-suspicious-deaths-custody (accessed 28 June 2011).

Hylton R (ed.) (2003) *Donald Rodney: Doublethink.* London: Autograph.

Ingold T (2000) *The Perception of the Environment.* London: Routledge.

Ingram VM (1957) Gene mutations in human haemoglobin: the chemical difference between normal and sickle cell haemoglobin. *Nature* 180(4581): 326–328.

Jain D, Warthe V, Dayama P, Sarate D, Colah R, et al. (2016) Sickle cell disease in Central India: a potentially severe syndrome. *The Indian Journal of Pediatrics* 83(10): 1071–1076.

Jain DL, Sarathi V, Upadhye D, Gulhane R, Nadkarni AH, et al. (2012) Newborn screening shows a high incidence of sickle cell anemia in Central India. *Hemoglobin* 36(4): 316–322.

Jans SMPJ, van El CG, Houwaart ES, Westerman MJ, Janssens RJPA, et al. (2012) A case study of haemoglobinopathy screening in the Netherlands: witnessing the past, lessons for the future. *Ethnicity and Health* 17(3): 217–239.

Jenerette CM and Brewer C (2010) Health-related stigma in young adults with sickle cell disease. *Journal of the National Medical Association* 102(11): 1050–1055.

Jewson ND (1974) Medical knowledge and the patronage system in 18th century England. *Sociology* 8(3): 369–385.

Jhally S (1984) The spectacle of accumulation: material and cultural factors in the evolution of the sports/media complex. *Critical Sociology* 12(3): 41–57.

Johnson AP and Iandoli K (2016) *Commissary Kitchen: My Infamous Prison Cookbook.* New York: Infamous Books.

Jones S (1994) *The Language of the Genes.* London: HarperCollins.

Jones S, Duncan, ER, Thomas N, Walters J, Dick MC, et al. (2005) Windy weather and low humidity are associated with an increased number of hospital admissions for acute pain and sickle cell disease in an urban environment with a maritime temperate climate. *British Journal of Haematology* 131(4): 530–533.

Jones SR, Binder RA and Donowho Jr, EM (1970) Sudden death in sickle-cell trait. *New England Journal of Medicine* 282(6): 323–325.

Jordan LB, Smith-Whitley K, Treadwell MJ, Telfair J, Grant AM, *et al.* (2011) Screening US college athletes for their sickle cell disease carrier status. *American Journal of Preventive Medicine* 41(6S4): S406–S412.

Joy DA, Feng X, Mu J, Furuya T, Chotivanich K, *et al.* (2003) Early origin and recent expansion of Plasmodium falciparum. *Science* 300(5617): 318–321.

Kadkhodaei Elyaderani M, Cinkotai KI, Hyde K, Waters HM, Howarth J, Goldstone S and Richards JT (1998) Ethnicity study and non-selective screening for haemoglobinopathies in the antenatal population of Central Manchester. *International Journal of Laboratory Haematology* 20(4): 207–211.

Kafando E, Nacoulma E, Ouattara Y, Ayéroué J, Cotton, F, Sawadogo, M and Gulbis, B (2009) Neonatal haemoglobinopathy screening in Burkina Faso. *Journal of Clinical Pathology* 62(1): 39–41.

Kai J, Ulph F, Cullinan T and Qureshi N (2009) Communication of carrier status information following universal newborn screening for sickle cell disorders and cystic fibrosis: qualitative study of experience and practice. *Health Technology Assessment* 13(57): 1–82.

Kalokairinou EM (2007) The experience of β-thalassaemia and its prevention in Cyprus. *Medicine and Law* 26(2): 291–307.

Kan YW and Dozy A (1978) Antenatal diagnosis of sickle-cell anaemia by DNA analysis of amniotic-fluid cells. *The Lancet* 312(8096): 910–912.

Kark JA (2000) Sickle cell trait. Available at: http://sickle.bwh.harvard.edu/sickle_trait.html.

Kark JA, Gardner JW, Ward FT and Virmani R (2008) Sickle cell trait and fatal exertional heat illness: implications for exercise-related death of young adults. Fort Belvoir, VA: Defense Technical Information Center. Available at: www.dtic.mil/dtic/tr/fulltext/u2/a500648.pdf.

Kark JA, Labotka RJ, Gardner JW and Ward FT (2010) Prevention of exercise-related death unexplained by pre-existing disease (EDU) associated with sickle cell trait (SCT) without hemoglobin (Hb) screening or Hb specific management. *Blood* 116(21): 945.

Kark JA, Posey DM, Schumacher HR and Ruehle CJ (1987) Sickle cell trait as a risk factor for sudden death in physical training. *New England Journal of Medicine* 317(13): 781–787.

Kato GJ, Gladwin MT and Steinberg MH (2007) Deconstructing sickle cell disease: reappraisal of the role of hemolysis in the development of clinical subphenotypes. *Blood Reviews* 21(1): 37–47.

Kawadler JM, Clayden JD, Clark CA and Kirkham FJ (2016) Intelligence quotient in paediatric sickle cell disease: a systematic review and meta-analysis. *Developmental Medicine & Child Neurology* 58(7): 672–679.

Kepron C, Somers GR and Pollanen MS (2009) Sickle cell trait mimicking multiple inflicted injuries in a 5-year-old boy. *Journal of Forensic Science* 54(5): 1141–1145.

Kerr A, Cunningham-Burley S and Amos A (1997) The new genetics: professionals' discursive boundaries. *Sociological Review* 45(2): 279–303.

Kerr A, Cunningham-Burley S and Amos A (1998) The new genetics and health: mobilizing lay expertise. *Public Understanding of Science* 7(1): 41–60.

Kerr-Ritchie J (2003) Forty acres, or an act of bad faith. *Souls* 5(3): 8–22.

Killeen GF, Smith TA, Ferguson HM, Mshinda H, Abdulla S, *et al.* (2007) Preventing childhood malaria in Africa by protecting adults from mosquitoes with insecticide-treated nets. *PLoS Med.* 4: e229.

King L, Fraser R, Forbes M, Grindley M, Ali S, *et al.* (2007) Newborn sickle cell disease screening: the Jamaican experience (1995–2006). *Journal of Medical Screening* 14(3): 117–122.

Kizito ME, Mworozi E, Ndugwa C and Serjeant GR (2007) Bacteraemia in homozygous sickle cell disease in Africa: is pneumococcal prophylaxis justified? *Archives of Disease in Childhood* 92(1): 21–23.

Konotey-Ahulu FID (1974) The sickle cell diseases: clinical manifestations including the 'sickle crisis'. *Archives of Internal Medicine* 133(4): 611–619.

Konotey-Ahulu FID (1980) Male procreative superiority index (MPSI): the missing coefficient in African anthropogenetics. *British Medical Journal* 281(6256): 1700–1702.

Konotey-Ahulu FID (1996) *Sickle Cell Disease Patient: Natural History from a Clinico-Epidemiological Study of the First 1550 Patients of Korle Bu Hospital Sickle Cell Clinic.* London and Basingstoke: Macmillan (1991) Watford: Tetteh-A'Domeno Company (T-AD Co) PO Box 189, Watford WD1 7NF (1996).

Konotey-Ahulu FID (2011) Blaming sudden death on sickle cell trait. Available at: www.sicklecell.md/blog/?p=105.

Koontz K, Short AD, Kalinyak K and Noll RB (2004) A randomized controlled pilot trial of a school intervention for children with sickle cell anaemia. *Journal of Paediatric Psychology* 29(1): 7–17.

Krieger N and Sidney S (1996) Racial discrimination and blood pressure: the CARDIA Study of young black and white adults. *American Journal of Public Health* 86(10): 1370–1378.

Kulozik AE, Wainscoat JS, Serjeant GR, Kar BC, Al-Awamy B, *et al.* (1986) Geographical survey of βs-globin gene haplotypes: evidence for an independent Asian origin of the sickle-cell mutation. *American Journal of Human Genetics* 39(2): 239–244.

Laird L, Dezateux C and Anionwu EN (1996) Neonatal screening for sickle cell disorders: what about the carrier infants? *British Medical Journal* 313(7054): 407–411.

Lainé A, Diallo D and Traoré B (2012) De Koloci à la drépanocytose. *Anthropologie et Santé* 4. Available at: http://anthropologiesante.revues.org/884.

Lane PA (2001) Cost-effectiveness and equity: an American perspective. *International Workshop on Haemoglobinopathy Screening to Inform the Screening Developments in England.* London: NHS Sickle Cell and Thalassaemia Screening Programme 10–14. Available at: http://sct.screening.nhs.uk/Researchdevelopment#fileid11009 (accessed 15 May 2014).

Lanzkron S, Carroll CP and Haywood Jr, C (2013) Mortality rates and age at death from sickle cell disease: US, 979–2005. *Public Health Reports* 128(2): 110–116.

Lapouniéroulie C, Dunda O, Ducrocq R, Trabuchet G, Mony-Lobe M, *et al.* (1992) A novel sickle cell mutation of yet another origin in Africa: the Cameroon type. *Human Genetics* 89(3): 333–337.

Lappé M, Gustafson JM and Roblin R (1972) Ethical and social issues in screening for genetic disease. *New England Journal of Medicine* 286(21): 1129–3112.

Latour B (1993) *We Have Never Been Modern.* Cambridge, MA: Harvard University Press.

Latour B (1999) *Pandora's Hope: Essays on the Reality of Science Studies.* Cambridge, MA: Harvard University Press.

Latour B (2000) When things strike back: a possible contribution of 'science studies' to the social sciences. *British Journal of Sociology* 51(1): 107–123.

Latour B (2013) *An Inquiry into Modes of Existence.* Cambridge, MA: Harvard University Press.

Latour B (2015) International relations at the time of Gaia-politics? Keynote address from the 2015 Millennium Conference, London School of Economics, 17 October 2015. Available at: http://mil.sagepub.com/site/Videos/Videos.xhtml [046:35].

Latour B (2016) Two bubbles of unrealism: learning from the tragedy of Trump. *Los Angeles Review of Books*, 17 November 2016. Available at: https://lareviewofbooks.org/article/two-bubbles-unrealism-learning-tragedy-trump/.

Lavinha J, Gonçalves J, Faustino P, Romão L, Osório-Almeida L, *et al.* (1992) Importation route of the sickle cell trait into Portugal: contribution of molecular biology. *Human Biology* 64(6): 891–901.

Layder D (1993) *New Strategies in Social Research.* Cambridge: Polity Press.

Leach E (1970) *Lévi-Strauss.* London: Fontana.

Lebby R (1846) A case of absence of the spleen. *Southern Journal of Medical Pharmacology* 1: 481–483.

Lee A, Thomas P, Cupidore L, Serjeant B and Serjeant G (1995) Improved survival in homozygous sickle cell disease: lessons from a cohort study. *British Medical Journal* 311(7020): 1600–1602.

Le Gallais D, Lonsdorfer J, Bogui P and Fattoum S (2007) Point: counterpoint: sickle cell trait should/should not be considered asymptomatic and as a benign condition during physical activity. *Journal of Applied Physiology* 103(6): 2137–2138.

Lehmann H (1963) Some medical problems of immigration into Britain: haemoglobinopathies. *Proceedings of the Royal Society of Medicine* 56(7): 569–572.

Lehmann H and Huntsman RG (1974) *Man's Haemoglobins.* Amsterdam: North-Holland Publishing.

Lewontin R, Rose S and Kamin L (1982) Bourgeois ideology and the origins of biological determinism. *Race and Class* 24(1): 1–16.

Lewontin R, Rose S and Kamin L (1984) *Not in Our Genes: Biology, Ideology and Human Nature.* New York: Pantheon Books.

Link BG and Phelan J (2014) Stigma power. *Social Science and Medicine* 103(2014): 24–32.

Little I, Vinogradova Y, Orton E, Kai J and Qureshi N (2017) Venous thromboembolism in adults screened for sickle cell trait: a population-based cohort study with nested case-control analysis. *BMJ Open* 7(3) p.e012665.

Livingstone FB (1958a) Anthropological implications of sickle cell gene distribution in West Africa. *American Anthropologist* 60(3): 533–562.

Livingstone FB (1958b) The distribution of the sickle cell gene in Liberia. *American Journal of Human Genetics* 10(1): 33–41.

Livingstone FB (1962) On the non-existence of human races. *Current Anthropology* 3(3): 279–281.

Livingstone FB (1985) *Frequencies of Hemoglobin Variants: Thalassemia, the Glucose-6-Phosphate Dehydrogenase Deficiency, G6PD Variants, and Ovalocytosis in Human Populations.* New York: Oxford University Press.

Lobel JS, Cameron BF, Johnson E, Smith D and Kalinyak K (1989) Value of screening umbilical cord blood for hemoglobinopathy. *Pediatrics* 83(5): 823–882.

Lorey FW, Arnopp J and Cunningham GC (1996) Distribution of hemoglobinopathy variants by ethnicity in a multi-ethnic state. *Genetic Epidemiology* 13(5): 501–512.

Lowe R (2002) A century of Local Education Authorities: what has been lost? *Oxford Review of Education* 28(2–3): 149–158.

Loy DE, Liu W, Li Y, Learn GH, Plenderleith LJ, *et al.* (2017) Out of Africa: origins and evolution of the human malaria parasites *Plasmodium falciparum* and *Plasmodium vivax. International Journal for Parasitology* 47(2): 87–97.

Lucas SB (2004) The morbid anatomy of sickle cell disease and sickle cell trait. In: I Okpala (ed.) *Practical Management of Haemoglobinopathies* Oxford: Blackwell, 45–62.

Lucas SB, Mason DG, Mason M and Weyman D (2008) *A Sickle Crisis? Report of the National Confidential Enquiry into Patient Outcome and Death* London: NCEPOD. Available at: www.ncepod.org.uk/2008report1/Downloads/Sickle_report.pdf.

Lukes S (1974) *Power: A Radical View.* London: Macmillan.

Lynch M (1985) *Art and Artifact in Laboratory Science.* London: Routledge and Kegan Paul.

Macauley S (2018) *Sikul Sel Song.* Available at: https://soundcloud.com/viv-rolfe/sikul-sel-song-sierra-leone.

Macharia AW, Mochamah G, Uyoga S, Ndila CM, Nyutu G, *et al.* (2018) The clinical epidemiology of sickle cell anemia in Africa. *American Journal of Hematology* 93(3): 363–370.

MacKenzie D (1979) Eugenics and the rise of mathematical statistics in Britain. In: J Irvine, I Miles and J Evans (eds) *Demystifying Social Statistics.* London: Pluto Press, 39–50.

Macpherson W (1999) *The Stephen Lawrence Inquiry: Report of an Inquiry by Sir William Macpherson* (Cm 4262–1). London: The Stationery Office.

Marin A, Cerutti N and Massa ER (1999) Use of the amplification refractory mutation system (ARMS) in the study of HbS in predynastic Egyptian remains. *Bollettino della Società Italiana di Biologia Sperimentale* 75(5–6): 27–30.

Markel H (1992) The stigma of disease: implications of genetic screening. *The American Journal of Medicine* 93(2): 209–215.

Markel H (1997) Scientific advances and social risks: historical perspectives of genetic screening programs for sickle cell disease, Tay-Sachs disease, neural tube defects, and Down syndrome, 1970–1997. *NIH-DOE Working Group on Ethical, Legal and Social Implications of Human Genome Research.* National Institutes of Health. Available at: www.ncbi.nlm.nih.gov/books/NBK231976.

Marlin L, Etienne-Julan M, Le Gallais D and Hue O (2005) Sickle cell trait in French West Indian elite sprint athletes. *International Journal of Sports Medicine* 26(8): 622–625.

Marmot MG and Wilkinson RG (2006) *Social Determinant of Health,* 2nd edn. New York: Oxford University Press.

Marsh VM, Kamuya DM and Molyneux SS (2011) 'All her children are born that way': gendered experiences of stigma in families affected by sickle cell disorder in rural Kenya. *Ethnicity and Health* 16(4–5): 343–359.

Marsh VM, Kombe F, Fitzpatrick R, Molyneux S and Parker M (2013) Managing mis-aligned paternity findings in research including sickle cell disease screening in Kenya: 'consulting communities' to inform policy. *Social Science and Medicine* 96(2013): 92–199.

Martin PH (1999) Genes as drugs: the social shaping of gene therapy and the reconstruction of genetic disease. *Sociology of Health and Illness* 21(5): 517–538.

Martin TW, Weisman IM, Zeballos RJ and Stephenson SR (1989) Exercise and hypoxia increase sickling in venous blood from an exercising limb in individuals with sickle cell trait. *The American Journal of Medicine* 87(1): 48–56.

Mason D (1982) After Scarman: a note on the concept of institutional racism. *Journal of Ethnic and Migration Studies* 10(1): 38–45.

Mason VR (1922) Sickle cell anemia. *Journal of the American Medical Association* 79(16): 1318–1320.

Mathur VA, Kiley KB, Haywood Jr C, Bediako SM, Lanzkron S, *et al.* (2016) Multiple levels of suffering: discrimination in health-care settings is associated with enhanced laboratory pain sensitivity in sickle cell disease. *The Clinical Journal of Pain* 32(12): 1076–1085.

Maxwell K, Streetly A and Bevan D (1999) Experiences of hospital care and treatment seeking for pain from sickle cell disease: qualitative study. *British Medical Journal* 318(7198): 1585–1590.

McAuley CF, Webb C, Makani J, Macharia A, Uyoga S, *et al.* (2010) High mortality from Plasmodium falciparum malaria in children living with sickle cell anemia on the coast of Kenya. *Blood* 116(10): 663–1668.

McDonald MA, Creary MS, Powell J, Daley LA, Baker C *et al.* (2017) Perspectives and practices of athletic trainers and team physicians implementing the 2010 NCAA Sickle Cell Trait Screening Policy. *Journal of Genetic Counseling* 26(6): 1292–1300.

McGann PT, Grosse SD, Santos B, de Oliveira V, Bernardino L, *et al.* (2015) A cost-effectiveness analysis of a pilot neonatal screening program for sickle cell anemia in the Republic of Angola. *Journal of Pediatrics* 167(6): 1314–1319.

Merton, RK (1936) The unanticipated consequences of purposive social action. *American Sociological Review* 1(6): 894–904.

Miles R (1982) *Racism and Migrant Labour.* London: Routledge and Kegan Paul.

Miller FA, Paynter M, Hayeems RZ, Little J, Carroll JC, *et al.* (2010) Understanding sickle cell carrier status identified through newborn screening: a qualitative study. *European Journal of Human Genetics* 18(3): 303–308.

Missirian A and Schlenker W (2017) Asylum applications respond to temperature fluctuations. *Science* 358 (6370): 1610–1614.

Mitchell BL (2007) Sickle cell trait and sudden death: bringing it home. *Journal of the National Medical Association* 99(3): 300–305.

Mittal H, Roberts L, Fuller GW, O'Driscoll S, Dick MC, *et al.* (2009) The effects of air quality on haematological and clinical parameters in children with sickle cell anaemia. *Annals of Haematology* 88(6): 529–533.

Modell B and Anionwu EN (1996) Guidelines for screening for haemoglobin disorders: service specifications for low- and high-prevalence district health authorities. In: NHS Centre for Reviews and Dissemination. *Ethnicity and Health: Reviews of Literature for Purchasers in the Areas of Cardiovascular Disease, Mental Health and Haemoglobin-opathies.* York: University of York, 127–178.

Modell B and Darlison M (2008) Global epidemiology of haemoglobin disorders and derived service indicators. *Bulletin of the World Health Organization* 86 (6): 417–428.

Modell B, Harris R, Lane B, Khan M, Darlison M, *et al.* (2000) Informed choice in genetic screening for thalassaemia during pregnancy: audit from a national confidential inquiry. *British Medical Journal* 320(7231): 337–341.

Modell B and Modell M (1992) *Towards a Healthy Baby: Congenital Disorders and the New Genetics in Primary Care.* New York: Oxford University Press.

Modell B, Petrou M, Layton M, Slater C, Ward RHT, *et al.* (1997) Audit of prenatal diagnosis for haemoglobin disorders in the United Kingdom: the first 20 years. *British Medical Journal* 315(7111): 779–784.

Modell B, Ward RHT, Rodeck C, Petrou M, Faireweather DVI, *et al.* (1984) Effect of fetal diagnostic testing on birth-rate of thalassaemia major in Britain. *The Lancet* 324(8416): 1383–1386.

Modi N (2011) Gujarat awarded Prime Minister Civil Services Award for successfully tackling sickle cell anemia in Gujarat. Available at: www.narendramodi.in/gujarat-awarded-prime-minister%E2%80%99s-civil-services-award-for-successfully-tackling-sickle-cell-anemia-in-gujarat-3939, 11 April 2011.

Modiano D, Luoni G, Sirima BS, Simporé J, Verra F, *et al.* (2001) Haemoglobin C protects against clinical Plasmodium falciparum malaria. *Nature* 414(6861): 305–308.

Moez P and Younan DNA (2016) High prevalence of haemoglobin S in the closed Egyptian community of Siwa Oasis. *Journal of Clinical Pathology* 69(7): 632–636.

Mol A (2008) *The Logic of Care: Health and the Problem of Patient Choice.* London: Routledge.

Molokie RE, Montminy C, Dionisio C, Farooqui MA, Gowhari M, *et al.* (2018) Opioid doses and acute care utilization outcomes for adults with sickle cell disease: ED versus acute care unit. *The American Journal of Emergency Medicine* 36(1): 88–92.

Montagu A (1998 [1942]) *Man's Most Dangerous Myth: The Fallacy of Race,* 6th edn. Walnut Creek, CA: Rowman Altamira.

Morning Call (2013) Lawsuit: Prison guards inflicted 'grave injuries' before inmate's death, 31 January 2013. Available at: http://articles.mcall.com/2013-01-31/news/mc-p-lehigh-prison-lawsuit-restraint-chair-20130130_1_restraint-chair-prison-guards-wrongful-death-lawsuit (accessed 8 October 2013).

Morton T (2017) *Humankind: Solidarity with Nonhuman People.* London: Verso Books.

Moskowitz JT, Butensky E, Harmatz P, Vichinsky E, Heyman MB *et al.* (2007) Caregiving time in sickle cell disease: psychological effects in maternal caregivers. *Pediatric Blood and Cancer* 48(1): 64–71.

Naik RP, Irvin MR, Judd S, Gutiérrez OM, Zakai NA, *et al.* (2017) Sickle cell trait and the risk of ESRD in blacks. *Journal of the American Society of Nephrology* 28(7): 2180–2187.

Nair V, Yanamandra U, Kapoor R, Kumar R, Das SR *et al.* (2017) Splenic infarct as an harbinger for sickle cell traits in high altitude. *Blood* 130 (Suppl 1): 4650.

Nalbandian RM (1972) Mass screening programs for sickle cell hemoglobin. *Journal of the American Medical Association* 221(5): 500–502.

National Athletic Trainers' Association (NATA) (2007) Consensus statement: sickle cell trait and the athlete. Available at: www.nata.org/statements/consensus/sicklecell.pdf (accessed 7 January 2008).

Nazroo JY (1999) The racialization of ethnic inequalities in health. In: D Dorling and S Simpson (eds) *Statistics in Society: The Arithmetic of Politics.* London: Arnold, 215–222.

NCAA (National Collegiate Athletic Association) (2011) Monster within. *Champion Magazine,* 29 November. Available at: www.ncaastudent.org/wps/wcm/connect/public/ncaa/resources/latest+news/2011/november/monster+within+-+eckerd+basketball+standout+kearse+proves+sickle+cell+trait+can+be+a+tamed+monster (accessed 14 April 2014).

Nelson A (2011) *Body and Soul: The Black Panther Party and the Fight Against Medical Discrimination.* Minneapolis, MN: University of Minnesota Press.

Nelson DA, Deuster PA, Carter III R, Hill OT, Wolcott VL, *et al.* (2016) Sickle cell trait, rhabdomyolysis, and mortality among US Army soldiers. *New England Journal of Medicine* 375(5): 435–442.

New C (2005) Sex and gender: a critical realist approach. *New Formations* 56: 54–70.

New York Times (2016) A pioneer in treating sickle cell anemia dies at 89. Available at: www.nytimes.com/2016/04/08/nyregion/yvette-fay-francis-mcbarnette-a-pioneer-in-treating-sickle-cell-anemia-dies-at-89.html?_r=0.

News Herald (2007) Author, pathologist supports Siebart, 3 August 2007. Available at: https://web.archive.org/web/20070928060624/www.newsherald.com/headlines/article.display.php?a=2622.

NICE (National Institute for Health and Care Excellence) (2012) *Sickle Cell Disease: Managing Acute Painful Episodes in Hospital.* Available at: www.nice.org.uk/guidance/cg143.

NIH (National Institutes of Health) (2014) *Evidence Based Management of Sickle Cell Disease.* National Heart Lung and Blood Institute. Available at: www.nhlbi.nih.gov/sites/www.nhlbi.nih.gov/files/sickle-cell-disease-report.pdf.

Nixon R (1972) Statement on Signing the National Sickle Cell Anemia Control Act May 16, 1972. Online by Gerhard Peters and John T Woolley. *The American Presidency Project.* Available at: www.presidency.ucsb.edu/ws/?pid=3413.

Noll RB, Ris MD, Davies WH, Bukowski WM and Koontz K (1992) Social interactions between children with cancer or sickle cell disease and their peers: teacher ratings. *Journal of Developmental and Behavioural Pediatrics* 13(3): 187–192.

Noll RB, Vannatta K, Koontz K, Kalinyak K, Bukowski WM *et al.* (1996) Peer relationships and emotional well-being of youngsters with sickle cell disease. *Child Development* 67(2): 423–436.

Nollan RH (2016) *LW Diggs, Sickle Cell Anaemia and the South's First Blood Bank.* Knoxville, TN: University of Tennessee Press.

Novitski E (2004) On Fisher's criticism of Mendel's results with the garden pea. *Genetics* 166(3): 1133–1136.

Nussbaum RL, Powell C, Graham HL, Caskey CT and Fernbach DJ (1984) Newborn screening for sickling hemoglobinopathies. *American Journal of Diseases of Children* 138(1): 44–48.

Nzewi E (2001) Malevolent ogbanje: recurrent reincarnation or sickle cell disease? *Social Science and Medicine* 52(9): 1403–1416.

Obaro S (2009) Pneumococcal infections and sickle cell disease in Africa: does absence of evidence imply evidence of absence? *Archives of Disease in Childhood* 94(9): 713–716.

Ogunjuyigbe P (2004) Under-five mortality in Nigeria: perception and attitudes of the Yorubas towards the existence of "Abiku". *Demographic Research* 11(2): 43–56.

Ohene-Frempong K and Nkrumah FK (1994) Sickle cell disease in Africa. In: SH Embury, RP Hebbel, N Mohandas, and MH Steinberg (eds) *Sickle Cell Disease: Basic Principles and Clinical Practice.* New York: Raven Press, 423–435.

Okany CC and Akinyanju OO (1993) The influence of socio-economic status on the severity of sickle cell disease. *African Journal of Medicine and Medical Sciences* 22(2): 57–60.

Okpuzor J, Adebesin A, Ogbunugafor H and Amadi I (2008) The potential of medicinal plants in sickle cell disease control: a review. *International Journal of Biomedical and Health Sciences* 4(2): 47–55.

Okumura JV, Silva DG, Torres LS, Belini-Junior E, Barberino WM, *et al.* (2016) Inheritance of the Bantu/Benin haplotype causes less severe hemolytic and oxidative stress in sickle cell anemia patients treated with hydroxycarbamide. *Journal of Human Genetics* 61(7): 605–611.

Ola BA, Coker R and Ani C (2013) Stigmatising attitudes towards peers with sickle cell disease among secondary school students in Nigeria. *International Journal of Child, Youth and Family Studies* 4(4): 391–402.

Ola BA, Yates SJ and Dyson SM (2016) Living with sickle cell disease and depression in Lagos, Nigeria: a mixed methods study. *Social Science and Medicine* 161(2016): 27–36.

Olakunle OS, Kenneth E, Olakekan AW and Adenike O-B (2013) Knowledge and attitude of secondary school students in Jos, Nigeria on sickle cell disease. *Pan African*

Medical Journal 15(127). Available at: www.panafrican-med-journal.com/content/article/15/127/full.

Oliver M (1992) Changing the social relations of research production. *Disability, Handicap and Society* 7(2): 101–114.

Oliver M (1998) Theories in health care and research: theories of disability in health practice and research. *British Medical Journal* 317(7170): 1446–1449.

Oliver M (2013) The social model of disability: thirty years on. *Disability and Society* 28(7): 1024–1026.

Orbach S (2009) *Bodies.* London: Profile Books.

Oredugba FA and Savage KO (2002) Anthropometric findings in Nigerian children with sickle cell disease. *Pediatric Dentistry* 24(4): 321–325.

Outram SM and Ellison GTH (2005) Anthropological insights into the use of race/ethnicity to explore genetic contributions to disparities in health. *Journal of Biosocial Science* 38(1): 83–102.

Owolabi RS, Alabi P and Olusoji D (2011) Knowledge and attitudes of secondary school students in Federal Capital Territory (FCT), Abuja, Nigeria towards sickle cell disease. *Nigerian Journal of Medicine: Journal of the National Association of Resident Doctors of Nigeria* 20(4): 479–485.

Pagnier J, Mears JG, Dunda-Belkhodja O, Schaefer-Rego KE, Beldjord C, *et al.* (1984) Evidence for the multicentric origin of the sickle cell hemoglobin gene in Africa. *Proceedings of the National Academy of Sciences* 81(6): 1771–1773.

Palermo TM, Riley CA and Mitchell BA (2008) Daily functioning and quality of life in children with sickle cell disease pain: relationship with family and neighborhood socioeconomic distress. *The Journal of Pain* 9(9): 833–840.

Panepinto JA, Pajewski NM, Foerster LM, Sabnis S and Hoffmann RG (2009) Impact of family income and sickle cell disease on the health-related quality of life of children. *Quality of Life Research* 18(1): 5–13.

Panigrahi S, Patra PK and Khodiar PK (2011) Neonatal screening of sickle cell anemia: a preliminary report. *Indian Journal of Paediatrics* 79(6): 747–750.

Parra FC, Amado RC, Lambertucci JR, Rocha J, Antunes CM *et al.* (2003) Color and genomic ancestry in Brazilians. *Proceedings of the National Academy of Sciences of the United States of America* 100(1): 177–182.

Parsons T (1951) *The Social System.* London: Routledge.

Patel AB and Pathan HG (2005) Quality of life in children with sickle cell haemoglobinopathy. *Indian Journal of Pediatrics* 72(7): 567–571.

Patra PK, Chauhan VS, Khodiar PK, Dalla AR and Serjeant GR (2011) Screening for the sickle cell gene in Chhattisgarh state, India: an approach to a major public health problem. *Journal of Community Genetics* 2(3): 147–151.

Pauling L (1967) Reflections on the new biology: foreword. *UcLA Law Review* 15(2): 267–272.

Pauling L, Itano HA, Singer SJ and Wells IC (1949) Sickle cell anemia, a molecular disease. *Science* 110(2865): 543–548.

Pawson R and Tilley N (1997) *Realistic Evaluation.* London: Sage.

Pearson M (1986) Racist notions of ethnicity and culture in health education. In: S Rodmell and A Watt (eds) *The Politics of Health Education.* London: Routledge and Kegan Paul, 38–56.

Pegelow CH, Colangelo L, Steinberg M, Wright EC, Smith J, *et al.* (1997) Natural history of blood pressure in sickle cell disease: risks for stroke and death associated with relative hypertension in sickle cell anemia. *The American Journal of Medicine* 102(2): 171–177.

Pemberton S (2008) Demystifying deaths in police custody: challenging state talk. *Social and Legal Studies* 17(2): 237–262.

Penman BS, Gupta S and Buckee CO (2012) The emergence and maintenance of sickle cell hotspots in the Mediterranean. *Infection, Genetics and Evolution* 12(7): 1543–1550.

Penman BS, Pybus OG, Weatherall DJ and Gupta S (2009) Epistatic interactions between genetic disorders of hemoglobin can explain why the sickle cell gene is uncommon in the Mediterranean. *Proceedings of the National Academy of Sciences* 106(50): 21242–21246.

Pennisi E (2003) Gene counters struggle to get the right answer. *Science* 301(5636): 1040–1041.

Piel FB, Adamkiewicz TV, Amendah D, Williams TN, Gupta S, *et al.* (2016) Observed and expected frequencies of structural hemoglobin variants in newborn screening surveys in Africa and the Middle East: deviations from Hardy-Weinberg equilibrium. *Genetics in Medicine* 18(3): 265–274.

Piel FB, Hay SI, Gupta S, Weatherall DJ, and Williams TN (2013b) Global burden of sickle cell anaemia in children under five, 2010–2050: modelling based on demographics, excess mortality, and interventions. *PLoS Med* 10(7): e1001484.

Piel FB, Patil AP, Howes RE, Nyangiri OA, Gething PW, *et al.* (2013a) Global epidemiology of sickle haemoglobin in neonates: a contemporary geostatistical model-based map and population estimates. *Lancet* 381(9861): 142–151.

Piel FB, Steinberg MH and Rees DC (2017) Sickle cell disease. *New England Journal of Medicine* 376(16): 1561–1573.

Piel FB, Tatem AJ, Huang Z, Gupta S, Williams TN and Weatherall DJ (2014) Global migration and the changing distribution of sickle hemoglobin: a quantitative study of global trends between 1960 and 2000. *The Lancet Global Health* 2(2): e80–e89.

Plath, S (2005 [1963]) *The Bell Jar.* London: Faber & Faber.

Pletcher MJ, Kertesz SG, Kohn MA and Gonzales R (2008) Trends in opioid prescribing by race/ethnicity for patients seeking care in US emergency departments. *Journal of the American Medical Association* 299(1): 70–78.

Polanyi, K (2001 [1944]) *The Great Transformation: The Political and Economic Origins of Our Time.* Boston: Beacon Books.

Powars D, Overturf G, Weiss J, Lee S and Chan L (1981) Pneumococcal septicemia in children with sickle cell anemia: changing trend of survival. *Journal of the American Medical Association* 245(18): 1839–1842.

Prabhakar H, Haywood Jr, C and Molokie R (2010) Sickle cell disease in the United States: looking back and forward at 100 years of progress in management and survival. *American Journal of Hematology* 85(5): 346–353.

Prashar U, Brozovic M and Anionwu EN (1985) *Sickle-Cell Anaemia: Who Cares?* London: Runnymede Trust.

Pretzlaff RK (2002) Death of an adolescent athlete with sickle cell trait caused by exertional heat stroke. *Pediatric Critical Care Medicine* 3(3): 308–310.

Pronger B (2002) *Body Fascism: Salvation in the Technology of Physical Fitness.* Toronto: University of Toronto Press.

Ragusa A, Frontini M, Amata S, Lombardo T, Labie D, *et al.* (1992) Presence of a β-globin gene cluster haplotype in normal chromosomes in Sicily. *American Journal of Hematology* 40(4): 313–315.

Rahimy MC, Gangbo A, Ahouignan G and Alihonou E (2009) Newborn screening for sickle cell disease in the Republic of Benin. *Journal of Clinical Pathology* 62(1): 46–48.

Rapp R (2000) *Testing Women, Testing the Fetus.* London: Routledge.

Reed K (2011) 'He's the dad isn't he?' Gender, race and the politics of prenatal screening. *Ethnicity and Health* 16(4–5): 327–341.

Rees DC, Williams, TN and Gladwin MT (2010) Sickle-cell disease. *The Lancet* 376(9757): 2018–2031.

Reverby SM (2000) *Tuskegee's Truths: Rethinking the Tuskegee Syphilis Study.* Chapel Hill, NC: University of North Carolina Press.

Robb J and Harris OJT (2013) *The Body in History.* Cambridge: Cambridge University Press.

Roberts D (1997) *Killing the Black Body.* New York: Vintage Books.

Roberts I and de Montalembert M (2007) Sickle cell disease as a paradigm of immigration haematology: new challenges for haematologists in Europe. *Haematologica* 92(7): 865–871.

Rodney W (1972) *How Europe Underdeveloped Africa.* London/Dar es Salaam: Bogle-L'Ouverture Publications.

Rose S (1997) *Lifelines.* Harmondsworth: Penguin.

Rose S and Rose H (1986) Less than human nature: biology and the new right. *Race and Class* 27(3): 47–66.

Roth JA (1966) Hired hand research. *American Sociologist* 1(4): 190–196.

Rothman BK (1994) *The Tentative Pregnancy*, rev. edn. London: Pandora Press.

Roulstone A and Barnes C (2005) *Working Futures: Disabled People, Policy and Social Inclusion.* Bristol: Policy Press.

Rouse CM (2009) *Uncertain Suffering: Racial Health Care Disparities and Sickle Cell Disease.* Berkeley, CA: University of California Press.

Royal CD, Novembre J, Fullerton SM, Goldstein DB, Long JC, *et al.* (2010) Inferring genetic ancestry: opportunities, challenges, and implications. *The American Journal of Human Genetics* 86(5): 661–673.

Royal CDM and Dunston GM (2004) Changing the paradigm from 'race' to human genome variation. *Nature Genetics* 36(11): S5–S7.

Rucknagel DL (2001) The role of rib infarcts in the acute chest syndrome of sickle cell diseases. *Paediatric Pathology and Molecular Medicine* 20(2): 137–154.

Rubin EM and Rowley PT (1979) Sickle cell trait/sickle cell hereditary persistence of fetal hemoglobin trait. *American Journal of Diseases of Children* 133(12): 1248–1250.

Sabatier R (1988) *Blaming Others: Prejudice, Race and Worldwide AIDS.* Washington, DC: Panos Institute.

Sallares R, Bouwman A and Anderung C (2004) The spread of malaria to Southern Europe in antiquity: new approaches to old problems. *Medical History* 48(3): 311–328.

Santos RV, Fry PH, Monteiro S, Maio MC, Rodrigues JC, *et al.* (2009) Color, race, and genomic ancestry in Brazil: dialogues between anthropology and genetics. *Current Anthropology* 50(6): 787–819.

Sassi F, Archard L and Le Grand J (2001a) Equity and the economic evaluation of health care. *Health Technology Assessment* 5(3): 1–138.

Sassi F, Le Grand J and Archard L (2001b) Equity versus efficiency: a dilemma for the NHS. *British Medical Journal* 323(7316): 762–763.

Savitt TL (1997) The second reported case of sickle cell anemia Charlottesville, Virginia, 1911. *Virginia Medical Quarterly* 124: 84–92.

Savitt TL (2002 [1981]) *Medicine and Slavery: Health Care of Blacks in Antebellum Virginia.* Chicago: University of Illinois Press.

Savitt TL (2010) Tracking down the first recorded sickle cell patient in Western medicine. *Journal of the National Medical Association* 102(11): 981–992.

Savitt TL (2014) Learning about sickle cell: the patient in early sickle cell disease case reports, 1910–1933. *Journal of the National Medical Association* 106(1): 31–41.

Savitt TL and Goldberg MF (1989) Herrick's 1910 case report of sickle cell anemia: the rest of the story. *Journal of the American Medical Association* 261(2): 266–271.

Savitt TL, Smith WR, Haywood Jr C and Creary MS (2014) Use of the word "crisis" in sickle cell disease: the language of sickle cell. *Journal of the National Medical Association* 106(1): 23–30.

Sayer A (2005) *The Moral Consciousness of Class.* Cambridge: Cambridge University Press.

SB Nation (2014) The right thing to do versus the State of Florida, 26 August 2014. Available at: www.sbnation.com/longform/2014/8/26/6065867/devaughn-darling-profile-florida-state-football (accessed 22 October 2018).

Schneider LT (2017) The ogbanje who wanted to stay: the occult, belonging, family and therapy in Sierra Leone. *Ethnography* 18(2): 133–152.

Schroeder WA, Munger ES and Powars DR (1990) Sickle cell anaemia, genetic variations, and the slave trade to the United States. *The Journal of African History* 31(2): 163–180.

Scott RB (1970) Health care priority and sickle cell anemia. *Journal of the American Medical Association* 214(4): 731–734.

Seabrook J (2016) How the lifestyle of the rich became anthropogenic activity in the climate change debate. *Race and Class* 57(4): 87–94.

Sen A (1981) Ingredients of famine analysis: availability and entitlements. *The Quarterly Journal of Economics* 96(3): 433–464.

Serjeant GR (1997) Sickle cell disease. *Lancet* 350(9079): 725–730.

Serjeant GR (2005) Mortality from sickle cell disease in Africa: interventions used to reduce mortality in non-malarial areas may be inappropriate. *British Medical Journal* 330(7489): 432–433.

Serjeant GR (2006) The case for dedicated sickle cell centres. *Indian Journal of Human Genetics* 12(3): 148–150.

Serjeant GR and Serjeant BE (2001) *Sickle Cell Disease,* 3rd edn. Oxford: Oxford University Press.

Serjeant GR, Serjeant BE, Mason KP, Gibson F, Gardner R, *et al.* (2017) Voluntary premarital screening to prevent sickle cell disease in Jamaica: does it work? *Journal of Community Genetics* 8(2): 133–139.

Shakespeare T (1995) Back to the future? New genetics and disabled people. *Critical Social Policy* 15(2/3): 22–25.

Shiao JL, Bode T, Beyer A and Selvig D (2012) The genomic challenge to the social construction of race. *Sociological Theory* 30(2): 67–88.

Shilling C (1993) *The Body and Social Theory.* London: Sage.

Shriner D and Rotimi CN (2018) Whole-genome-sequence-based haplotypes reveal single origin of the sickle allele during the Holocene Wet Phase. *The American Journal of Human Genetics* 102(4): 547–556.

Sickle Cell Society (2018) *Standards for the Clinical Care of Adults with Sickle Cell Disease in the UK.* London: Sickle Cell Society.

Sim J (2004) The victimized state and the mystification of social harm. In: P Hillyard, C Pantazis, D Gordon and S Tombs (eds) *Beyond Criminology: Taking Harm Seriously.* London: Pluto Press.

Simien EM and Clawson RA (2004) The intersection of race and gender: an examination of black feminist consciousness, race consciousness, and policy attitudes. *Social Science Quarterly* 85(3): 793–810.

Simonnet C, Elanga N, Joly P, Vaz T and Nacher M (2016) Genetic modulators of sickle cell disease in French Guiana: markers of the slave trade. *American Journal of Human Biology* 28(6): 811–816.

Singer R (1954) The origin of the sickle cell. *Suid-Afrikaanse Joernal van Wetenskap* 50(11): 287–291.

Sivanandan A (1985) Racism awareness training and the degradation of black struggle. *Race and Class* 26(4): 1–33.

Skeggs B (2014) Values beyond value? Is anything beyond the logic of capital? *British Journal of Sociology* 65(1): 1–20.

Skloot R (2010) *The Immortal Life of Henrietta Lacks.* New York: Random House.

Sledge D and Mohler G (2013) Eliminating malaria in the American South: an analysis of the decline of malaria in 1930s Alabama. *American Journal of Public Health* 103(8): 1381–1392.

Smith JA, Epseland M, Bellevue R, Bonds D, Brown AK, *et al.* (1996) Pregnancy in sickle cell disease: experience of the cooperative study of sickle cell disease. *Obstetrics and Gynaecology* 87(2): 199–204.

Smith WR, Bauserman RL, Ballas SK, McCarthy WF, *et al.* and Investigators of the Multicenter Study of Hydroxyurea in Sickle Cell Anemia (2009) Climatic and geographic temporal patterns of pain in the Multicenter Study of Hydroxyurea. *Pain* 146(1): 91–98.

Smith WR, Penberthy LT, Bovbjerg VE, McClish DK, Roberts JD, *et al.* (2008) Daily assessment of pain in adults with sickle cell disease. *Annals of Internal Medicine* 148(2): 94–101.

Sobota A, Neufeld EJ, Sprinz P and Heeney MM (2011) Transition from pediatric to adult care for sickle cell disease: results of a survey of pediatric providers. *American Journal of Hematology* 86(6): 512–515.

Soren D and Soren N (1995) What killed the babies of Lugnano? *Archaeology* 48(5): 43–48.

Spracklen K (2008) The Holy Blood and the Holy Grail: myths of scientific racism and the pursuit of excellence in sport. *Leisure Studies* 27(2): 221–227.

Steinberg MH (2005) Predicting clinical severity in sickle cell anaemia, *British Journal of Haematology* 129(4): 465–481.

Stenhouse L (1974) *The Evolution of Intelligence: A General Theory and Some of Its Implications* London: George Allen and Unwin.

St Louis B (2003) Sport, genetics and the natural athlete: the resurgence of racial science. *Body and Society* 9(2): 75–95.

Street P (2003) Color blind: prisons and the new American racism. In: T Herivel and P Wright (eds) *Prison Nation: The Warehousing of America's Poor.* New York: Routledge, 30–40.

Streetly A, Latinovic R, and Henthorn J (2010) Positive screening and carrier results for the England-wide universal newborn sickle cell screening programme by ethnicity and area for 2005–7. *Journal of Clinical Pathology* 63(7): 626–629.

Stuart J, Schwartz FCM, Little AJ and Raine DN (1973) Screening for abnormal haemoglobins: a pilot study. *British Medical Journal* 4(5887): 284–287.

Sweet FW (2005) *Legal History of the Color Line.* Palm Coast, FL: Backintyme.

Sydenstricker VP (1924a) Sickle cell anemia. *Southern Medical Journal* 17(3): 177–183.

Sydenstricker VP (1924b) Further observations on sickle cell anemia. *Journal of the American Medical Association* 83(1): 12–17.

Sykes B (2001) *The Seven Daughters of Eve.* London: Bantam Press.

Tamedu O (2005) *Menace in My Blood: My Affliction with Sickle Cell Anaemia.* Victoria, BC: Trafford Publishing.

Tanabe K, Mita T, Jombart T, Eriksson A, Horibe S, *et al.* (2010) Plasmodium falciparum accompanied the human expansion out of Africa. *Current Biology* 20(14): 1283–1289.

Tapper M (1999) *In the Blood: Sickle Cell Anaemia and the Politics of Race.* Philadelphia, PA: University of Pennsylvania Press.

Tarini BA, Brooks MA and Bundy DG (2012) A policy impact analysis of the mandatory NCAA sickle cell trait screening program. *Health Services Research* 47(1, Part 2): 446–461.

Telfer P, Coen P, Chakravorty S, Wilkey O, Evans J, *et al.* (2007) Clinical outcomes in children with sickle cell disease living in England: a neonatal cohort in East London. *Haematologica* 92(7): 905–912.

Tewari S, Brousse V, Piel FB, Menzel S and Rees, DC (2015) Environmental determinants of severity in sickle cell disease *Haematologica* 100(9): 1108–1116.

Tewari S and Rees DC (2013) Morbidity pattern of sickle cell disease in India: a single centre perspective. *Indian Journal of Medical Research* 138(3): 288–290.

Thogmartin JR (1998) Sudden death in police pursuit. *Journal of Forensic Sciences* 43(6): 1228–1231.

Thomas VJ and Taylor LM (2002) The psychosocial experience of people with sickle cell disease and its impact on quality of life: qualitative findings from focus groups. *British Journal of Health Psychology* 7(3): 345–363.

Times of India (2014) Modi's Japan visit gives hope to sickle cell patients, 3 September 2014. Available at: https://timesofindia.indiatimes.com/india/Modis-Japan-visit-gives-hope-to-sickle-cell-patients/articleshow/41586759.cms.

Timmann C and Meyer CG (2010) Malaria, mummies, mutations: Tutankhamun's archaeological autopsy. *Tropical Medicine and International Health* 15(11): 1278–1280.

Todd J and Ruane J (2004) The roots of intense ethnic conflict may not in fact be ethnic: categories, communities and path dependence. *European Journal of Sociology* 45(2): 209–232.

Todd Z (2016) An indigenous feminist's take on the ontological turn: 'ontology' is just another word for colonialism. *Journal of Historical Sociology* 29(1): 4–22.

Truth About Zane (2018) Available at: www.truthaboutzane.com (accessed 22 October 2018).

Tshilolo L, Aissi LM, Lukusa D, Kinsiama C, Wembonyama S, *et al.* (2009) Neonatal screening for sickle cell anaemia in the Democratic Republic of the Congo: experience from a pioneer project on 31,204 newborns. *Journal of Clinical Pathology* 62(1): 35–38.

Turner BS (2008) *The Body and Society,* 3rd edn. London: Sage.

Ulph F, Cullinan T, Qureshi N and Kai J (2011) Familial influences on antenatal and newborn haemoglobinopathy screening. *Ethnicity and Health* 16(4–5): 361–375.

Ulph F, Cullinan T, Qureshi N and Kai J (2015) Parents' responses to receiving sickle cell or cystic fibrosis carrier results for their child following newborn screening. *European Journal of Human Genetics* 23(4): 459–465.

UNESCO (1950) *The Race Question.* Text of the statement issued 18 July 1950. Paris: UNESCO. Available at: http://unesdoc.unesco.org/images/0012/001282/128291eo.pdf.

United Nations (1997) Economic and Social Council Commission on Human Rights 53rd Session E/CN.4/1997/7 10 January 1997. Item 8a Provisional Agenda. Available at: www.refworld.org/pdfid/3b00f4158.pdf (accessed 22 October 2018).

Upadhye DS, Jain DL, Trivedi YL, Nadkarni AH, Ghosh K, *et al.* (2016) Neonatal screening and the clinical outcome in children with sickle cell disease in central India. *PLoS One* 11(1): p.e0147081.

Valier, H and Bivins, R (2002) Organization, ethnicity and the British National Health Service. In: J Stanton (ed.) *Innovations in Health and Medicine.* London: Routledge, 37–64.

van Baelen H, Vandepitte J and Eeckels R (1969) Observations on sickle-cell anaemia and haemoglobin Bart's in Congolese neonates. *Annales de la Société Belge de Médecine Tropicale* 49(2): 157–164.

Vandepitte J and Stijns J (1963) Hemoglobinopathies in the Congo (Leopoldville) and Rwanda-Burundi. *Annales de la Société Belge de Médecine Tropicale* 43: 271–281.

Vichinsky E, Hurst D, Earles A, Kleman K, and Lubin B (1988) Newborn screening for sickle cell disease: effect on mortality. *Pediatrics* 81(6): 749–755.

Vitzhum VJ, Fix AG and Livingstone A (2006) The four-field anthropology and multifaceted life of Frank B Livingstone. *Retrospectives: Works and Lives of Michigan Anthropologists* 16(1): 136–174. Available at: http://quod.lib.umich.edu/m/mdia/0522508.001 6.107?rgn=main;view=fulltext (accessed 22 October 2018).

Wailoo K (1997) *Drawing Blood: Technology and Disease Identity in Twentieth-Century America.* Baltimore, MD: Johns Hopkins University Press.

Wailoo K (2001) *Dying in the City of the Blues: Sickle Cell Anemia and the Politics of Race and Health.* Chapel Hill, NC: University of North Carolina Press.

Wailoo K and Pemberton S (2006) *The Troubled Dream of Genetic Medicine.* Baltimore, MD: Johns Hopkins University Press.

Waltz X, Romana M, Hardy-Dessources MD, Lamarre Y, Divialle-Doumdo L, *et al.* (2013) Hematological and hemorheological determinants of the six-minute walk test performance in children with sickle cell anemia. *PLoS One* 8(10): p.e77830.

Washburn RE (1911) Peculiar elongated and sickle-shaped red blood corpuscles in a case of severe anemia. *Virginia Medical Semi-Monthly* 15: 490–493.

Waters AP, Higgins DG and McCutchan TF (1991) Plasmodium falciparum appears to have arisen as a result of lateral transfer between avian and human hosts. *Proceedings of the National Academy of Sciences* 88(8): 3140–3144.

Watts CP (2011) The 'Wind of Change': British decolonisation in Africa, 1957–1965. *History Review* 71: 12–17.

Weatherall D (2010) *Thalassaemia: The Biography.* Oxford: Oxford University Press.

Whitten CF (1967) Innocuous nature of the sickling (pseudosickling) phenomenon in deer. *British Journal of Haematology* 13(5): 650–655.

Wilkinson RG (1996) *Unequal Societies: The Afflictions of Inequality.* London: Routledge.

Wilkinson RG and Pickett K (2009) *The Spirit Level: Why More Equal Societies Almost Always do Better.* London: Allen Lane.

Williams G (1984) The genesis of chronic illness: narrative re-construction. *Sociology of Health and Illness* 6(2): 175–200.

Williams TN, Mwangi TW, Wambua S, Peto TE, Weatherall DJ, *et al.* (2005) Negative epistasis between the malaria-protective effects of α+-thalassemia and the sickle cell trait *Nature Genetics* 37(11): 1253–1257.

Williams TN and Obaro SK (2011) Sickle cell disease and malaria morbidity: a tale with two tails. *Trends in Parasitology* 27(7): 315–320.

Williams TN, Uyoga S, Macharia A, Ndila C, McAuley CF, *et al.* (2009) Bacteraemia in Kenyan children with sickle-cell anaemia: a retrospective cohort and case-control study. *Lancet* 374(9698): 1364–1370.

Wilson JMG and Jungner G (1968) *Principles and Practice of Screening for Disease.* Public Health Papers #34 Geneva: World Health Organization Available at: www.who.int/bulletin/volumes/86/4/07-050112BP.pdf.

Winsor T and Burch GE (1945) Sickle cell anemia, a great masquerader: easily recognizable with routine use of diagnostic parameter. *Journal of the American Medical Association* 129(12): 793–796.

Witzig R (1996) The medicalization of race: scientific legitimization of a flawed social construct. *Annals of Internal Medicine* 125(8): 675–679.

Word Press (2008) *Claude N'Deh.* Available at: https://ndeh.wordpress.com/ (accessed 4 April 2018).

WHO (World Health Organization) (1988) *The Haemoglobinopathies in Europe: Combined Report of Two WHO Meetings,* document EUR/ICP/MCH 110. Copenhagen: WHO Regional Office for Europe.

WHO (World Health Organization) (2006) *Sickle-Cell Anaemia.* 59th World Health Assembly Document A59/9, 24 April 2006.

WHO (World Health Organization) (2012) Genes and human disease. Available at: www.who.int/genomics/public/geneticdiseases/en/index2.html (accessed 7 November 2018).

WHO/TIF (World Health Organization/Thalassaemia International Federation) (2008) *Management of Haemoglobin Disorders: Report of a Joint WHO/TIF Meeting.* Nicosia, Cyprus, 16–18 November 2007.

Yalcindag E, Elguero E, Arnathau C, Durand P, Akiana J, *et al.* (2012) Multiple independent introductions of *Plasmodium falciparum* in South America. *Proceedings of the National Academy of Sciences* 109(2): 511–516.

Yallop D, Duncan ER, Norris E, Fuller GW, Thomas N, *et al.* (2007) The associations between air quality and the number of hospital admissions for acute pain and sickle-cell disease in an urban environment. *British Journal of Haematology* 136(6): 844–848.

Yanni E, Grosse SD, Yang QH and Olney RS (2009) Trends in pediatric disease-related mortality in the United States, 1983–2002. *Journal of Pediatrics* 154(4): 541–545.

Yudell M, Roberts D, DeSalle R and Tishkoff S (2016) Taking race out of human genetics. *Science* 351(6273): 564–565.

Zeuner D, Ades AE, Karnon J, Brown J, Dezateux C, *et al.* (1999) Antenatal and neonatal haemoglobinopathy screening in the UK: review and economic analysis. *Health Technology Assessment* 3(11): 1–186.

Zborowski M (1952) Cultural components in responses to pain. *Journal of Social Issues* 8(4): 16–30.

Index

Page numbers in **bold** denote tables, those in *italics* denote figures.

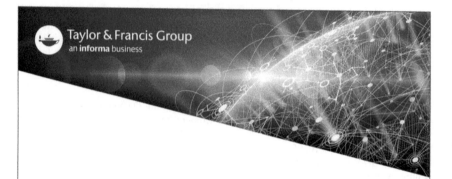

Milton Keynes UK
Ingram Content Group UK Ltd.
UKHW040105071024
449327UK00019B/827